ANNUAL REVIEW OF NURSING RESEARCH

VOLUME 28, 2010

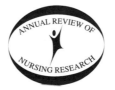

Annual Review of Nursing Research

Nursing Workforce Issues

VOLUME 28, 2010

Series Editor

CHRISTINE E. KASPER, PhD, RN, FAAN

Volume Editors

ANNETTE TYREE DEBISETTE, PhD, RN, CAPT, USPHS

JUDITH A. VESSEY, PhD, CRNP, MBA, FAAN

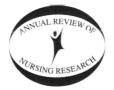

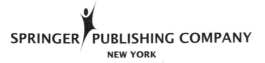

SPRINGER PUBLISHING COMPANY

NEW YORK

Copyright © 2011 Springer Publishing Company, LLC

Springer Publishing Company, LLC
11 West 42nd Street
New York, NY 10036
www.springerpub.com

Acquisitions Editor: Allan Graubard
Senior Editor: Rose Mary Piscitelli
Composition: Newgen Imaging

ISBN: 978-0-8261-1902-5
E-book ISBN: 978-0-8261-1903-2
ISSN: 0739-6686
Online ISSN: 1944-4028

11 12 13 14/ 5 4 3 2 1 $95.00

The author and the publisher of this Work have made every effort to use sources believed to be reliable to provide information that is accurate and compatible with the standards generally accepted at the time of publication. Because medical science is continually advancing, our knowledge base continues to expand. Therefore, as new information becomes available, changes in procedures become necessary. We recommend that the reader always consult current research and specific institutional policies before performing any clinical procedure. The author and publisher shall not be liable for any special, consequential, or exemplary damages resulting, in whole or in part, from the readers' use of, or reliance on, the information contained in this book. The publisher has no responsibility for the persistence or accuracy of URLs for external or third-party Internet Web sites referred to in this publication and does not guarantee that any content on such Web sites is, or will remain, accurate or appropriate.

Special discounts on bulk quantities of our books are available to corporations, professional associations, pharmaceutical companies, health care organizations, and other qualifying groups.

If you are interested in a custom book, including chapters from more than one of our titles, we can provide that service as well.

For details, please contact:
Special Sales Department, Springer Publishing Company, LLC
11 West 42nd Street, 15th Floor, New York, NY 10036-8002
Phone: 877-687-7476 or 212-431-4370; Fax: 212-941-7842
Email: sales@springerpub.com

Printed in the United States of America by Hamilton Printing

Contents

The Nursing Environment

Nursing Workforce Studies and the Future

About the Volume Editors

Annette Tyree Debisette, PhD, RN, CAPT, USPHS, is currently a Senior Nurse Officer and responsible for two national training programs for Medical Devices and Radiological Health in the U.S. Food and Drug Administration, Office of Regulatory Affairs, ORA-U, in Rockville, MD. She has direct responsibility for training Consumer Safety Officers, Investigators, and Analysts that conduct inspections of domestic and international manufacturers who make medical devices.

From 2006 to 2008, she was the Director for the Division of Nursing, Department of Health and Human Services, Health Resources and Services Administration, Bureau of Health Professions, Rockville, MD. The Division of Nursing implements nursing workforce legislation authorized under Title VIII of the Public Health Service Act and in FY 2007 administered programs totaling 149.8 million dollars. She received her BSN and MS degrees in nursing from Syracuse University, Syracuse, NY, and PhD from the Catholic University of America, Washington, DC.

From 2004 to 2006, she was Senior Advisor to the Associate Administrator for Health Professions, Health Resources and Services Administration (HRSA), Department of Health and Human Services, Rockville, MD. From 2002 to 2004, she was Chief for Advanced Nurse Education in HRSA's Division of Nursing. Practice roles for Dr. Debisette have included that of an adult nurse practitioner, medical-surgical clinical nurse specialist, nurse consultant, nursing educator, and nursing administrator. Teaching in associate's, baccalaureate, master's and doctoral degree, and practical nursing programs, Dr. Debisette served on the faculties of Syracuse University, HMI Regency School of Practical Nursing, Washington, DC, Catonsville Community College, Baltimore, MD, Marymount University, Arlington, VA, and the Catholic University of America. She was the Director of Medical-Surgical Services at National Hospital for Orthopedics and Rehabilitation, and Interim Director for Medical-Surgical Services at Northern Virginia Community Hospital, both in Arlington, VA.

She serves as an Associate Investigator for the U.S. Public Health Service in a Tri-Service Nursing Research Study of nursing deploying to uncontrolled nursing environments. Dr. Debisette is former President of Sigma Theta Tau,

Kappa Chapter (twice winning the coveted Key Award under her leadership), and serves as a Captain in the Commissioned Corps of the U.S. Public Health Service. Commissioned Corps Awards include the PHS Citation, Special Assignment, Crisis Response, and Unit Commendation Awards. In 2005, she graduated from the DHHS Primary Health Care Policy Fellowship Program. She has deployed to Bethel, AK, the regional health center for the Yukon Kuskokwim Health Corporation, and recently contributed in setting up a field hospital in Baton Rouge, LA, during Hurricane Katrina. Dr. Debisette has written several publications and resides in Gaithersburg, MD.

Judith A. Vessey, PhD, CRNP, MBA, FAAN, currently holds the Lelia Holden Carroll Professor in Nursing in the Boston College, William F. Connell School of Nursing. She received her BSN from Goshen College, a certificate as a Developmental Pediatric Nurse Practitioner for the University of Miami, her MSN and PhD from the University of Pennsylvania, and was a Robert Wood Johnson Nurse Scholar at the University of California, San Francisco. More recently, she received her MBA in Medical Services from Johns Hopkins University, recognizing the need to understand how the economics and business practice of health care were essential in order to contribute to policy determinations regarding care delivery systems for to pediatric populations.

Dr. Vessey's current research and policy activities focus on bullying—from the schoolyard to the workplace. Of particular interest is the role that intraprofessional and interprofessional bullying, harassment, and horizontal violence play in patient safety and patient care outcomes. Her research has been funded through the National Institute of Nursing research, professional organizations, and private foundations. Dr. Vessey has authored more than 100 articles, chapters, and books, presented widely, and consulted with numerous academic and service organizations. She is actively involved in the American Academy of Nurses.

Contributors

Catherine R. Davis, PhD, RN
Director, Global Research and Test
  Administration
CGFNS International
Philadelphia, PA

Annette Tyree Debisette, PhD, RN
CAPT, USPHS
Senior Nurse Officer
Gaithersburg, MD

Rosanna DeMarco, PhD, PHCNS-BC,
  ACRN, FAAN
Associate Professor
Boston College, William F. Connell
  School of Nursing
Chestnut Hill, MA
Pediatric Nurse Practitioner
Children's Hospital
Boston, MA

Rachel DiFazio, PhDc, RN, PNP
Boston College
William F. Connell School of Nursing
Chestnut Hill, MA
Pediatric Nurse Practitioner
Children's Hospital
Boston, MA

Barbara Easterling, MS, CNS, RN
Nurse Consultant
Health Resources and Services
  Administration, Bureau of Primary
  Health Care
Rockville, MD

M. Christina R. Esperat, RN, PhD,
  FAAN
Associate Dean for Clinical Services and
  Community Engagement
Anita Thigpen Perry School of Nursing
Texas Tech University Health Sciences
  Center
Lubbock, TX

DiJon R. Fasoli, PhD, MSN, MBA, RN
Research Health Scientist
Department of Veterans Affairs
Bedford, MD

Jeanne Geiger-Brown, PhD, RN
Associate Professor
Work & Health Research Center
University of Maryland School
  of Nursing
Baltimore, MD

Alexia Green, RN, PhD, FAAN
Professor and Dean Emeritus
Anita Thigpen Perry School
  of Nursing
Texas Tech University Health Sciences
  Center
Lubbock, TX

Anne H. Gross, PhD, RN, NEA-BC
Vice President, Adult Nursing and
  Clinical Services
Dana-Farber Cancer Institute
Boston, MA

Kathlyn Sue Haddock, PhD, RN
Associate Chief of Staff for Research
Department of Veterans Affairs
Columbia, SC

Dorothy Jones, EdD, RNC, FAAN
Professor
Boston College
William F. Connell School of Nursing
Chestnut Hill, MA

Gail Keenan, RN, PhD
Associate Professor
University of Illinois at Chicago
   College of Nursing
Chicago, IL

Patricia A. Watts Kelley, PhD, RN, CAPT, NC, USN
Associate Professor
Uniformed Services University of
   Health Sciences
Bethesda, MD

Aileen Kishi, PhD, RN
Program Director, Texas Center for
   Nursing Workforce Studies Dept. of
   State Health Services—Center for
   Health Statistics
Austin, TX

Kara Lacey, BA
Communications Manager
Nursing and Patient Care Services
Dana-Farber Cancer Institute
Boston, MA

Jane Lipscomb, PhD, RN, FAAN
Professor
Work & Health Research Center
University of Maryland School of Nursing
Baltimore, MD

Margaret Lunney, RN, PhD
Professor
College of Staten Island
City University of New York (CUNY) &
   Doctoral Faculty, CUNY DNS Program
Staten Island and New York City, NY

Angela Martinelli, PhD, RN, CNOR
CAPT, USPHS
Senior Nurse Officer
Gaithersburg, MD

Robert Martiniano, MPH, MPA
Center for Health Workforce Studies
University at Albany School of Public
   Health
Rensselaer, NY

Sandra McGinnis, PhD
Formerly with the Center for Health
   Workforce Studies
University at Albany School of Public
   Health
Rensselaer, NY

Patricia R. Messmer, PhD, BC, RN, FAAN
Consultant Nursing Education & Research
School of Nursing Medical Center
   Campus
Miami Dade College
Miami, FL

Yolanda J. Milliman-Richard, RN, BSN
Nursing Director Radiology
Children's Hospital Boston
Boston, MA

Jean Moore, RN, MSN
Center for Health Workforce Studies
University at Albany School of Public
   Health
Rensselaer, NY

Sue Moorhead, RN, PhD
Associate Professor
The University of Iowa College of Nursing
Iowa City, IA

Barbara L. Nichols, DHL, MS, RN, FAAN
Chief Executive Officer
CGFNS International
Philadelphia, PA

Patricia Reid Ponte, RN, DNSc, NEA-BC, FAAN
Senior Vice President, Patient Care
   Services and Chief Nursing Officer
Dana-Farber Cancer Institute
Boston, MA
Executive Director, Oncology Nursing &
   Clinical Services
Brigham and Women's Hospital
Boston, MA

Donna R. Richardson, JD, RN
Director, Governmental Affairs and
   Professional Standards
CGFNS International
Philadelphia, PA

Irene Sandvold, DrPH, CNM, FACNM
Nurse Consultant
Health Resources and Services
   Administration, Bureau of Health
   Professions
Rockville, MD

Joanne Spetz, PhD
Professor
Departments of Community Health
   Systems & Social and Behavioral
   Sciences
UCSF School of Nursing
Faculty Researcher
Center for the Health Professions, UCSF
San Francisco, CA

Marian C. Turkel, RN, PhD, NEA-BC
Director of Professional Nursing Practice
Albert Einstein Healthcare Network
Philadelphia, PA

Judith A. Vessey, PhD, CRNP, MBA, FAAN
Lelia Holden Carroll Professor
   in Nursing
Boston College
William F. Connell School of Nursing
Chestnut Hill, MA

George A. Zangaro, PhD, RN
Associate Professor
The Catholic University of America
Washington, DC

Preface

This 28th volume in the *Annual Review of Nursing Research* (ARNR) series examines the timely and important topic of the nursing workforce. Drs. Nettye Debisette and Judith Vessey, well-known scholars and researchers in this field, have served as the volume editors. They selected the content for the chapters and edited them into this in-depth book.

The volume comprises five sections. Part I focuses on the nursing workforce and the United States and includes four chapters. Joanne Spetz addresses the crucial need for accurate and good data and its role in policy in Chapter 1. George A. Zangaro and Patricia A. Watts Kelley examine the interplay between job satisfaction and the retention of nurses in the military in Chapter 2. In Chapter 3, Robert Martiniano, Sandra McGinnis, and Jean Moore examine the supply and distribution of registered nurses. In Chapter 4, Alexia Green, Aileen Kishi, and M. Christina R. Esperat review current state policies and initiatives focused on improving the nursing workforce.

In Part II the focus is on global nursing workforce issues lead by an in-depth review by Barbara L. Nichols, Catherine R. Davis, and Donna R. Richardson in Chapter 5. Part III includes two chapters. Judith A. Vessey, Rosanna DeMarco, and Rachel DiFazio address the crucial issue of bullying, harassment, and horizontal violence in the nursing workforce and examine the status of research in this important and emerging field in Chapter 6. Patricia Reid Ponte, Anne H. Gross, Yolanda J. Milliman-Richard, and Kara Lacey explore positive practice environments, collaboration, and teamwork in nursing practice in Chapter 7.

Part IV discusses various aspects of the nursing environment and its influence on practice. In Chapter 8 the work environment and professional safety are presented by Jeanne Geiger-Brown and Jane Lipscomb. Patricia R. Messmer and Marian C. Turkel discuss the advent and evolution of the Magnet hospital on nursing practice in Chapter 9. In Chapter 10, Dorothy Jones, Margaret Lunney, Gail Keenan, and Sue Moorhead explore the use of standardized nursing languages. In Chapter 11, DiJon R. Fasoli and Kathlyn Sue Haddock review patient classification systems.

The final section examines nursing workforce studies and the future. In Chapter 12, Annette Tyree Debisette, Irene Sandvold, Barbara Easterling, and

Angela Martinelli apply their considerable expertise in reviewing the area of nursing workforce studies. Together, these thoughtful scholarly discussions highlight what is known, what needs to be studied, and areas for future action. It is expected that this issue will lead the way for setting the foundation for the important research that needs to be accomplished in the near future. It will also guide the way for students who are drawn to establish their research careers in these areas of study.

The aging of the nursing workforce as well as the retirement of a large sector of our educators and researchers has continued to heighten our collective concern and sense of unease as to the future of our profession. Cogent planning has been further complicated by recent economic failures, which drove large numbers of inactive and retired nurses back into the workforce. An economic recovery is certain to rapidly expose the gaps in the nursing education and employment pipeline. Clearly, many have met and counseled together pondering the various tactics and strategies that the academic and governmental institutions can use to bolster the predicted shortfalls in the nursing workforce. The education of the nursing workforce has been addressed this year in two significant publications, "Educating Nurses: A Call for Radical Transformation" by the Carnegie Foundation for the Advancement of Teaching and "The Future of Nursing: Leading Change, Advancing Health" by the Institute of Medicine of the National Academies of Science. Both have served to bring to public awareness significant issues in educating the nursing workforce and the need for reform.

In times of crisis it is understandable that we focus on issues of creating and deploying an educated and skilled nursing workforce. However, we now need to carefully consider what does "educated" mean in terms of the intellectual capacity and flexibility of those nurses we have produced. The past decade has seen the regrettable loss of those courses in programs that create the educated human in favor of those focusing on the popular dogma or theory of the day. Often we unintentionally deliver the dreaded technical training of years past under the guise of higher education. Our students rarely are able to take courses in the humanities and arts that are the hallmark of the educated person. Where is the math and undiluted basic sciences forming the core of understanding of all of the physiology central to nursing practice? The loss of these may eventually affect our ability to care as well as to act for the protection and betterment of our patients.

Study abroad is a hallmark of higher education today with large numbers of students from all colleges and universities experiencing firsthand the global community. Nursing students need not be deprived of this important, intellectually formative experience. It can and has been done. The University of Evansville will shortly be celebrating the 40th anniversary of sending undergraduate nursing students to Harlaxton College in England.

Luckily our best universities still insist on a rigorous and well-rounded curriculum for their students. Rigor of thought underpins the entire profession and every action we take on behalf of our patients. There are no shortcuts or easy ways. We cannot default to utilitarian actions in educating our nursing workforce. We sorely need to "up our game" and carefully reflect on how we can personally promote intellectual rigor in our students and in our selves. Do we select our education based on excellence or what is convenient, easy, and gets that next career "box" checked off? It is a slippery slope and ultimately damaging to the future of our profession.

Christine E. Kasper, PhD, RN, FAAN
Series Editor

Acknowledgments

Suzanne L. Feetham, PhD, RN, FAAN
Visiting Professor
University of Wisconsin, Milwaukee

Ada Sue Hinshaw, PhD, RN, FAAN
Dean
Uniformed Services University of the Health Sciences
Graduate School of Nursing
Bethesda, MD
Boston College, William F. Connell School of Nursing
Chestnut Hill, MA
The Catholic University of America School of Nursing
Washington, DC

CHAPTER 1

The Importance of Good Data

How the National Sample Survey of Registered Nurses Has Been Used to Improve Knowledge and Policy

Joanne Spetz

ABSTRACT

In 1977, the federal government launched the nation's largest and most significant program to collect data on the registered nurse (RN) workforce of the United States—the National Sample Survey of Registered Nurses (NSSRN). This survey is conducted by the U.S. Health Resources and Services Administration, first in 1977 and then every 4 years since 1980. This article offers the history of the NSSRN and a review of the ways in which the NSSRN data have been used to examine education, demographics, employment, shortages, and other aspects of the RN workforce. The influence this body of research has had on policymaking is explored. Recommendations for future research are offered, in the hope that future waves of the NSSRN will continue to be used to their fullest potential.

The United States has experienced shortages of licensed nurses—particularly registered nurses (RNs)—since the end of World War II. The most recent shortage started in the late 1990s (Buerhaus, 1999), with other serious shortages reported in the late 1940s, the late 1970s, and the late 1980s (Aiken, 1982; Aiken & Mullinix, 1987; Friss, 1994; Yett, 1970, 1975). These shortages often have been interspersed with perceived oversupply of RNs, such as that occurred in the mid-1990s when the growth of managed care insurance programs reduced hospital utilization and thus pushed down demand for nurses (Aiken, Sochalski, & Anderson, 1996; Buerhaus & Staiger, 1996).

Federal and state policymakers have sought solutions to nursing shortages for decades, with one of the earliest federal interventions being the Nurse Training Act of 1964 (Yett, 1966). However, it was difficult to assess the impact of the Nurse Training Act and other programs on the nursing workforce due to a lack of data and information. Sporadic data collection had been conducted by the American Nurses Association (ANA) since 1949, primarily consisting of inventories of RNs obtained as part of license renewal (Reichelt & Young, 1985). These data focused on education and employment status. As the shortage of the 1970s commenced, it became apparent that better data were needed to understand the causes of shortages and evaluate policies to remedy them.

Thus, in 1977, the federal government launched the nation's largest and most significant program to collect data on the RN workforce of the United States—the National Sample Survey of Registered Nurses (NSSRN). This survey is conducted by the U.S. Health Resources and Services Administration (HRSA), first in 1977 and then ever 4 years since 1980. The survey questionnaires have been included about 15 pages of questions, producing a comprehensive set of information from a large sample of RNs. The most recent survey was completed in 2008. These data have been analyzed by both HRSA and scholars throughout the United States, yielding a deep understanding of the characteristics of the RN workforce.

This article offers the history of the NSSRN and a review of the ways in which the NSSRN data have been used to examine education, demographics, employment, shortages, and other aspects of the RN workforce. The influence this body of research has had on policymaking is explored. Recommendations for future research are offered, in the hope that future waves of the NSSRN will continue to be used to their fullest potential.

THE NATIONAL SAMPLE SURVEY OF REGISTERED NURSES

The HRSA is an agency of the U.S. Department of Health and Human Services (HHS), with responsibility for ensuring that there are adequate resources—workforce, physical capital, and services—to ensure that all Americans can receive the health care they need. Within HRSA is the Bureau of Health Professions, which focuses on the health workforce of the United States. At the time the first NSSRN was launched in 1977, the U.S. Public Health Service's (PHS's) Health Resources and

Services Administration, and later HRSA, housed the Bureau of Health Manpower, which was charged with conducting a survey of nurses (US DHHS, 2010b).

The mandate to collect data on the nursing workforce arose from the Nurse Training Act of 1975 (Title IX, Public Law 94–63, Section 951), which requires the gathering of data that will provide national and state level estimates on the number and distribution of nurses, type of employment and practice location, numbers working full-time and part-time, average rates of compensation by type of practice and location of practice, employment and activities of nurses with advanced training and graduate degrees, and immigration of nurses from other nations. Section 792 of the PHS Act (42 USC 295k, enacted 1992) called for a program to collect, compile, and analyze data on health professions, including nurses. The Health Professions Education Partnerships Act of 1998 (Public Law 105–392, Section 806(f)) added the requirement that information about workforce diversity and more education and practice data be obtained.

The NSSRN is designed to gather data about RNs who have active licenses and live in the 50 states and the District of Columbia (which is hereafter included as a "state" for brevity). The number of respondents has to be sufficient to enable estimates of the population and characteristics of the workforce for the United States as a whole and for each state. The survey has used a multimode data collection strategy since its inception, although the methods have been modified over time. The questionnaire also has been revised with each cycle of the survey.

Survey Management

The HRSA has contracted with outside organizations to conduct the survey. The first survey contract was initiated in 1975 with Westat, and the survey was cosponsored by the ANA. The contractors for subsequent surveys were Research Triangle Institute (1980, 1988, 1992, 1996, and 2000), Gallup (2004), and Westat (1984 and 2008). For the surveys conducted from 1977 through 2000, the contractor designed the sampling strategy and managed the data collection, producing a data file. Researchers at HRSA then performed the data analysis and wrote reports summarizing the findings. In 2004 and 2008, the contractor was responsible for the analysis of the survey data and writing preliminary and final reports.

Sample Selection and Data Collection

The population eligible to receive the NSSRN is all nurses with active licenses in one of the 50 states or the District of Columbia. Lists of licensed nurses are obtained from each State Board of Nursing. Because nurses can be licensed in multiple states, the NSSRN used a nested cluster design in which RNs were clustered alphabetically by last name and then selected in each state based on their alphabetically based cluster. This design is referred to as the "alpha-segment design" and was used from 1977 through 2004. This was an innovative way to address the possibility of nurses having licenses in more than one state, especially when many states did not have sophisticated computer databases of license records. In all cycles of the NSSRN, the sampling rate has been different for each state, to ensure there would be a sufficient number of respondents from each state to produce state-level estimates of the RN population and its characteristics.

The alpha-segment design was rather cumbersome to implement, and constructing an alpha-segment sampling frame is a time-consuming task. Perhaps more importantly, because RNs of the same racial/ethnic background may have names that are clustered alphabetically, the alpha-segment design may have resulted in larger variation for some estimates, such as racial and ethnic composition of the RN workforce. Thus, the 2008 NSSRN sample design was based on independent systematic random samples selected from state-based strata, with equal probability of selection within each stratum. This design was straightforward to implement and eliminated the clustering that could increase variability to survey estimates, particularly for survey results associated with race/ethnicity.

The NSSRN is primarily conducted by mail, with mail and telephone follow-up to increase response. The telephone follow-up serves two purposes: first, nonrespondents are contacted to encourage them to complete the survey, and second, respondents who skip key questions or provide inconsistent data are asked to provide complete information. Two innovations were added to the 2004 administration of the survey: the option to respond through a web-based version of the survey as offered, and the third mailing was shipped by Priority Mail through the U.S. Postal Service. The 2008 survey also included the option to respond to a web-based survey. Final mailings were sent through Federal Express for the nonrespondents who could not be contacted by telephone.

The first National Sample Survey was mailed to 20,417 RNs throughout the country. Using mail and telephone follow-up, a response rate of 82.2% was achieved, yielding 16,267 observations. Response rates have dropped over time, to 62.4% in 2008, which is consistent with trends for other surveys (Biener, Garrett, Gilpin, Roman, & Currivan, 2004; Dillman & Carley-Baxter, 2000). Because the number of RNs selected to receive the survey has increased, the number of nurses represented in the data files has been approximately 30,000 since 1980 (Bentley, Jones, Kendall, Moulton, & Savia, 1982). Table 1.1 summarizes the NSSRN sample sizes and responses for each year in which the survey was conducted.

Variables

Each time the NSSRN has been conducted, the survey has been based on the preceding survey. The first part of the survey focuses on the educational

TABLE 1.1

*Sample Sizes, Number of Respondents, and Response Rates for the
National Sample Surveys of Registered Nurses*

Survey Year	Sample Size	Respondents	Response Rate (%)
1977	20,417	16,267	82.2
1980	39,573	30,535	80.0
1984	44,268	32,100	79.8
1988	42,371	33,272	80.7
1992	43,629	32,489	79.7
1996	45,000	29,908	72.3
2000	54,000	35,579	71.7
2004	50,691	35,724	70.5
2008	55,151	33,549	62.4

Source: Adapted from Moses (1994, 1998), Roth, Graham, & Schmittling (1979),
Spratley, Johnson, Sochaski, Fritz, & Spencer (2002), and US DHHS (1983, 1986,
1990, 2006, 2010a).

background of the respondent. The questions include initial nursing education, education preceding nursing education, postlicensure education, preparation in advanced practice fields, and current enrollment in a degree or certificate program. Information about licensure, including when the RN first obtained an RN license and the number of states in which the respondent is licensed, is requested. The 2004 and 2008 surveys included questions about disaster preparedness training.

Detailed questions about employment are in the survey, with a focus on what the respondent considers to be his or her "principal" nursing position—the position in which the greatest number of working hours is spent. These questions are asked with respect to a specific date; for example, the 2008 survey asked "On March 10, 2008, were you employed or self-employed in nursing," and subsequent questions referred to March 10. The 1977 survey referred to September 15, 1976. The work setting (industry), job title, and clinical areas in which the respondent works are requested for the principal position. The questions about the clinical settings and patient populations with whom the nurse works have been revised over the years, including a substantial restructuring of these questions in 2008. Respondents are asked to report the percent of their work time spent on each of set of activities, including direct patient care, teaching, and management.

If the nurse has multiple positions, the setting of these is requested. Respondents are asked to report the number of weeks they work per year, and hours per week, for their principal and other nursing positions. In some years, the survey has asked for information about hours worked on an overtime basis and on-call hours. The location of the principal nursing position is requested, to enable analysis of the employment of nurses within each state or region.

In 2000, a question was added to the survey asking whether the nurse's satisfaction had improved in the previous year. This question was revised in 2004 to ask about job satisfaction in general (not compared to a previous year). Also starting in 2000, the survey asked for the number of years of experience in nursing. The survey requests the nurse's annual earnings and, after 1980, the income received from the nurse's primary job is reported separately from that of secondary nursing employment.

Respondents are asked about their employment in the previous year, using a reference date 1 year prior. They also are asked about their employment intentions—whether they plan to continue working in nursing in the near future. Questions about non-nursing employment are asked, and there is a set of questions for nurses who are not employed in nursing to report how many years have passed since they last worked in nursing, the reasons for not working in nursing, and their intentions to return to nursing employment.

Nurses are asked to provide demographic information, including their age, gender, race/ethnicity, marital status, whether children are present in the home, and whether there are dependent adults in the home. In 2004, a question was added about language fluency. In 1977, the survey asked for the employment status of the nurse's spouse (if the nurse was married); this question did not appear in any other survey. Total household income is reported after 1984.

Weighting and Imputation

A weight is computed for each respondent, based on the probability of a nurse being sampled in and responding from each state, so that analyses can ensure the results represent the full U.S. (or state) population of RNs, rather than only those who responded to the survey. These weights are developed in accordance with the sampling method used for the NSSRN. For the 2000 and 2004 surveys, the weights also accounted for lower response weights of nurses under age 26 years. In 2008, the weights accounted for differential response for multiple age groups. When analyzing the data, weights must be used so that the resulting statistics represent the full U.S. (or state) population.

To estimate the variability of the estimates from the NSSRN, replicate weights are computed. These replicates can be used to assess the precision of sample estimates as well as to compare estimates either within the 2008 NSSRN database or between estimates from various years.

A survey response is considered complete if a specified set of key questions are completed by the respondent. In 2008, when complete data could not be obtained from the sampled RN, statistical imputation was used to generate likely responses for missing values for individual questions within completed cases. Imputation of this type had not been used previously for the NSSRN. The imputation method was based on regression modeling, which is a powerful statistical method when used appropriately.

Data Access

After HRSA publishes a report summarizing the key findings from the NSSRN, a public-use file (PUF) is made available. The PUF contains the individual-level data, with specific variables omitted to ensure that individual respondents cannot be identified and their privacy is maintained. For example, detailed educational information collected in the survey is aggregated into summary variables in the PUF. The locations in which the nurse lives and works are provided at a regional level, rather than with a zip code. In one version of the file, the county of residence is provided, but some demographic variables are aggregated to protect individual identities. The other version omits the county indicators and instead has an indicator for metropolitan residence and more demographic characteristics. Documentation is included with the PUFs, and the PUFs are accompanied with SAS programs to prepare the data for analysis with that statistical analysis software. The 2008 PUF includes indicators for which variables have been imputed; thus, analysts can choose to omit imputed values if they choose.

RESEARCH THAT HAS USED THE NSSRN

The NSSRNs are used by HRSA to provide an integrated, in-depth picture of the total RN population, to assess the impact of federal programs for nursing and to evaluate the need for future federal interventions. Findings from each wave of the NSSRN have been reported in a significant publication about 2 years after the survey is fielded. The NSSRN data also have been incorporated into reports and recommendations from the National Advisory Council on Nurse Education and Practice (NACNEP). NACNEP has produced reports on nurse education and employment since 2001, as required under Section 845 of Title VIII of the PHS Act when it was amended by the Nurse Education and Practice Improvement Act of 1998 (Public Law 105–392). NACNEP's reports have focused on nursing shortages, educational needs, and the employment of RNs (NACNEP, 2002).

The NSSRN data have been used by many nongovernment researchers to study the RN workforce because the NSSRN data contain a rich array of variables, are readily available, and are free. Many articles and reports that have used the NSSRN are difficult to identify because "National Sample Survey of Registered Nurses" is usually not identified as a keyword or phrase. Some articles do not cite the NSSRN data among the references, but rather note the data source in the text. Finally, articles have been published in a variety of types of journals, including nursing, medicine, health policy, and economics. Searches of single databases, such as PubMed, will not identify articles published in different disciplines.

The articles discussed here provide a sense of the types of studies that have been conducted using the NSSRN. They were identified by searching the Social Science Citation Index, PubMed, CINAHL, and Google Scholar. References in each article were examined to identify other articles that used the NSSRN. Despite this broad search strategy, the review presented here should not be considered comprehensive. There are likely many other reports and articles that used the NSSRN, but were not identified for this article.

Because the report published by HRSA provides comprehensive descriptive statistics about the RN workforce, most articles published in academic journals focus on specific topics and utilize detailed statistical methods. This section reviews the key topics that have been considered in research articles that used the NSSRN.

Education of Nurses

The NSSRN contains detailed information about RN education and has been used to assess educational capacity and policy. These studies range from descriptive to theoretical and have been conducted by nursing researchers, economists, policy researchers, and scholars in other disciplines. The data can be used to assess educational trends, as well as relationships between education and employment, earnings, and demographics.

A few studies have considered whether education affects employment rates of RNs. For example, Schoen and Schoen (1985) found a positive relationship between employment and a nurse's highest level of educational preparation with 2000 NSSRN data. Nurses with graduate degrees were most likely to work, and RNs with associate degrees also had high employment rates. Nurses with diplomas and baccalaureate degrees had comparatively low rates of employment. Using multivariate regression methods, Buerhaus (1991) also found that RNs with an associate degree in nursing worked more hours than those with a diploma certificate. These findings suggest that efforts to expand the overall labor supply of RNs should invest more in AD education because AD graduates are more likely to work more hours.

A large number studies have examined the relationship between nurse education and earnings. Many of these studies use multivariate regression equations to estimate the effect of education while holding other RN characteristics constant. Nearly all these studies have found that nurses receive a small, statistically significant wage premium for the Bachelor of Science in Nursing (BSN; Booton & Lane, 1985; Lehrer, White, & Young, 1991; Link, 1988, 1992; Mennemeyer & Gaumer, 1983; Schumacher, 1997; Seago & Spetz, 2002; Spetz, 2002). Many of these studies also have found that the higher earnings received by baccalaureate-educated nurses are not high enough to make up for the additional years of educational expense required to obtain a BSN (Booton & Lane, 1985; Lehrer et al., 1991; Link, 1988; Mennemeyer & Gaumer, 1983; Seago & Spetz, 2002; Spetz, 2002). Seago and Spetz (2002) note that the lack of a substantial income differential between BSN nurses and those with associate degrees or diplomas is likely part of the reason most RNs receive their initial nursing education outside a baccalaureate program.

Spetz (2002) examined the impact of education on the probability of a nurse holding a managerial or other advanced job title and found that the BSN and graduate degrees are significantly associated with professional advancement. She hypothesizes that nurses who intend to pursue promotions and advanced opportunities will be more likely to see the BSN, even if the average return to the BSN is small. She also notes that the average age at graduation of AD-educated nurses is older than that of BSN graduates, suggesting that the associate degree is comparatively more attractive to returning, "second-career" students.

Pan and Straub (1997) used the 1992 NSSRN to examine whether the returns to education are different for nurses employed in rural areas as compared to urban areas. They found that nurses with higher education have higher earnings, but this gain is smaller for nurses who work in rural areas. They also find that work experience and employment setting are associated with the lower earnings for rural practice.

Demographics

The NSSRN has been used to examine changes in the age distribution of the U.S. nursing workforce and the implications of aging for current and future RN employment. It is well-documented HRSA's reports from the NSSRN that the age distribution of RNs is moving toward older age groups; independent studies have delved into the implications of aging and employment patterns for future labor supply. For example, using multiple years of the NSSRN, Sochalski (2002) reported that employment of young nurses had declined in 2000 relative to previous years and concluded that this could portend a lower supply of RNs in the future.

A number of studies have found that male nurses have higher earnings than female RNs, even when controlling for education, experience, and other factors that affect wages. Kalist (2002) used the NSSRN from 1992 and 1996 to study gender and earnings. He found that male nurses earned 2% more because they were more likely to work in administration—this job title difference explained 16% of the wage gap. Link's (1988) and Schumacher's (1997) studies of the return to nursing education using the NSSRN also found that the earnings of female nurses were lower than those of men.

Differences in rates of employment of male and female nurses have been studied. For example, Buerhaus (1991) found that male RNs worked 11 weeks more than married female RNs. More recently, Rajapaksa and Rothstein (2009) used the 2000 NSSRN and found that men were 2.5 times more likely than women to cite better salaries as a reason for leaving the nursing profession. There was no difference in the odds of citing more convenient hours or to state that the non-nursing position was more professionally rewarding.

The 2000, 2004, and 2008 NSSRNs included a question about language fluency. Kalist (2005) used the 2000 NSSRN to study the value of bilingualism. He hypothesizes that employers will pay a higher wage to bilingual nurses to improve patient care, meet government requirements, and limit legal liability. Using multivariate regression methods, he finds that bilingual RNs received wage premiums of up to 7% and that the premium was associated with the fraction of the population that spoke Spanish in the RN's county of employment.

The number of internationally educated nurses (IENs) living in the United States has increased over time. IENs accounted for 5.4% of licensed RNs in 2008 (US DHHS, 2010a, 2010b), which was an increase from 3.5% in 2004 (US DHHS, 2006). A number of studies have focused on this population, including Brush's descriptive article that used multiple data sources, including the NSSRN (Brush, Sochalski, & Berger, 2004). More recently, Xu and colleagues have examined the demographics and employment of internationally educated RNs. They have compared multiple waves of the NSSRN (Xu & Kwak, 2006), as well as provided more detailed analyses from single years of data (Xu & Kwak, 2007; Xu, Zaikina-Montgomery, & Shen, 2010).

Employment

The NSSRN is well suited to studying the decisions of nurses to work and the changes in employment patterns of nurses. Schoen and Schoen (1985) used NSSRN data from 1977 and 1980, along with data from the preceding surveys conducted by the ANA, to study nurse employment in a life table format. They found an increase in the labor force participation of nurses, as a nurse aged 20 could be expected to spend 28.5 years in the labor force in 1949 and 34.1 years in the labor force in 1980. Much of that rise was attributable to higher rates of full-time employment.

The factors that determine employment have been examined in many studies. For example, Buerhaus (1991) used the 1984 NSSRN to analyze the effects of economic and sociodemographic variables on the number of hours worked annually by RNs. Using multivariate regression analyses, he found that higher wages lead to only modest increases in the number of annual hours worked among unmarried RNs. Wages did not have a significant effect on the number of hours worked by married RNs, or RNs who were widowed, divorced, or separated. He also found that male and non-White nurses worked more hours per year, and the presence of young children at home had a substantial negative effect on the number of hours RNs worked.

A series of articles published by Charles Link, some with colleagues, has examined the impact of wages on the labor supply of nurses. Some of these studies have found that wage increases tend to reduce the number of hours nurses work, probably because nurses can attain a desired income with fewer hours of work. For example, Link and Settle (1980) found that wage increases have little effect on the number of nurses working and have a negative effect on the number of hours worked per week by married RNs. More recently, Chiha and Link (2003) used data from the 1992, 1996, and 2000 NSSRNs to examine labor supply. As in previous studies, they found that the wages have minor effects on both labor force participation and hours.

Several studies have focused on RNs who are not employed in nursing. Black, Spetz, and Harrington (2010) used the 2004 NSSRN to study the factors that predict nurses' decisions to not work in nursing and to work in other fields. Black, Spetz, and Harrington (2008) examined in more detail the reasons nurses work in non-nursing positions. Nooney, Unruh, and Yore (2010) analyzed the timing of attrition using survival analysis. With the 2004 NSSRN, they considered the exit path taken (career change vs. labor force separation) and the major socioeconomic, family structure, and demographic variables predicting attrition. They found that the rate of labor force separation is highest after the age of 60 and that early labor force separation is associated with marriage and providing care to dependents in the home.

Because the NSSRN has a large number of observations, analysis of specific subpopulations can be conducted. Goodman-Bacon and Ono (2007) used the surveys from 1980 through 2000 to study the demographic characteristics that predict temporary employment of nurses. Thompson (2010) also used multiple NSSRN surveys (1992–2004) to focus on occupational health nurses. He focused on characteristics that influence entry and retention in occupational health nursing practice. Schumacher (2007) focused on nursing faculty, using the NSSRNs from 1988 through 2004. He focused on the wages of RN instructors relative to RNs working in other positions, finding that the wages of RN instructors have been declining relative to other fields of nursing work.

Regional Analyses

The NSSRN provides information about the locations in which RNs live and work and thus can be used for regional analyses. The characteristics of nurses living in rural communities have been a topic of much study. Movassaghi, Kindig, Juhl, and Geller (1992) provided a descriptive study of the demographics and supply of nurses working in nonmetropolitan areas using the 1988 NSSRN. They found important differences in the ratio of RNs per population across county sizes and regions of the country and also found differences in the educational background and work activities of rural nurses as compared with those working in urban areas.

More recently, Skillman and colleagues examined the rural RN workforce using NSSRNs from 1980 through 2004 (Skillman, Palazzo, Hart, & Butterfield, 2007; Skillman, Palazzo, Keepnews, & Hart, 2006). They found that the number of rural RNs grew by 216%, which was a higher rate of growth when compared with urban RNs. However, a growing proportion of rural RNs commuted to larger rural towns and urban areas for work, resulting in a lower number of working RNs per capita in rural regions as compared to urban areas. Rural RNs have less nursing education on average than urban RNs. The salaries of RNs who live in rural areas are significantly lower than those living in cities, regardless of where they work, and the salary gap increased between 1980 and 2004. This is consistent with the finding of Pan and Straub (1997) that nurses employed in rural practices receive a lower income gain for education than do urban-employed RNs.

Brewer, Feeley, and Servoss (2003) used the 1996 and 2000 NSSRN to focus on the workforce of New York State. They compared characteristics of New York nurses to those of the United States as a whole. They found differences, particularly in the racial/ethnicity diversity of New York RNs and the share educated in other countries. They also determined that nurses in the eastern part of the state had different characteristics than those living in the western part of the state. Rosenfeld and Adams (2008) used the 1996, 2000, and 2004 NSSRNs to compare the RN workforce of the New York City metropolitan area with New York State as a whole. RNs working in New York City were less likely to have children living in the home, were more likely to have never married, had higher education and earnings levels, and were more likely to have been educated in another country. They also were more likely to work in hospitals and full-time.

Shortages

The NSSRN has been used to forecast the supply of RNs, which is important to assessing the current and future adequacy of the RN workforce. In 2002, the HRSA published forecasts of supply and demand of RNs through 2020, predicting that there would be a growing shortfall in the supply of RNs. The data also have been used to develop nursing labor market forecasts for single states; for example, Coffman and Spetz (1999) and Spetz (2009) have used the NSSRN data as part of forecasting California's workforce.

THE INFLUENCE THIS BODY OF RESEARCH HAS HAD ON POLICYMAKING

The forecasts of future nursing shortages published by HRSA (2002) provided the impetus for many states and the federal government to invest in expansions of nursing education to increase the long-term supply of RNs. Similarly, forecasts developed in California were a factor that led California nursing schools to expand 55% between 2003–2004 and 2007–2008 (Spetz, 2009). Subsequent waves of the NSSRN enable policymakers to assess the effectiveness of their efforts to increase RN supply; the 2008 NSSRN found that the number of RNs below 40 years of age increased substantially between 2004 and 2008, suggesting that investments in nursing education are leading to a measurably larger population of younger RNs (US DHHS, 2010a, 2010b).

Research that has demonstrated that the short-term supply of RNs is not very responsive to increases in wages also has played a role in leading states to expand the nursing education pipeline. If nurse supply increased significantly in response to wage growth, policymakers could assume that shortages would be brief, as wage increase would quickly bring more nurses into the labor market. Because this is not the case, policymakers know that RN supply increases primarily through the growth of the total number of licensed nurses, which requires enough educational capacity to ensure net growth.

Title VIII of the PHS Act authorizes programs that are administered by HRSA to support the RN workforce. The programs under Title VIII include grants to schools for master's and postmaster's nursing education, workforce diversity grants, loan repayment for nurses who practice in facilities with a critical shortage of nurses, loans for nurses pursuing master's and doctoral degrees, and grants to support geriatric nursing education. The NSSRN allows policymakers to identify the areas of greatest need, target Title VIII programs to those areas, and assess the impact of programs. Data on the diversity and education level of the RN workforce are particularly important to evaluation of Title VIII.

Researchers have consistently found that baccalaureate-educated nurses receive only a small increase in earnings relative to RNs with associate degrees or diplomas. This finding has helped to explain why associate degree RN programs are comparatively attractive to potential nurses. Policymakers and nursing leaders know that if they want to increase the share of RNs with baccalaureate and higher education, the cost of BSN education must be reduced, or the earnings of BSN nurses must be increased.

The NSSRN also has been used to evaluate other programs that affect nursing, such as California's minimum nurse-to-patient regulation for acute-care hospitals, which were implemented in 2004. Mark, Harless, and Spetz (2009) compared wage growth in California to that in other states, using the NSSRN and other data sources. They found that wages increased substantially faster in California than in other states, reflecting the higher demand for RNs spurred by California's law.

As the Patient Protection and Affordable Care Act of 2010—often called "health reform"—is implemented over the next decade, the NSSRN will provide important data to assess the adequacy of the RN workforce to meet health care needs in hospitals, ambulatory care, and other settings. The act created a National Health Workforce Commission to evaluate whether the demand for health workers is being met and to evaluate the need to engage in efforts to increase the supply of health workers. The first Chair of the Commission, Peter Buerhaus, PhD, RN, is deeply familiar with the NSSRN, having published a number of the articles cited in this review.

RECOMMENDATIONS FOR FUTURE RESEARCH

The NSSRN has been used to enrich our understanding of the RN workforce. While the data have been used to analyze many aspects of nursing in the United States, many other topics can and should be studied. These include more analysis of nurses who work as faculty and instructors, the characteristics and employment of newly licensed RNs, employment of men and minorities in nursing, and the work of nurses prepared in advanced practice fields. Topics that have been studied in the past can be reassessed as new data are available and the health care system of the United States changes.

The Institute of Medicine Committee on the Future of Nursing used the NSSRN to obtain data to inform their recommendations and also made specific recommendations regarding the need for better data on the health care workforce (Institute of Medicine, 2010). The committee recommends that HRSA increase the sample size of the NSSRN and conduct the survey every 2 years, in addition to developing a national repository for a "minimum data set" of information collected by state boards of nursing as part of their license renewal process.

If implemented, these recommendations would greatly enhance our ability to understand our RN workforce.

REFERENCES

Aiken, L. H. (1982). *Nursing in the 1980s: Crises, opportunities, challenges.* Philadelphia, PA: J.B. Lippincott Co.

Aiken, L. H., & Mullinix, C. F. (1987). The nursing shortage: Myth or reality? *New England Journal of Medicine, 317*(10), 641–646.

Bentley, B. S., Jones, D. C., Kendall, E. M., Moulton, S., & Savia, J. (1982). *National Sample Survey of Registered Nurses, II: Status of nurses, November, 1980.* Research Triangle Park, NC: Research Triangle Institute.

Biener, L., Garrett, C. A., Gilpin, E. A., Roman, A. M., & Currivan, D. B. (2004). Consequences of declining survey response rates for smoking prevalence estimates. *American Journal of Preventive Medicine, 27*(3), 254–257.

Black, L., Spetz, J., & Harrington, C. (2008). Nurses working outside of nursing: Societal trend or workplace crisis? *Policy, Politics, and Nursing Practice, 9*(3), 143–157.

Black, L., Spetz, J., & Harrington, C. (2010). Nurses who do not nurse: Factors that predict non-nursing work in the U.S. registered nursing labor market. *Nursing Economics, 28*(4), 245–254.

Booton, L. A., & Lane, J. I. (1985). Hospital market structure and the return to nursing education. *Journal of Human Resources, 20*(1), 183–195.

Brewer, C. S., Feeley, T. H., & Servoss, T. J. (2003). A statewide and regional analysis of New York state nurses using the 2000 National Sample Survey of Registered Nurses. *Nursing Outlook, 51*(5), 220–226.

Brush, B. L., Sochalski, J., & Berger, A. M. (2004). Imported care: Recruiting foreign nurses to U.S. health care facilities. *Health Affairs, 23*(3), 78–87.

Buerhaus, P. I. (1991). Economic determinants of annual hours worked by registered nurses. *Medical Care, 29*(12), 1181–1195.

Buerhaus, P. I. (1999). Is a nursing shortage on the way? *Nursing Management, 30*(2), 54–55.

Buerhaus, P. I., & Staiger, D. O. (1996). Managed care and the nurse workforce. *Journal of the American Medical Association, 276*(18), 1487–1493.

Chiha, Y. A., & Link. C. R. (2003). The shortage of registered nurses and some new estimates of the effects of wages on registered nurses labor supply: A look at the past and a preview of the 21st century. *Health Policy, 64,* 349–375.

Coffman, J., & Spetz, J. (1999). Maintaining an adequate supply of registered nurses in California: The case for increased public investment in nursing education. *Image: The Journal of Nursing Scholarship, 31*(4), 389–393.

Dillman, D. A., & Carley-Baxter, L. R. (2000). Structural determinants of mail survey response rates over a 12 year period, 1988–1999. *Proceedings of the Section on Survey Methods, American Statistical Association.* Alexandria, VA: American Statistical Association.

Friss, L. (1994). Nursing studies laid end to end form a circle. *Journal of Health Politics Policy and Law 19,* 597–631.

Goodman-Bacon, A., & Ono, Y. (2007). Who are temporary nurses? *Economic Perspectives Federal Reserve Bank of Chicago, Q1,* 2–13.

Health Resources and Service Administration. (2002). *Projected supply, demand, and shortage of registered nurses, 2000–2020.* Rockville, MD: Health Resources and Service Administration, U.S. Department of Health and Human Services.

Institute of Medicine. (2010). *The future of nursing: Leading change, advancing health.* Washington, DC: National Academies Press.

Kalist, D. E. (2002). The gender earnings gap in the RN labor market. *Nursing Economics, 20*(4), 155–162.

Kalist, D. E. (2005). Registered nurses and the value of bilingualism. *Industrial and Labor Relations Review, 59*(1), 101–118.

Lehrer, E. L., White, W. D., & Young, W. B. (1991). The three avenues to a registered nurse license: A comparative analysis. *Journal of Human Resources, 26,* 362–379.

Link, C. R. (1988). Returns to nursing education: 1970–1984. *Journal of Human Resources, 23*(3), 372–387.

Link, C. R. (1992). Labor supply behavior of registered nurses: Female labor supply in the future? *Research in Labor Economics, 13,* 287–320.

Link, C. R., & Settle, R. F. (1980). Financial incentive and labor supply of married professional nurses: An economic analysis. *Nursing Research, 29*(4), 238–243.

Mark, B., Harless, D. W., & Spetz, J. (2009). California's minimum-nurse-staffing legislation and nurses' wages. *Health Affairs, 28*(2), w326–w334.

Mennemeyer, S. T., & Gaumer, G. (1983). Nursing wages and the value of educational credentials. *Journal of Human Resources, 18*(1), 32–48.

Moses, E. B. (1994). *The registered nurse population: Findings from the National Sample Survey of Registered Nurses, March 1992.* Rockville, MD: Health Resources and Service Administration, U.S. Department of Health and Human Services.

Moses, E. B. (1998). *The registered nurse population: Findings from the National Sample Survey of Registered Nurses, March 1996.* Rockville, MD: Health Resources and Service Administration, U.S. Department of Health and Human Services.

Movassaghi, H., Kindig, D. A., Juhl, N., & Geller, J. M. (1992). Nursing supply and characteristics in the nonmetropolitan areas of the United States: Findings from the 1988 National Sample Survey of Registered Nurses. *Journal of Rural Health, 8*(4), 276–282.

National Advisory Council on Nurse Education and Practice (NACNEP). (2002). *Second report to the Secretary of Health and Human Services and the Congress.* Rockville, MD: U.S. Department of Health and Human Services.

Nooney, J. G., Unruh, L., & Yore, M. M. (2010). Should I stay or should I go? Career change and labor force separation among registered nurses in the U.S. *Social Science and Medicine, 70*(12), 1874–1881.

Pan, S., & Straub, L. (1997). Returns to nursing education: Rural and nonrural practice. *Journal of Rural Health, 13*(1), 78–85.

Rajapaksa, S., & Rothstein, W. (2009). Factors that influence the decisions of men and women nurses to leave nursing. *Nursing Forum, 44*(3), 195–206.

Reichelt, P. A., & Young, W. B. (1985). Professional nursing personnel: Data-based policy formulation. *Journal of Professional Nursing, 1*(3), 164–171.

Rosenfeld, P., & Adams, R. E. (2008). Factors associated with hospital retention of RNs in the New York City metropolitan area: An analysis of the 1996, 2000, and 2004 National Sample Survey of Registered Nurses. *Policy, Politics, & Nursing Practice, 9*(3), 158–172.

Roth, A., Graham, D., & Schmittling, G. (1979). *1977 National Sample Survey of Registered Nurses: A report on the nurse population and the factors affecting their supply.* Kansas City, MO: American Nurses Association.

Schoen, D. C., & Schoen, R. (1985). A life table analysis of the labor force participation of U.S. nurses, 1949 to 1980. *Research in Nursing and Health, 8*(2), 105–116.

Schumacher, E. J. (1997). Relative wages and the returns to education in the labor market for registered nurses. In S. Polochek (Ed.), *Research in labor economics,* Vol. 16. London: JAI Press.

Schumacher, E. J. (2007). *Relative wages and the market for nursing instructors.* Manuscript, Trinity University, San Antonio, Texas.

Seago, J. A., & Spetz, J. (2002). Registered nurse pre-licensure education in California. *Nursing Economics, 20*(3), 113–117

Skillman, S. M., Palazzo, L., Hart, L. G., & Butterfield, P. (2007). *Changes in the rural registered nurse workforce from 1980 to 2004. Final Report #115.* Seattle, WA: University of Washington Rural Health Research Center.

Skillman, S. M., Palazzo, L., Keepnews, D., & Hart, L. G. (2006). Characteristics of registered nurses in rural versus urban areas: Implications for strategies to alleviate nursing shortages in the United States. *Journal of Rural Health, 22*(2), 151–157.

Sochalski, J. (2002). Nursing shortage redux: Turning the corner on an enduring problem. *Health Affairs, 21*(5), 157–164.

Spetz, J. (2002). The value of additional education in a licensed profession: The choice of associate or baccalaureate degrees in nursing. *Economics of Education Review, 21*, 73–85.

Spetz, J. (2009). *Forecasts of the registered nurse workforce in California.* Sacramento, CA: California Board of Registered Nursing.

Spratley, E., Johnson, A., Sochaski, J., Fritz, M., & Spencer, W. (2002). *The registered nurse population: Findings from the National Sample Survey of Registered Nurses, March 2000.* Rockville, MD: Health Resources and Service Administration, U.S. Department of Health and Human Services.

Thompson, M. C. (2010). Review of occupational health nurse data from recent national sample surveys of registered nurses-part I. *AAOHN Journal, 58*(1), 27–39.

U.S. Department of Health and Human Services (US DHHS). (1983). *The registered nurse population: An Overview from National Sample Survey of Registered Nurses, November, 1980.* Rockville, MD: Health Resources and Service Administration, U.S. Department of Health and Human Services.

U.S. Department of Health and Human Services (US DHHS). (1986). *National Sample Survey of Registered Nurses, November 1984.* Rockville, MD: Health Resources and Service Administration, U.S. Department of Health and Human Services.

U.S. Department of Health and Human Services (US DHHS). (1990). *The registered nurse population: Findings from the National Sample Survey of Registered Nurses, March 1988.* Rockville, MD: Health Resources and Service Administration, U.S. Department of Health and Human Services.

U.S. Department of Health and Human Services (US DHHS). (2006). *The registered nurse population: Findings from the National Sample Survey of Registered Nurses, March 2004.* Rockville, MD: Health Resources and Service Administration, U.S. Department of Health and Human Services.

U.S. Department of Health and Human Services (US DHHS). (2010a). *The registered nurse population: Findings from the 2008 National Sample Survey of Registered Nurses.* Rockville, MD: Health Resources and Service Administration, U.S. Department of Health and Human Services.

U.S. Department of Health and Human Services (US DHHS). (2010b). *Organization/History.* Rockville, MD: Health Resources and Service Administration, U.S. Department of Health and Human Services. Retrieved October 31, 2010, from http://www.hrsa.gov/about/organi zation/history.html

Xu, Y., & Kwak, C. (2006). Trended profile of internationally educated nurses in the United States: Implications for the nursing shortage and beyond. *Journal of Nursing Administration, 36*(11), 522–525.

Xu, Y., & Kwak, C. (2007). Comparative trend analysis of characteristics of internationally educated nurses and U.S. educated nurses in the United States. *International Nursing Review, 54*(1), 78–84.

Xu, Y., Zaikina-Montgomery, H., & Shen, J. J. (2010). Characteristics of internationally educated nurses in the United States: An update from the 2004 National Sample Survey of Registered Nurses, *Nursing Economics, 28*(1), 19–43.

Yett, D. E. (1966). The nursing shortage and the Nurse Training Act of 1964, *Industrial and Labor Relations Review, 19*(2), 190–200.

Yett, D. E. (1970). Causes and consequences of salary differentials in nursing. *Inquiry, 7,* 78–99.

Yett, D. E. (1975). *An economic analysis of the nurse shortage.* Lexington, MA: Lexington Books.

CHAPTER 2

Job Satisfaction and Retention of Military Nurses

A Review of the Literature

George A. Zangaro and Patricia A. Watts Kelley

ABSTRACT

Job satisfaction is an extremely important concept that influences a nurse's decision to stay in an organization, as well as the cost of turnover and the nursing shortage. The purpose of this review is to identify published research studies that have assessed job satisfaction and retention (intent to stay) in military nurses serving in the Army, Navy, or Air Force. The available literature was searched from 1980 to 2010 and the review resulted in 21 studies. The majority of the studies used a descriptive correlational design and was specific to one particular service. The researchers reported several satisfiers such as strong sense of teamwork, favorable work environments, pay and benefits, promotional opportunities, leadership and management experiences offered to junior officers. One of the major dissatisfiers was the lack of support from leadership. Nurse researchers must expand the retention science with robust longitudinal interventional studies. Nurse researchers are well positioned to provide military nurse leaders with the best possible evidence to address issues and make decisions regarding nurse retention.

© 2011 Springer Publishing Company
DOI: 10.1891/0739-6686.28.19

Job satisfaction has been studied for decades and is perhaps one of the most widely studied concepts in the nursing and organizational literature. Job satisfaction intuitively influences retention rates of nurses in all organizations. The purpose of this review is to identify published research studies that have assessed job satisfaction and retention (intent to stay) in military nurses serving in the Army, Navy and Air Force.

Job satisfaction is defined as the degree to which employees like their job (Price & Mueller, 1986), and is extremely important to nursing for three main reasons. First and most importantly is the direct, positive relationship between job satisfaction and an employee's intent to stay in an organization. Intent to stay is defined as the degree of likelihood of an employee maintaining membership in the organization (Price & Mueller, 1986). Job satisfaction is an employee attitude, which refers to an employee's orientation toward their work, whereas intent to stay is a behavior that refers to an employee maintaining membership in the organization. Therefore, satisfied employees are more likely to remain in an organization.

The second reason is related to the cost of turnover in organizations. Evidence exists that provides substantial support for the position that nurse turnover is costly (Jones, 2004, 2005; Jones & Gates, 2007; O'Brien-Pallas et al., 2006; Waldman, Kelly, Arora, & Smith, 2004). Nursing administrators have both economic and non-economic concerns regarding the turnover of nurses. Economic concerns include the cost of turnover, quality of care being provided to patients and the loss of human capital with many years of experience. Cost projections for filling a nurse vacancy are between $82,000 and $88,000 per nurse (Jones, 2008). In addition to recruitment and training costs, this includes the cost of filling the vacancy through premium pay and bonuses, and the use of agency nurses and overtime. Non-economic concerns include increased workload of existing staff, which may trigger greater absenteeism and increased turnover due to job dissatisfaction, job stress, and inadequate staffing to provide safe care to patients.

The final reason that job satisfaction is important to nursing is the perpetuation of the chronic nursing shortage in the United States. The most recent shortage of nurses has become the longest lasting shortage in nursing history (Buerhaus, Donelan, Ulrich, Norman, & Dittus, 2005). While the current global recession has eased the shortage, it is projected that the shortfall of nurses in the US could reach 500,000 by 2025 (Buerhaus, Staiger, & Auerbach, 2009). The report by Buerhaus and colleagues also projects that the demand for nurses will increase by 2% to 3% each year. The federal government has increased funding and also initiated programs such as the Nurse Reinvestment Act (2002), in an effort to alleviate the shortage of nurses. However, the average age of a registered nurse is 46.8 years (Buerhaus et al., 2009) reflecting the high probability that many currently practicing nurses will not be in the workforce 20 years from now.

Buerhaus and colleagues also project that nurses in their 50s will become the largest segment of the nursing workforce by 2012.

The U.S. military is also competing for the same shrinking pool of registered nurses. In contrast to the private sector, there are unique aspects related to military recruitment and retention. A military nurse is required to sign a contract for a fixed number of years which prevents the service member from leaving the military to take other jobs. This may be one reason that the current shortage of nurses is not demonstrating as much of an immediate effect on the military. In all the military services, there are set recruitment goals that recruiters are required to meet in order to ensure that the end strength (required number of FTEs) does not fall below a critical level. The age of the military nurse has remained relatively constant due to the age restrictions on military service members. Military nurses tend to be significantly younger than nurses who work in civilian hospitals. Finally, the military offers attractive recruiting packages, robust pay and health care benefits, outstanding educational benefits, housing allowances and on-base facilities for childcare. These are factors that contribute to a lessening of the shortage of military nurses (Cooper & Parsons, 2002). Each of the military services are well prepared and experienced in the rapid mobilization and deployment of large volumes of personnel, equipment, and supplies. During a wartime crisis, one of the most crucial groups of individuals to be deployed are military nurses. Operational readiness is affected if Nurse Corps officers are not retained, especially in the critical specialties such as certified registered nurse anesthetists (CRNAs), nurse practitioners (NPs), and peri-operative and critical care nurses.

Although the impacts of the nursing shortage are not as severe in the military, as compared to the private sector, military hospitals are vulnerable to the nursing shortage because of the increased demand for acute care services for service members recently sustaining injuries in Iraq and Afghanistan. Additionally, military hospitals are unique because the staffing is a mix of both military and civilian personnel. Civilian nursing personnel complement active-duty military nursing staff and serve as "back-fill" for military nurses during humanitarian and wartime operations. Civilian nurses are an integral part of the mission in military hospitals and are especially critical to achieving the hospital mission due to the increased demand for acute care services. However, due to the shortage of nurses nationwide and the increasing opportunities in the civilian sector for nurses, it is becoming more difficult to recruit and retain civilian nurses in military facilities.

JOB SATISFACTION AND INTENT TO STAY

The conceptual distinction between job satisfaction and intent to stay is that job satisfaction is an employee attitude and intent to stay is a behavior. In the nursing and organizational literature, models frequently specify job satisfaction as an intervening variable between work-related, organizational and individual factors and intent to stay (Kim, Price, Mueller, & Watson, 1996; Kovner, Brewer, Greene, & Fairchild, 2009; Kovner et al., 2007; Price, 2001; Price & Mueller, 1986; Zangaro, 2004). A substantial body of empirical evidence supports a positive relationship between job satisfaction and intent to stay (Hinshaw, Smeltzer, & Atwood, 1987; Ingersoll, Olsan, Drew-Cates, DeVinney, & Davies, 2002; Kovner et al., 2007, 2009; Larrabee et al., 2003; Price & Mueller, 1981; Zangaro, 2004). Job satisfaction is a determinant of intent to stay (Coomber & Barriball, 2007; Hayes et al., 2006; Ingersoll et al., 2002; Kim et al., 1996; Larrabee et al., 2003; Lu, While & Barriball, 2005; Price, 2001; Price & Mueller, 1986; Rambur, Palumbo, McIntosh, & Mongeon, 2003; Yin & Yang, 2002).

The nursing literature on retention indicates that several factors affect the retention of nurses: (1) work environment, (2) job dissatisfaction, (3) job-related stress, (4) personal commitments and career opportunities, and (5) lack of recognition of professional status (Aiken et al., 2001; Coomber & Barriball, 2007; Fletcher, 2001; Greiner, Krause, Ragland, & Fisher, 2004; Kovner et al., 2009; Ma, Lee, Yang, & Chang, 2009). In a review of the nursing literature on turnover, Hayes et al. (2006) reported that job satisfaction and intent to stay were consistently found to affect nurse retention.

These factors are not unique to the civilian community. Zangaro and Johantgen (2009) conducted a study which assessed nurses' job satisfaction of Navy Nurses ($n = 283$) and Civil Service ($n = 213$) nurses employed at three federal facilities on the east coast using a descriptive correlational, survey design. They concluded that there were some differences in the satisfiers for both military and civilian personnel, and therefore suggested tailoring retention strategies specific to each group to enhance retention. Military nurses were not satisfied with the support they received from their supervisors, whereas the civilian nurses perceived a lack of coworker support and role ambiguity. Pagliara (2003) conducted a secondary data analysis of Navy Nurses who were surveyed over a 3-year period (1998, $n = 522$; 1999, $n = 377$; 2000, $n = 391$) and found decreased job stress and increased satisfaction were related to intent to stay. Using a descriptive, survey design, Allgood, O'Rourke, VanDerslice, and Hardy (2000) conducted a study in an Army hospital in the southwestern United States that assessed job satisfaction among both military ($n = 144$) and civilian ($n = 57$) nursing staff. They found that military personnel were no less dissatisfied than civil service staff; both groups indicated frustration with staff shortages, hospital policies, scheduling, and lack of administrative support. In a study of job satisfaction among Navy NPs ($n = 45$), the most important dissatisfiers were work overload and being placed in a billet outside of one's specialty (Chung-Park, 1998). All of these studies were conducted at military hospitals and therefore have limited general application.

METHODS

This review of the literature uses studies published in English that were available in the literature from 1980 to June 2010. The population of interest for this literature review consists of studies of registered nurses in the Army, Navy, and Air Force. Studies were reviewed by the authors and included if they met the following criteria: (1) the study was published between 1980 and June 2010, (2) the study was a quantitative or qualitative analysis of data, (3) the study sample included military nurses, and (4) the study was published in English. Studies were excluded if they did not meet the above eligibility criteria.

An exhaustive literature search technique was performed to reduce the risk of biasing the results of the review. Extensive searching of electronic databases and footnote chasing was performed to locate published studies meeting the inclusion criteria. In June 2010, computerized database searches were conducted using Medline (1980–2010), CINAHL (1980–2010), PubMed (1980–2010), PsycINFO (1980–2010), and ProQuest (1980–2010). The searches included keywords that were based on the constructs being analyzed in this review, job satisfaction and intent to stay. The keywords used in the searches were job satisfaction, military nursing, intent to stay, intent to leave, retention, and military nurse retention. A Boolean strategy using operators "AND" and "OR" was utilized to refine the searches and ensure an exhaustive search was completed.

RESULTS

Fourteen articles, five dissertations and two master's theses, for a total of 21 studies, were found that met the inclusion criteria for the review (Table 2.1).

The quantitative studies across all services varied in sample selection, data collection techniques, methods, and job satisfaction and intent to stay instruments. Due to the variability in the studies and the lack of statistics reported in the majority of the studies, a meta-analysis examining the magnitude of the relationship between job satisfaction and intent to stay is not possible. However, the findings from these studies consistently identified models that demonstrated a relationship between various work related, organizational and/or individual factors and job satisfaction, which serves as an intervening variable between these factors and intent to stay in the military. Additionally, the studies consistently reported a positive relationship between job satisfaction and intent to stay.

TABLE 2.1

Summary of Research on Job Satisfaction and Intent to Stay of Military Nurses

Author/Year	Purpose	Sample	Design	Findings
Allgood et al. (2000)	To identify factors associated with job satisfaction among nursing staff at an Army hospital.	Army (*n* = 144) and civil service (*n* = 57) nursing staff in a military hospital in the Southwestern United States.	Descriptive; cross-sectional survey	50.4% response rate; overall satisfaction score 4.1 and there was no difference in satisfaction between military and civil service. All nurses rated professional status and autonomy as the most important job components.
Chung-Park (1998)	To describe the perceptions of the Navy Nurse Practitioner's (NP) roles by leadership and measure the level of job satisfaction among Navy NPs.	NPs (*n* = 45) and leadership (*n* = 402) (Commanding Officers, Directors of Nursing, Physicians in the US Navy in hospitals and clinics in the US and overseas)	Descriptive survey	Response rates were 64% from NPs; 40% from leadership; Overall NPs were satisfied with their job (Personal satisfaction had the highest mean score). Leadership was very satisfied with NPs. Dissatisfiers were: 1) lack of bonuses, 2) command taking precedence over professional needs, 3) increased administrative tasks, 4) not being fully accepted by other Nurse Corps officers, 5) being pulled between physicians and Nurse Corps, and 6) limited contact with other NPs.

Cox et al. (2010)	To identify factors that contribute to the retention of United States Navy Nurse Corps reservists called to active duty in 2003.	Navy Nurse Corps Reservists (n = 264)	Retrospective, cross-sectional survey	Nurses were asked what their retention intentions were and 73% will probably to definitely stay until retirement Job satisfaction had the strongest influence on one's intent to stay in the Navy Reserves.
Foley et al. (2002)	To describe characteristics of nurses and their work environment at two military hospitals.	Military Nurses (n = 59) and Civil Service nurses (n = 41)	Descriptive, cross-sectional	Both military and civilian nurses reported a very positive, satisfying work environment. No differences were noted on sub-scale scores between military and civilian nurses. The findings all reflect favorably on the military work environment.
Janelli & Jarmuz (1987)	To identify motivational factors which contribute to the retention of reserve flight nurses in an aeromedical evacuation unit.	United States Air Force Reserve Nurses (n = 69)	Descriptive, cross-sectional, survey	Overall nurses were satisfied with their job. 48% indicated that their greatest satisfaction was flying and the chance to fly actual missions. Dissatisfiers were work conditions (amount of work expected), inadequate management, and quality of policies.
Kocher et al. (1994)	To identify factors that explain turnover behavior of Army Nurses making career choices to stay or leave the military.	Female Army Officers (n = 158) at the rank of 2nd Lieutenant, 1st Lieutenant and Captain	Longitudinal analysis of retention behaviors	Satisfaction with work and military life, location / assignment stability, race-ethnic group, and family status all had significant effects on retention decisions.

(Continued)

TABLE 2.1

Summary of Research on Job Satisfaction and Intent to Stay of Military Nurses   *(Continued)*

Author/Year	Purpose	Sample	Design	Findings
LaRocco et al. (1989)	To examine the perceptions of military physicians, dentists, and nurses of dimensions of the work environment pertinent to stress and well-being.	Navy Physicians ($n = 86$), Dentists ($n = 40$), and Nurses ($n = 94$) all stationed at one large US Naval Hospital.	Descriptive correlational; cross-sectional survey	Nurses reported the most satisfaction with control over others, influence on decisions, self-determination on the job, and understanding of events in the work environment. Nurses reported the lowest job satisfaction, growth satisfaction, satisfaction with work hours, and professional satisfaction as compared to physicians and dentists.
Patrician et al. (2010)	To examine organizational determinants of work outcomes and quality of care ratings.	Army Nurses ($n = 353$), Civilian Nurses ($n = 602$) who worked in Army's 23 U.S. hospitals	Descriptive correlational; cross-sectional survey	Response rate 53%; Unfavorable nursing practice environments were associated with job dissatisfaction, emotional exhaustion, intent to leave, and fair to poor quality of care.
Prevosto (2001)	To examine the impact of mentoring on job satisfaction and intent to stay.	U.S. Army Reserve Nurses ($n = 171$)	Quasi-experimental	Response rate 57%; Mentored nurses reported a higher level of job satisfaction and intent to stay as compared to non-mentored nurses.
Robinson et al. (1993)	To compare military and civilian nurses' perceptions of work life.	Navy Nurses ($n = 37$) and civilian nurses ($n = 37$)	Descriptive correlational; cross-sectional survey	Response rate 89%; Military nurses felt less supported by supervisors and peers, but more satisfied with pay and fringe benefits as compared to civilian nurses.

Savage et al. (1993)	To report the findings of the extended research and the discovery of significant levels of work excitement.	Navy Nurses ($n = 201$)	Descriptive correlational; cross-sectional survey	Navy nurses were excited about the variety of their job, leadership / management experiences, and opportunities for teaching and learning. They were not satisfied or excited about the level of support provided from management.
Stuckey et al. (2006)	To examine job satisfaction among U.S. Air Force Certified Registered Nurse Anesthetists (CRNAs).	Air Force CRNAs ($n = 83$)	Descriptive correlational; cross-sectional survey	Response rate 60.1%; Most CRNAs (75.9%) satisfied with their job and believed the military was a good company to work for. U.S. Air Force CRNAs perceive inadequate pay and compensation and lack of promotion opportunities as the primary issues affecting their intent to stay.
Yoder (1995)	To investigate the career development relationships (CDRs) experienced by staff nurses in relation to professionalism, job satisfaction, and intent to stay.	Army Nurses ($n = 390$)	Descriptive correlational; cross-sectional survey	Job satisfaction and intent to stay were significant outcomes of having a CDR (positive correlations). Army nurses placed most importance on quality of leadership. However, Army staff nurses desire more support from leadership at the immediate supervisor level, more flexible schedules, more support services, and better staffing.

(Continued)

TABLE 2.1

Summary of Research on Job Satisfaction and Intent to Stay of Military Nurses (Continued)

Author/Year	Purpose	Sample	Design	Findings
Zangaro (2009)	To expand knowledge of satisfaction of Navy and Civil Service Nurses.	Navy Nurses (n = 283) and Civil Service (n = 213)	Descriptive correlational, cross-sectional survey	Response rate 42%; Supervisor support, promotional opportunity, and resource adequacy had a significantly positive association with job satisfaction of Navy Nurses. Routinization has the strongest negative association with satisfaction for both Navy and Civil Service Nurses. Higher levels of routinization were associated with less job satisfaction.
Dissertations and Theses				
House* (2007)	To examine forces impacting career longevity of Army nurses.	Army Nurses (n = 6)	Qualitative: semi-structured interviews	The interviews revealed that job satisfaction, leadership, availability of education, personal life events, and presence of children all influenced retention of Army Nurses.
Lang (2008)	To examine the validity and measurement properties of the Practice Environment Scale, Maslach Burnout Inventory, and a proposed intent to leave model.	Army Nurses (n = 333) and Civil Service Nurses (n = 408)	Secondary data analysis	The SEM findings did not support the hypothesis that individual attributes, job dissatisfaction, practice environment, or burnout are causal underpinnings of intent to leave.

Moorhead (1993)	To develop and estimate a causal model of job satisfaction, commitment, search behavior, and intent to leave the Air Force.	Air Force Nurses (n = 256)	Descriptive correlational; cross-sectional survey	Variance explained in the causal model is: job satisfaction (58%), commitment (56%), search behavior (38%) and intent to leave (68%). Job satisfaction (-.456) and commitment (-.455) had the greatest total effect on intent to leave. Promotional opportunity (-.304) had the third largest effect.
Owings* (1999)	To assess factors affecting job satisfaction among Family Nurse Practitioners (FNPs) in the U.S. Air Force.	Air Force FNPs (n = 32)	Descriptive correlational; cross-sectional survey	Overall, Air Force FNPs report a high level of satisfaction with their jobs. Autonomy, sense of accomplishment, and time spent in patient care were the top 3 factors contributing to job satisfaction. Lack of opportunity to utilize their skills as an NP, lack of supervisor and coworker support, heavy workload, and salary were all dissatisfiers.
Pagliara (2003)	To use secondary data to examine levels of job satisfaction, job stress, importance of career needs of Navy Nurses.	Navy Nurses - 1998 (n = 522); 1999 (n = 377); 2000 (n = 391).	Descriptive correlational; Secondary analysis	Overall, Navy Nurses reported intent to stay on active duty, moderate levels of job satisfaction, and low levels of stress on the job. In each year of the study, job satisfaction had the highest significant positive correlation with intent to stay and job stress had a negative correlation with intent to stay. In the regression model, job satisfaction was the most significant predictor of intent to stay.

(Continued)

TABLE 2.1

Summary of Research on Job Satisfaction and Intent to Stay of Military Nurses   (Continued)

Author/Year	Purpose	Sample	Design	Findings
Roach (1991)	To determine if correlations existed between six factors of work satisfaction.	Army Reserve Nurses (n = 144)	Descriptive correlational; cross-sectional survey	Overall job satisfaction, role conflict, and years of prior active service were the most significant predictors of intent to leave the reserves. In addition, as role conflict and role ambiguity increase, job satisfaction decreases.
Stewart (2002)	To assess levels of job stress and job satisfaction and their relation to intent to stay in the Army.	Army Nurses (n = 136)	Descriptive correlational; cross-sectional survey	Response rate 60%; Overall, nurses reported a low stress level and low satisfaction level. Neither variable was significantly correlated with intent to stay.

*Indicates thesis.

The majority of the studies were conducted by nurses using a descriptive, correlational design. Typically, a survey approach was utilized to elicit nurses' attitudes, beliefs, perceptions and behaviors concerning job satisfaction and intent to stay. The surveys were handed out in the workplace, placed in a work mailbox, or mailed to nurses' homes. All studies used a convenience sample of nurses in one or more facilities. There were two dissertations that utilized secondary data (Lang, 2008; Pagliara, 2003) and one master's thesis that used a qualitative approach (House, 2007). Of the 21 studies, the samples consisted of nine Army, seven Navy, four Air Force and one study that did not identify the service being studied. Not all studies reported a response rate, but of those that did (8/21), response rates were all 42% or higher.

One of the major challenges assessing job satisfaction is the inconsistent use of a particular instrument to measure job satisfaction. Job Satisfaction was measured by many different instruments across the 21 studies, with multiple independent variables being correlated with job satisfaction. In addition, job satisfaction was used as both an independent and dependent variable in studies. The most consistent measures of job satisfaction noted across the studies were Price and Mueller's (1986) measure of job satisfaction (Cox et al., 2010; Moorhead, 1993; Stewart, 2002; Zangaro & Johantgen, 2009) and a version of the Nurse Work Index (Allgood et al., 2000; Foley et al., 2002; Lang, 2008; Patrician, Shang, & Lake, 2010; Stewart, 2002; Yoder, 1995). There was no justification provided for the use of a particular measure of job satisfaction over another measure, which makes it difficult to determine if the measure was selected out of convenience or because of high reliability coefficients in prior studies. Intent to stay was measured using multiple measures with a number of different items on each measure. The reliability for both job satisfaction and intent to stay instruments was reported in most of the studies. The reliability was estimated using Cronbach's alpha and the estimates were all acceptable with a score of .70 or higher (Nunnally & Bernstein, 1994). Sample specific validity was reported in a few studies, but the majority of the studies reported validity being established using other samples.

Several of the studies only used basic statistics (e.g., t-tests and analysis of variance) when conducting their analyses. Seven studies used multivariate analysis and reported the variance explained in job satisfaction and/or intent to stay (Cox et al., 2010; Lang, 2008; LaRocco et al., 1989; Moorhead, 1993; Pagliara, 2003; Patrician et al., 2010; Roach, 1991; Zangaro & Johantgen, 2009). The percent of variance among both variables: job satisfaction and intent to stay, varied between studies. The variation noted between these variables could be related to several factors such as the variables being added into and/or controlled in the model, study designs and methods used when conducting the study. Typically, researchers reported correlations among variables and alpha coefficients as a measure of reliability of all scales.

Six studies examined the factors affecting job satisfaction and/or retention of both military and civil service nurses (Allgood et al., 2000; Foley et al., 2002; Lang, 2008; Patrician et al., 2010; Robinson, Sammons, & Keim, 1993; Zangaro & Johantgen, 2009). The inclusion of civil service nurses is extremely important because in most military facilities they comprise at least 45% to 55% of the nursing staff. When military staff are deployed for a wartime or peacetime mission the civil service nurses are relied on to continue operations as usual. The findings across the majority of the studies indicate that the level of job satisfaction did not differ between military and civil service personnel. Patrician and colleagues (2010) indicated that there was no difference in intent to leave between military and civil service nurses. One of the more relevant findings from this study was the fact that poor work environments were significantly associated with job dissatisfaction, emotional exhaustion, intent to leave and fair to poor quality of care. Additionally, military and civil service nurses rated nurse manager ability and support as 2.58 and 2.57, respectively. These ratings are just above the midpoint on a four-point response scale that was used in this study.

Robinson and colleagues (1993) identified a statistically significant ($p < .01$) difference in job satisfaction between military ($n = 37$) and civil service nurses ($n = 37$). Civil service nurses reported a significantly higher level of job satisfaction as compared to military nurses. After conducting post-hoc testing, it was noted that civil service nurses were significantly less satisfied with their pay and benefits as compared to military nurses. Additionally, military nurses perceived less supervisor support and less peer cohesion as compared to civil service nurses. The lack of supervisor support and peer cohesion may result in decreased teamwork and cooperation from the staff. Savage and colleagues (1993) compared Navy nurses to civilian nurses in a non-military setting. Navy nurses reported a higher level of satisfaction as compared to civilian counterparts in a non-military setting. Navy nurses were excited about the variety of jobs offered, leadership and management experience gained and teaching and learning experience obtained while in the military. However, in this study, work excitement was negatively correlated with inadequate support from nursing management. Again, nurses were asking for more support from leadership.

Zangaro and Johantgen (2009) identified factors associated with job satisfaction of military and civil service nurses. Using a linear regression approach, the models explained 51% of the variance in job satisfaction for Navy Nurses and 55% for civilian nurses. For both Navy and civil service nurses, routinization has the strongest significant relationship with job satisfaction. Moreover, promotional opportunity, supervisor support and resource adequacy were significant predictors for military nurses. Additional significant predictors for civil service nurses were promotional opportunity, coworker support and role ambiguity.

Allgood et al. (2000) identified a significant difference between military and civil service nurses on the concept of professional interaction. Military nurses reported more satisfaction with professional interactions. When asked to list what they liked least about their jobs, both military and civil service nurses listed military structure, staff shortages, scheduling, and lack of administrative support. Interestingly, organization politics does not only provide high levels of satisfaction, but it had the lowest mean score when ranked against the other variables used to measure job satisfaction. Foley et al. (2002) found no differences in level of job satisfaction between military and civil service nurses, but reported that military nurses had a significantly higher autonomy score as compared to civil service nurses. Another interesting finding was a significant difference in professional certifications (i.e., Emergency Room, Medical / Surgical, CCRN, or CNS/NP), with civil service nurses having more certifications as compared to military nurses.

In the studies by Moorhead (1993) and Pagliara (2003), both found that job satisfaction was the most significant predictor of intent to stay. Organizational commitment and promotional opportunity had also had a moderately large effect on intent to stay (Moorhead). Pagliara analyzed data from nurses across a 3-year period, and her findings supported the positive relationship between job satisfaction and intent to stay, and the negative relationship between job stress and intent to stay that has been identified in several studies. Overall, Pagliara found that Navy nurses reported low levels of job stress, moderate levels of satisfaction and an intention to stay on the job.

There were four studies conducted with Army, Navy and Air Force reserve nurses (Cox et al., 2010; Janelli & Jarmuz, 1987; Prevosto, 2001; Roach, 1991). Cox et al. (2010) reported that job satisfaction had the strongest influence on intent to stay in the reserves. Job satisfaction was also noted to be a significant mediator between environmental, employee and work-related factors and intent to stay. Seventy-three percent of the nurses indicated that they would probably-to-definitely stay in the reserves. Janelli and Jarmuz (1987) studied nurses in an aeromedical evacuation unit. The authors reported that 48% of the flight nurses indicated that their work itself provided them with the greatest satisfaction. Interestingly, the work conditions, defined as the amount of work expected, was the greatest dissatisfier. Roach (1991) reported that the strongest predictor of intent to stay was overall job satisfaction followed by years of prior service. The longer someone was in the service the more likely he or she is to stay. She also concluded that there was a negative relationship between role conflict and job satisfaction ($r = .28$), and role ambiguity and job satisfaction ($r = .20$).

There was one quasi-experimental study (Prevosto, 2001) in this group of reserve nurse studies. The study randomly selected a sample of reserve nurses who had mentors as compared to a control group of nurses who did not have a mentor. The researchers hypothesized that reserve nurses who had a mentor would report a higher level of job satisfaction and would be more likely to stay as compared to reserve nurses who are not mentored. The hypothesis was supported for both job satisfaction and intent to stay. In addition, there was a significantly strong correlation ($r = .62$) between job satisfaction and intent to stay. A similar study by Yoder (1995) compared a group of Army nurses ($n = 236$) who experienced a career development relationship (CDR), to a group ($n = 154$) who did not have a CDR. A CDR was defined as precepting, peer-strategizing, coaching, sponsoring, and mentoring. When the two groups were compared across these five variables, there was no difference between the groups. However, there was a significant difference in job satisfaction and intent to stay, favoring the CDR group.

Another aspect of Yoder's study compared the CDR and non-CDR groups with Magnet hospital counterparts from a study conducted by Kramer and Schmalenberg (1991). The comparison was conducted using the subscales of the Nurse Work Index (management style, quality of leadership, organizational structure, professional practice, and professional development). The scores indicated that the CDR group of Army nurses reported more satisfaction on all subscales except professional development. The non-CDR group was only slightly more satisfied than their Magnet counterparts were. This study signifies that Army staff nurses had been asking for better staffing, flexible scheduling, more support services and most importantly improved leadership at all levels.

NPs' and CRNAs' perceptions of job satisfaction were assessed (Chung-Park, 1998; Owings, 1999; Stuckey et al., 2006). Two of the studies (Chung-Park, 1998; Owings, 1999) were conducted with samples of NPs and one study (Stuckey et al., 2006) was with a sample of CRNAs. Across all three studies inadequate pay and compensation through bonuses was a primary dissatisfier and most often cited variable as their reason to leave military service. Despite dissatisfaction with some elements of their job, the NPs and CRNAs all reported overall satisfaction with the military and 66% of the CRNAs surveyed ($n = 83$) indicated they would stay on active duty for 20 or more years.

The only study comparing military nurses to military physicians and dentists was conducted by La Rocco et al. (1989). Of particular interest in this study was that as compared to physicians and dentists, nurses reported the lowest overall job satisfaction scores. Additionally, subscale scores on professional growth potential, satisfaction with work hours and professional satisfaction were low among nurses. However, nurses reported having more administrative responsibilities and having more control and decision making authority in the work environment. This may be related to the military rank structure, which can provide nurses with positional authority. In addition, the increased administrative duties may lead to more job stress, which might explain the lower satisfaction scores for nurses.

Kocher and Thomas (1994) conducted the only longitudinal study in this review to determine female Army officers' turnover behavior. In this study, the authors assessed the effect of external market conditions, personal factors and work-related satisfaction factors on junior officers' decision to stay or leave the military. The findings indicated that a nurse who was married with children was 70% less likely to remain on active duty as compared to a single female without children. In addition, as satisfaction with work / military life and flexibility in location of assignments increased nurses were 80% and 70%, respectively, more likely to remain in the military. While these factors were significant predictors in the regression model, they were common factors reported anecdotally or in descriptive studies as major dissatisfiers. This is an excellent study for use in developing recruitment and retention policies that reflect changes in the requirements for frequent transfers to duty stations located outside particular geographical areas. While frequent transfers have been a tradition in the military allowing personnel to remain in a particular geographical location for extended periods of time may enhance retention. This is specifically important to married couples with school-aged children.

The qualitative study (House, 2007) explored factors contributing to Army nurse retention and understanding how certain life events impact a nurse's decision to remain on active duty. The retention of Army nurses was influenced by job satisfaction, the work environment, supervisory leadership, availability of education, personal life events, spousal support and the presence of children. This study demonstrated that job satisfaction, along with other factors, is an important factor in deciding on whether or not to remain on active duty.

DISCUSSION

This review of the literature on military nurses' job satisfaction and intent to stay represents the first attempt at analyzing a body of research on these variables. For the past 30 or more years, the same or similar work-related, organizational and individual variables have been studied in relation to job satisfaction and intent to stay. Similar results have been reported across all the military services. The most consistent result is that job satisfaction has a positive relationship with intent to stay. The more satisfied an employee is the more likely he or she is to stay in the organization. However, the studies that have been conducted reflect attitudes from several years ago and need to be updated to be consistent with today's market. Additionally the previously conducted studies have not measured the Global War on Terror's effect either positive or negative on retention of the military nurse workforce. This is of particular importance today given the increased frequency of active duty deployments and activation of the reservists.

The majority of the studies in this review used a descriptive design and basic statistics to conduct the analysis. Multivariate approaches have become more common in the nursing literature. More studies with military samples using this approach need to be conducted. Longitudinal studies need to be conducted to determine the causal relationships between variables in multi-level models. This multivariate approach will enable the joint effect of variables to be studied and provide more precise assumptions about the causal impact of work-related, organizational and individual factors on job satisfaction and intent to stay (Tabachnick & Fidell, 2007). While this method will not address all the limitations of previously used study designs, it will provide a more comprehensive understanding of research on retention issues in military nursing. For example, in the study by Cox et al. (2010), job satisfaction had the strongest influence on a nurse's intent to stay in the military. The causal model in her study identified work-related, organizational and individual factors that influenced job satisfaction, which supports the notion that job satisfaction is a major factor in retention of nurses. This finding is consistent with nursing literature (Hayhurst, Saylor, & Stuenkel, 2005; Ingersoll et al., 2002; Kovner, Brewer, Wu, Cheng, & Suzuki, 2006; Zangaro & Soeken, 2007).

This review has indicated that overall, military nurses are satisfied with their jobs and a good majority plan to stay on active duty. However, there is also a fairly large percentage of nurses who intend to leave military service due to dissatisfaction or retirement. There were multiple factors that contributed to satisfaction and dissatisfaction identified in this review. The major satisfiers for military nurses were health care benefits, educational opportunities, pay, promotional opportunities, job variety and leadership and management experiences offered. In general, the findings across studies in this review reflect positively on the military work environment, which may be a result of the strong sense of teamwork among military members. Military nurses provided a more favorable rating of their work environments as compared to what has been reported in the literature. High levels of satisfaction with nurse-physician relationships and collaboration between professionals was reported across studies (Allgood et al., 2000; Foley et al., 2002; Janelli & Jarmuz, 1987; Patrician et al., 2010) . This finding may be due to the rank structure in the military as it serves as an equalizer among different professional groups. Nursing leaders should continue to promote and capitalize on these satisfiers to continue to ensure a strong workforce.

The dissatisfiers included lack of support from leadership, rigid scheduling, work hours, assignment stability, and workload. The scheduling, work hours, and workload are unit specific issues that can be managed locally. However, of particular importance is the lack of support from leadership, which was identified in multiple studies as a dissatisfier (Allgood et al., 2000; House, 2007; Patrician et al., 2010; Robinson et al., 1993; Savage et al., 1993; Zangaro, 2009). Lack of support from leadership is an extremely important factor that has been identified for at least 17 years in military nursing studies. Nursing leaders should find this result to be very informative. This finding may be explained by the fact that nurses in their early stages of their careers are likely to recognize the benefit of a more senior nurse as a mentor to help them navigate their career.

One of the benefits of being a military nurse is the career management and guidance that is offered to junior officers from senior nursing leadership. In two studies of U.S. Army nurses (Prevosto, 2001; Yoder, 1995) it was reported that when junior nurses had a mentor they were more satisfied and more likely to remain in the military. A mentor may help the nurses acclimate to the military environment and provide them with support when dealing with challenging situations. Robinson and colleagues (1993) recommend encouraging innovation in junior officers, providing more opportunities to be involved in decision-making and increased autonomy may enhance nurses' perceptions of supervisor support. Additional supervisor support will improve teamwork and enforce positive behaviors in future leaders. Nursing leadership should consider a more aggressive approach at ameliorating some of the factors identified as dissatisfiers in this review in an attempt to increase retention rates.

NPs and CRNAs could be considered a separate cohort because they provide a unique service as compared to the staff nurse. The NPs and CRNAs are both critical specialties, which are being utilized by all services to augment limited physician and physician assistant resources. Both specialties' perceptions were that pay and compensation through bonuses were not equivalent to their peers in the civilian sector. However, the military has partly addressed this issue and the compensation for both of these specialties has been improved over the years.

Assignment stability and family status both were significant predictors of retention in the study by Kocher and Thomas (1994). Nurses who were married and had children were less likely to be retained, but if there could be more stability in geographical locations, nurses were more likely to stay in the military. Traditionally, military officers are reassigned every 3 or 4 years to a new duty station, which may be in the same or a different geographical area. The relocation for nurses with children in school is difficult for the family and the child who has to adjust and make new friends every few years. The military is aware of these challenges and have been exploring options to meet the needs of the service members and their families. Moving military service members every 2, 3, or 4 years becomes expensive, especially in times when funding is limited and during an economic recession. Therefore, a solution to this situation would likely benefit both the service member and the government.

While the focus of this review was on military nurses, it is also important to mention the civil service nurses as well. There were six studies that compared military and civil service nurse satisfaction and/or intent to stay. Five of the six studies did not find a significant difference between military and civil service nurses' job satisfaction. This may be explained by the fact that several of the civilian nurses were prior military nurses on active duty or in the reserves. The civil service nurses may be spouses of military members and therefore have experience with the military norms and the military health care system. This understanding of the military norms and values provides an environment that fosters a shared cultural orientation between military and civilian staff and patients. Therefore, their perspectives and perceptions on the work environment would likely be similar. Foley et al. (2002) shares this view concerning military and civil service nurses.

Finally, a study is needed that uses an updated measurement instrument to assess job satisfaction and retention of Army, Navy and Air Force nurses. This is especially important since Army, Navy and Air Force military health care facilities are becoming Joint facilities where all services will be working together as a single entity. Using the same instrument across all three services will enable nursing leaders to identify similarities across the services and also isolate specific factors within a particular service. Zangaro and colleagues have received funding from the TriService Nursing Research Program and will be conducting such a study in the near future. The measurement instrument for this study will be a modified version of Price and Mueller's (1986) instrument. The researchers have reviewed applicable literature and updated the instrument to reflect the concerns being expressed by military personnel today.

As the nursing shortage continues to escalate, nurse leaders must examine their nursing workforce needs and consider strategies to retain military and civil service nurses. Military nurse researchers must work across services and with their civilian counterparts to address nurse retention factors in order to ensure the next and future generations of military nurses, as well as civil service nurses, are retained. Past science in the area of nurse retention has been descriptive in nature. As a result of this review—as well as advances made in design methodology and statistics—nurse researchers must expand the retention science with robust longitudinal intervention and evaluation studies. These studies should be based upon the work of previous researchers and the current TriService funded study being conducted by Zangaro and colleagues. Future studies must be rigorous, inclusive of all services, and targeted to the current work environment.

Military and civilian nurse researchers must conduct research that will provide the best possible evidence to prepare nurse leaders to make change. Military nurse leaders must be prepared to apply the best evidence when addressing issues and making decisions regarding military nurse retention. This will provide military nurse leaders with the best tools and approaches to maximize the retention of a stable and competent nursing workforce that is providing care to our nation's service members, veterans and families.

REFERENCES

Aiken, L. H., Clarke, S. P., Sloane, D. M., Sochalski, J. A., Busse, R., Clarke, H.,...Shamian, J. (2001). Nurses' reports on hospital care in five countries. *Health Affairs (Project Hope), 20*(3), 43–53.

Allgood, C., O'Rourke, K., VanDerslice, J., & Hardy, M. A. (2000). Job satisfaction among nursing staff in a military health care facility. *Military Medicine, 165*(10), 757–761.

Buerhaus, P. I., Donelan, K., Ulrich, B. T., Norman, L., & Dittus, R. (2005). Is the shortage of hospital registered nurses getting better or worse? Findings from two recent national surveys of RNs. *Nursing Economics, 23*(2), 61–71, 96, 55.

Buerhaus, P. I., Staiger, D. O., & Auerbach, D. I. (2009). *The future of the nursing workforce in the United States: Data, implications, and future trends.* Sudbury, MA: Jones and Bartlett, Inc.

Chung-Park, M. S. (1998). Perception of the nurse practitioner's role and job satisfaction in the United States Navy. *Military Medicine, 163*(1), 26–32.

Coomber, B., & Barriball, K. L. (2007). Impact of job satisfaction components on intent to leave and turnover for hospital-based nurses: A review of the research literature. *International Journal of Nursing Studies, 44*(2), 297–314.

Cooper, C. E., & Parsons, R. J. (2002). The nursing shortage. Implications for military nurses. *The Journal of Nursing Administration, 32*(3), 162–166.

Cox, C. W., Relf, M. V., Chen, R., & Zangaro, G. A. (2010). The retention of recalled United States Navy nurse reservists. *Nursing Outlook, 58*(4), 214–220.

Fletcher, C. E. (2001). Hospital RNs' job satisfactions and dissatisfactions. *The Journal of Nursing Administration, 31*(6), 324–331.

Foley, B. J., Kee, C. C., Minick, P., Harvey, S. S., & Jennings, B. M. (2002). Characteristics of nurses and hospital work environments that foster satisfaction and clinical expertise. *The Journal of Nursing Administration, 32*(5), 273–282.

Greiner, B. A., Krause, N., Ragland, D., & Fisher, J. M. (2004). Occupational stressors and hypertension: A multi-method study using observer-based job analysis and self-reports in urban transit operators. *Social Science & Medicine (1982), 59*(5), 1081–1094.

Hayes, L. J., O'Brien Pallas, L., Duffield, C., Shamian, J., Buchan, J., Hughes, F.,...Stone, P. W. (2006). Nurse turnover: A literature review. *International Journal of Nursing Studies, 43*(2), 237–263.

Hayhurst, A., Saylor, C., & Stuenkel, D. (2005). Work environmental factors and retention of nurses. *Journal of Nursing Care Quality, 20*(3), 283–288.

Hinshaw, A. S., Smeltzer, C. H., & Atwood, J. R. (1987). Innovative retention strategies for nursing staff. *The Journal of Nursing Administration, 17*(6), 8–16.

House, C. L. (2007). *Army nurse officer retention: A qualitative examination of forces influencing the career longevity of Army nurses.* Retrieved from ProQuest Dissertations and Theses. UMI No. AAT1443222.

Ingersoll, G. L., Olsan, T., Drew-Cates, J., DeVinney, B. C., & Davies, J. (2002). Nurses' job satis-faction, organizational commitment, and career intent. *The Journal of Nursing Administration,* *32*(5), 250–263.

Janelli, L. M., & Jarmuz, P. A. (1987). Motivational factors that affect the retention of reserve nurses in eight aeromedical evacuation flights. *Aviation, Space, and Environmental Medicine, 58*(4), 375–378.

Jones, C. B. (2004). The costs of nurse turnover, part 1: An economic perspective. *The Journal of Nursing Administration, 34*(12), 562–570.

Jones, C. B. (2005). The costs of nurse turnover, part 2: Application of the Nursing Turnover Cost Calculation Methodology. *The Journal of Nursing Administration, 35*(1), 41–49.

Jones, C. B. (2008). Revisiting nurse turnover costs: Adjusting for inflation. *The Journal of Nursing Administration, 38*(1), 11–18.

Jones, C. B., & Gates, M. (2007). The costs and benefits of nurse turnover: A business case for nurse retention. *Online Journal of Issues in Nursing, 12*(3), 1–17.

Kim, S. W., Price, J. L., Mueller, C. W., & Watson, T. W. (1996). The determinants of career intent among physicians at a U.S. Air Force hospital. *Human Relations, 49*(7), 947–976.

Kocher, K. M., & Thomas, G. W. (1994). Retaining Army nurses: A longitudinal model. *Research in Nursing & Health, 17*(1), 59–65.

Kovner, C. T., Brewer, C. S., Greene, W., & Fairchild, S. (2009). Understanding new registered nurses' intent to stay at their jobs. *Nursing Economics, 27*(2), 81–98.

Kovner, C. T., Brewer, C. S., Fairchild, S., Poornima, S., Kim, H., & Djukic, M. (2007). Newly licensed RNs' characteristics, work attitudes, and intentions to work. *The American Journal of Nursing, 107*(9), 58–70; quiz 70.

Kovner, C., Brewer, C., Wu, Y. W., Cheng, Y., & Suzuki, M. (2006). Factors associated with work satisfaction of registered nurses. *Journal of Nursing Scholarship: An Official Publication of Sigma Theta Tau International Honor Society of Nursing / Sigma Theta Tau, 38*(1), 71–79.

Kramer, M., & Schmalenberg, C. (1991). Job satisfaction and retention. Insights for the '90s. Part 1. *Nursing, 21*(3), 50–55.

Lang, G. M. (2008). *The work environment of Army hospital nurses: Measurement and construct validity.* Retrieved from ProQuest Dissertations and Theses. UMI No. AAT 3261586.

LaRocco, J. M., Tetrick, L. E., & Meder, D. (1989). Differences in perceptions of work environment conditions, job attitudes, and health beliefs among military physicians, dentists, and nurses. *Military Psychology, 1*(3), 135–151.

Larrabee, J. H., Janney, M. A., Ostrow, C. L., Withrow, M. L., Hobbs, G. R., & Burant, C. (2003). Predicting registered nurse job satisfaction and intent to leave. *The Journal of Nursing Administration, 33*(5), 271–283.

Lu, H., While, A. E., & Barriball, K. L. (2005). Job satisfaction among nurses: A literature review. *International Journal of Nursing Studies, 42*(2), 211–227.

Ma, J. C., Lee, P. H., Yang, Y. C., & Chang, W. Y. (2009). Predicting factors related to nurses' intention to leave, job satisfaction, and perception of quality of care in acute care hospitals. *Nursing Economics, 27*(3), 178–84, 202.

Moorhead, S. A. (1993). *Nurses' job satisfaction, commitment, search behavior and intent to leave the Air Force: A test of a causal model.* Retrieved from ProQuest Dissertations and Theses. UMI No. AAT 9334638.

Nunnally, J. C., & Bernstein, I. H. (1994). *Psychometric theory* (3rd ed.). New York, NY: McGraw-Hill.

Obrien-Pallas, L., Griffin, P., Shamian, J., Buchan, J., Duffield, C., Hughes, F., ... Stone, P. W. (2006). The impact of nurse turnover on patient, nurse and system outcomes: A pilot study and focus for a multicenter international study. *Policy, Politics, & Nursing Practice, 7*(3), 169–179.

Owings, J. E. (1999). *Job satisfaction among family nurse practitioners in the United States Air Force.* Retrieved from ProQuest Dissertations and Theses. UMI No. AAT 1399530.

Pagliara, C. M. (2003). *The impact of job satisfaction, stress and career needs on Navy Nurses intent to stay on active duty.* Retrieved from ProQuest Dissertations and Theses. UMI No. AAT 3108639.

Patrician, P. A., Shang, J., & Lake, E. T. (2010). Organizational determinants of work outcomes and quality care ratings among Army Medical Department registered nurses. *Research in Nursing & Health, 33*(2), 99–110.

Prevosto, P. (2001). The effect of "mentored" relationships on satisfaction and intent to stay of company-grade U.S. Army Reserve nurses. *Military Medicine, 166*(1), 21–26.

Price, J. L. (2001). Reflections on the determinants of voluntary turnover. *International Journal of Manpower, 22*(7), 600–624.

Price, J. L., & Mueller, C. W. (1986). *Absenteeism and turnover of hospital employees.* Greenwich: JAI Press, Inc.

Price, J. L., & Mueller, C. W. (1981). *Professional turnover.* Bridgeport, CT: Luce.

Rambur, B., Palumbo, M. V., McIntosh, B., & Mongeon, J. (2003). A statewide analysis of RNs' intention to leave their position. *Nursing Outlook, 51*(4), 182–188.

Roach, C. L. W. (1991). *Perceived role conflict, role ambiguity, and work satisfaction of the Army Reserve nurse.* Retrieved from ProQuest Dissertations and Theses. UMI No. AAT 9218401.

Robinson, S. E., Rodriguez, E. R., Sammons, M. T., & Keim, J. (1993). Does being in the military affect nurses' perceptions of work life? *Journal of Advanced Nursing, 18*(7), 1146–1151.

Savage, S., Simms, L. M., Williams, R. A., & Erbin-Roesemann, M. (1993). Discovering work excitement among navy nurses. *Nursing Economics, 11*(3), 153–161.

Stewart, D. W. (2002). *The relationship of job stress to job satisfaction and the intent to Army Nurse Corps officers to stay in active military service.* Retrieved from ProQuest Dissertations and Theses. UMI No. AAT 3059617.

Stuckey, C. A., Martinez, L. M., Gablehouse, A. S., Sylvia, B. M., Hartgerink, A. G., Watts, D. D., & Murray, J. (2006). Job satisfaction and retention of active duty Air Force Certified Registered Nurse Anesthetists. *AANA, 74*(5), 369–397.

Tabachnick, B. G., & Fidell, L. S. (2007). *Using multivariate statistics* (5th ed.). New York, NY: Harper Collins College Publishers.

Waldman, J. D., Kelly, F., Arora, S., & Smith, H. L. (2004). The shocking cost of turnover in health care. *Health Care Management Review, 29*(1), 2–7.

Yin, J. C., & Yang, K. P. (2002). Nursing turnover in Taiwan: A meta-analysis of related factors. *International Journal of Nursing Studies, 39*(6), 573–581.

Yoder, L. H. (1995). Staff nurses' career development relationships and self-reports of professionalism, job satisfaction, and intent to stay. *Nursing Research, 44*(5), 290–297.

Zangaro, G. A. (2004). *Factors associated with retention of nurses: Phase I instrument testing.* TSNRP funded study, MDA-905-02-1-TS10.

Zangaro, G. A., & Johantgen, M. (2009). Registered nurses' job satisfaction in Navy hospitals. *Military Medicine, 174*(1), 76–81.

Zangaro, G. A., & Soeken, K. L. (2007). A meta-analysis of studies of nurses' job satisfaction. *Research in Nursing & Health, 30*(4), 445–458.

CHAPTER 3

Understanding the Supply and Distribution of Registered Nurses

Where Are the Data and What Can They Tell Us?

Robert Martiniano, Sandra McGinnis, and Jean Moore

ABSTRACT

Health workforce researchers routinely conduct studies to determine whether a profession is currently in short supply and whether future shortages are likely. This is particularly important for registered nursing since the profession has experienced periodic shortages over the past three decades. Registered nurse (RN) forecast studies can be valuable in quantifying supply and demand gaps and identifying the most appropriate strategies to avert future shortages. In order to quantify RN supply/demand gaps, it is important to have accurate data on RNs, including the number of active RNs as well as their demographic, education, and practice characteristics, and work location(s). A lack of relevant and timely data on the nursing workforce is a significant barrier to identifying where nursing shortages exist, where they are most severe, and determining the factors that contribute to them. This lack of understanding impedes the development of effective health workforce programs and policies to mitigate shortages and the ability to evaluate these programs and policies for effectiveness. This study describes the national data sources available to nursing researchers to study the supply and distribution of the RN workforce and assesses the sources' strengths and limitations. This study also explores the potential for using state-level data for nursing workforce research.

© 2011 Springer Publishing Company
DOI: 10.1891/0739-6686.28.43

INTRODUCTION

The health of our country's population depends on the availability of a health care workforce that is both well trained and adequate in number. A health care system is only as good as its workforce and the workforce directly impacts quality, cost, and access to health care. Health policies designed to expand access, improve quality, and control costs must take into account the supply, distribution, education, and utilization of the health workforce in order for these policies to succeed. While the passage of the Patient Protection and Affordable Care Act has the potential to expand access to basic health services, it has heightened concerns about potential shortages of many types of health care professionals, including registered nurses (RNs).

Health workforce researchers routinely conduct studies to determine whether a profession is currently in short supply and whether future shortages are likely. This is particularly important for registered nursing since the profession has experienced periodic shortages over the past three decades. RN forecast studies can be valuable in identifying the most appropriate strategies to avert future shortages.

The purpose of this study is to review the available national datasets that are commonly used in nursing research and assess their value in describing RN supply and distribution. Further, this study explores the potential for using state-level data for nursing workforce research.

RESEARCH ON RN SUPPLY AND DISTRIBUTION: WHAT DO WE NEED TO KNOW?

Fluctuations in nursing workforce labor markets can lead to workforce imbalances, either shortages or surpluses. These imbalances can take many forms and include:

- Profession imbalances, such as shortages of RNs; or specialty imbalances within the profession, such as shortages of public health nurses;
- Geographic imbalances or differences in the supply of RNs between rural and urban areas or between economically disadvantaged and affluent communities;
- Institutional and service-based imbalances or differences in the supply of RNs in different health care settings, for example, acute care compared to long-term care;
- Public and private imbalances or differences in the supply of RNs between publicly and privately sponsored health care providers; and
- Gender or racial and ethnic imbalances in nursing, terms that refer to differences in the representation of men and certain racial and ethnic groups in nursing, compared to their presence in the community (Moore, 2008).

There are a number of variables that have substantial impacts on the supply of and demand for RNs that contribute to shortages in the profession. One important factor is age. RNs are one of the oldest health professions in the United States. In 2008, the average age of all licensed RNs in the United States was 47 (Health Resources and Services Administration [HRSA], 2010). Over the next 10–20 years, large numbers of RN retirements are expected, and there are concerns that too few young RNs will enter the profession to offset these losses (Buerhaus, 2008). Second, RNs are predominantly non-Hispanic White and female, while the U.S. population is becoming increasingly racially and ethnically diverse. Thus, the demographic pool from which RNs have been traditionally drawn is becoming a smaller proportion of the population and participation in nursing remains limited for some minority groups (especially Hispanics/Latinos) and men. Unless the profession can successfully increase its diversity, RN shortages could persist and worsen (Moore, 2008).

At the same time that the RN workforce is facing the demographic challenges described above, there are unprecedented pressures on the educational pipeline for RNs. Many RN education programs report difficulty recruiting nurse faculty and obtaining a sufficient number of placement sites for clinical rotations (Cleary, McBride, McClure, & Reinhard, 2009; Kuehn, 2007). This can limit the number of qualified candidates admitted to nursing education programs. In addition, some states are considering requiring RNs to have a 4-year nursing degree, which could affect the overall supply of RNs, particularly in rural areas with limited access to baccalaureate nursing programs.

Finally, new health policies have the potential to increase demand for RNs. Some states, such as California, have implemented mandated nurse staffing ratios in hospitals and nursing homes. Additionally, the passage of the Patient Protection and Affordable Care Act is expected to increase demand for primary care services and result in greater demand for more RNs in ambulatory settings as more individuals obtain health insurance coverage.

An important question that nursing researchers endeavor to answer is how many active RNs are there and is the available supply sufficient to meet demand for their services? In order to quantify RN supply/demand gaps, it is important to have accurate data on RNs, including the number of active RNs as well as their demographic, education, and practice characteristics, and work location(s).

WHAT DATA ARE NEEDED TO UNDERSTAND RN SUPPLY AND DISTRIBUTION?

Although many data sources are available to understand RN supply and demand, the data collected may not supply enough information to effectively assess

RN workforce issues. There has been much discussion nationally by nursing researchers about the key variables needed to understand the RN workforce, that is, which variables are necessary to describe supply, demand, distribution, and the educational pipeline for RNs. A number of key variables that researchers could use to evaluate the supply and distribution of RNs are described.

Demographics

Demographic information collected on RNs should include year of birth, gender, and race/ethnicity. These variables can be used to describe the current RN workforce and estimate what tomorrow's nursing workforce may look like. Additionally, these data elements can be used to identify potential racial/ethnic imbalances between the nursing workforce and the population as well as the impact of population aging on the nursing workforce. Finally, these demographic variables can be used to understand potential variations in RN education or practice characteristics, such as differences in hours or shifts worked or initial RN degree.

Nursing Education

For RNs, education tends to be a complex question. Entry-level RNs join the RN workforce with various degrees, ranging from diplomas conferred by 3-year hospital-based programs, 2-year associate degrees, 4-year bachelor's degrees, or master's degrees. Collecting information about the initial degree (the degree held at entry into the RN workforce) helps researchers to understand the type of nursing education programs that are available to the individuals interested in becoming RNs and where those programs are located geographically. For example, it may not be appropriate for a hospital in a specific rural area to require 4-year nursing degrees for newly trained RNs entering their workforce when the major supplier of RNs in that area is the local community college.

Likewise, data on the highest RN degree allow for an analysis of potential upward job mobility within the profession and the potential for RNs with advanced nursing degrees to serve as faculty. Analyzing the characteristics of particular RNs at substate levels who continue their education may help to explain why a smaller percentage of RNs have bachelor's degrees in nursing or other advanced degrees, especially in rural areas where there may be less opportunity to obtain such degrees.

Employment Status

In order to understand RN supply, data on employment status are needed. For example, it was estimated that in 2002 slightly more than one-quarter of the licensed RNs in New York were not actively practicing nursing in the state

(New York State Education Department, 2003); a significant number when one considers the persistent nursing shortages in many communities across the state. It is critical to ascertain whether an RN is working or not (either unemployed or retired), working in a position that requires an RN license, or serving as an unpaid RN volunteer. Since many RNs work in more than one nursing position or work a second job outside of nursing, information on both principal and secondary employment for working or volunteering allows for broader understanding of the potential workforce capacity of RNs.

Hours and Shifts Worked

It is necessary to understand the current patient care capacity of the RN workforce to determine whether the capacity can be expanded. This is accomplished by collecting data on hours worked, including hours spent in non-patient activities, such as administration, teaching, and clinical research. Assuming that RNs working part time in patient care can increase their hours may be erroneous without assessing time spent on other activities within nursing or outside of nursing. Hours worked can also be used to calculate RN full-time equivalents (FTEs) in total by dividing hours worked by the usual work week, typically 40 hours.

The shifts worked (weekends, weekdays, days, nights, evenings) can also be helpful to describe the nursing workforce and can be used to understand potential variations in salary, job satisfaction, and education. For example, salary differences for RNs with similar work experience and educational background may be explained by shift differentials. Further, an inability to acquire advanced degrees may be related to working conditions such as hours or shifts worked rather than accessibility to educational programs or family commitments.

Practice Setting

RNs work in many different health care settings and knowing the differences in practice settings is important to understanding current nursing capacity for patient care and the structure of the community's health care system in which RNs work. For example, more RNs may work in hospitals in a certain community due the presence of large hospitals in that area. Practice settings for RNs can include hospital inpatient, hospital outpatient, hospital emergency departments, physician offices, offices of other health practitioners, clinics and health centers, nursing homes, schools, home health agencies, public health agencies, and a myriad of non-patient care settings such as insurance companies, government, and universities conducting research. Practice settings can be used to explain differences in salary, education, job satisfaction, and hours and shifts worked.

Practice Address

Knowing the practice setting, however, may not be enough. Within geographic areas, RNs may not be well distributed or RNs may live in one area but commute to another area for work. Additionally, RNs may be licensed in multiple states while only actively practicing in one state. For example, in 2002 a New York state survey of RNs estimated that 10% of RNs licensed in New York were practicing in another state (New York State Education Department, 2003).

An RN's practice address, or at a minimum the practice zip code, can assist in understanding the issues as described above if both the home and work addresses or zip codes are collected. The full practice address can be geocoded, linked to specific census tracts or towns, plotted on a map, and used to describe the distribution of practicing RNs within a community, allowing for small area analysis of RN characteristics. If it is not feasible to collect the full practice address, requesting the practice zip code allows for similar small area analysis. Using either the complete address or the zip code allows for analysis of active RN characteristics at substate levels.

Job Title

Job title is useful in further understanding an RN's role in a specific practice setting. Various options for job titles include staff RN, nurse manager/supervisor, nurse executive, researcher, faculty, home health nurse, dean or chair of a nursing education program, insurance/claims reviewer, and public health nurse. RNs working in hospital settings have markedly different responsibilities based on their job title, such as staff nurse, vice president of nursing, quality assurance RN, nurse educator, among others. Identifying a job title provides the researcher an understanding of basic job duties, and when used in conjunction with other variables, such as practice setting (hospital, physician's office, health clinic, nursing home, etc.) or hours worked by activity (research, administration, etc.) it can provide researchers with a broad understanding of how RNs spend their time within and outside of patient care.

Future Plans

The aging of the population and, consequently, the aging of the nursing workforce will create potential issues in meeting future demand for RNs. The extent to which RNs leave the field for other occupations impacts on overall availability of RNs for patient care within a community. A basic question around future plans, usually asked in increments of 1, 2, or 3 years, including whether the RN plans to retire, leave the nursing field altogether, return to school for an advanced nursing degree, or continue to practice nursing but at another location (job setting, state, etc.) allows researchers to understand movement out of the profession and mobility within the profession, for example, to faculty, administration, or research.

NATIONAL DATASETS TO ASSESS RN SUPPLY

An important starting point for nursing workforce research, including RN forecast studies, is the ability to describe the supply and distribution of active RNs. There are a number of data sources available that can be used for this purpose. Ultimately, these data sources influence both the questions that can be answered as well as the geographic level of analysis.

There are positive and negative aspects for these data sources, such as certain datasets cannot be used below the state level and other datasets capture information on the number of jobs but not on RNs themselves. For example, the National Sample Survey of Registered Nurses is focused solely on RNs, while others such as the American Community Survey (ACS) and the Current Population Survey (CPS) provide information on the entire U.S. population, including RNs. Others such as the Occupational Employment Survey (OES) provide information on jobs, including RN jobs, rather than the individuals. A summary of these datasets are discussed in more detail below.

National Sample Survey of Registered Nurses

The National Sample Survey of Registered Nurses (NSSRN) is one of the most detailed sources of RN data available (http://datawarehouse.hrsa.gov/nursingsurvey.aspx). This survey of slightly more than 1% of all licensed RNs in the United States has been conducted approximately every 4 years since 1977 with the most recent survey completed in 2008. Response rates for these surveys range from 60% to 70%, depending on the survey year. The sampling methodology entails oversampling RNs in less populated states and undersampling RNs in more populous states that have large metropolitan areas.

The NSSRN has perhaps the best available information on the practice settings of RNs at national and state levels, with detail on not only the type of setting, but also the type of unit that hospital RNs work in. Data on hours worked, education, job title, and demographics are also collected. Employment information is available on up to two nursing jobs as well as work outside of the field of nursing.

While data on the number of licensed RNs in the United States are available through the NSSRN, the sampling methodology precludes using these data for substate analyses. Consequently, while NSSRN data have been used to estimate state-level supply and distribution of RNs (HRSA, 2010), it would not be appropriate to analyze geographic variation (i.e., county or subcounty levels) in the supply and distribution of RNs within a state. Sampling is conducted at the state level, and substate analysis using this dataset may not be reliable due to the sampling strategy.

However, a number of geographic indicators included in the NSSRN could be used to conduct broader analysis of RNs at a national level based on certain geographic differences. The NSSRN dataset could be linked to other sources of substate data to examine, for example, whether RNs in federally defined "persistent poverty" counties practice differently than other RNs, or whether RNs in metropolitan statistical areas (MSAs) with more hospital beds have changed jobs more frequently compared to those in MSAs with fewer hospitals beds.

When analyzing NSSRN data, it is important to recognize that cross-tabulation of variables at sublevels of analysis can create unreliable results due to small sample size. For example, in many states, determining the race/ethnicity of RNs working in ambulatory settings by age may yield a small result (prior to applying any sample weights) and may not truly represent the number of individuals in the practice setting for the age and race/ethnicity cohort in that state.

The NSSRN sampling methodology may also influence state-level estimates of RNs using certain variables such as race/ethnicity and setting. The undersampling of more populous states with large metropolitan areas that have a more racially/ethnically diverse RN workforce and larger numbers of RNs in hospital settings may underestimate diversity and RN employment by setting.

American Community Survey

The U.S. Census Bureau collects detailed data on a large sample of individuals throughout the country (approximately 1% of the population annually) as part of their ACS (http://www.census.gov/acs/www/). The ACS is carried out on an annual basis and contains all of the information formerly collected only on the "long form" of the decennial U.S. Census. While smaller pilot versions of the survey were administered in 2003 and 2004, the first year the full ACS survey was conducted was in 2005.[1] ACS data are available as 1- or 3-year estimates, that is, combining consecutive years to create one dataset. Three-year ACS estimates represent 3% of the U.S. population.

Out of the approximately three million people who are surveyed in each year's ACS, 32,000–33,000 report their occupation as "registered nurse." By downloading the Public Use Microdata Sample file, individual data files can be evaluated, and a sample of RNs can be extracted for analysis. Topics included in the ACS are demographic, social, economic, and housing characteristics. Of

---

[1] Except for the U.S. population living in group quarters, which was not surveyed until 2006.

particular interest to nursing workforce researchers, the data include level of education, employment status, sector of employment, setting of employment, location of employment, hours worked, and salary.

Perhaps the most useful feature of the ACS is the geographical variables. ACS data are available at the substate level, although the geographic unit is an area unique to the Census Bureau, called a Public Use Microdata Area (PUMA). The ACS includes data on PUMA of residence, PUMA of employment, and PUMA where the respondent lived the previous year. In theory, PUMAs do not correspond to any geographical unit other than states, although in practice they frequently share boundaries with counties or groups of counties or can be aggregated up to county boundaries.

Because the ACS is not meant to be an in-depth study of the American workforce, there are a few caveats. First, occupation is self-reported and there are a small number of respondents who report their occupation as "RN" but have less than a high school education. These respondents should be removed from any analysis because it is highly unlikely that they are, in fact, RNs. Second, the survey asks level of education but not field of education. There is no guarantee that an RN with a bachelor's degree earned that bachelor's degree in nursing, so researchers should avoid making that assumption. Finally, those who were employed in the past year and are no longer employed are asked their occupation the last time they worked, giving researchers a useful look at RNs who have left the paid workforce in the past year. But those who left nursing to work in another occupation will be listed under their new occupation, so researchers should recognize that not all of those who have left the field of nursing can be identified through these data.

The ACS gives a reasonable distribution of practice settings and good data on location, although, as previously discussed, it can be difficult to crosswalk the ACS geography with counties and MSAs. Hours worked do not differentiate between patient care and non-patient care, and education is limited to the highest degree respondents hold, with no data on the discipline in which the degree was earned. There is no job title information available in the ACS and, as previously noted, occupation is self-reported.

The ACS is strong on demographic information, with data available not only about the individual, but also about family and household. Employment status is more limited, with information only available about the RN's primary job. No data are available from the ACS about RNs working second RN jobs or working second jobs outside of nursing. RNs who are working in another occupation as their primary job cannot be identified by the ACS. Recent retirements from nursing (within the past year) can be identified using the ACS, but only if the retirees are not working for pay in any other job.

Current Population Survey

The CPS is jointly administered by the Bureau of Labor Statistics and the U.S. Census Bureau (http://www.census.gov/cps/ or http://www.bls.gov/cps/). It is a monthly sample survey of 60,000 households throughout the United States and is the main source of labor and unemployment information in the country. Information is collected on all of the individuals in the surveyed households who are 16 years of age and older, regardless of their employment status. Individuals in the military and in institutional settings such as prisons, nursing homes, and long-term care hospitals are excluded from the survey.

The sampling frame is developed at a state level to ensure that state-specific labor market conditions are accounted for, and CPS data are available at both the state and national levels, except in California and New York, where Los Angeles and New York City, respectively, are broken out from the remainder of the state. Households are in the sample for four consecutive months, out of the sample for eight consecutive months, in the sample for another four consecutive months, then out of the sample permanently. By using this method of sampling, one-eighth of the households are new each month, one-eighth of the households have been in the sample for 2 months, one-eighth of the households have been in the sample for 3 months, and so on. This arrangement ensures continuity of the results.

Data collected through the CPS include age, disability status, educational attainment, marital status, employment status (including self-employed), race/ethnicity, hours of work, full- and part-time status, and industry and occupation codes using the North American Industry Classification System (NAICS) and Standard Occupational Classifications (SOC). Survey respondents are also asked if they work more than one job and asked to identify the occupation and industry of their second job for individuals in the fourth and eighth month of the survey. Additionally, information is collected on individuals who are unemployed, if applicable, including reasons for unemployment and duration of unemployment.

Similar to the ACS, the CPS is strong on collecting employment, demographic, and education information. Unlike the ACS, employment information is collected on the primary and secondary place of employment. Additionally, characteristics of RNs who are unemployed can be determined. The limited sample size of the CPS, especially at the state level, may make it difficult to conduct occupation-specific analyses. For example, in 2007, there were too few RNs in the New York sample to make valid estimates of the breakdown of RNs by race/ethnicity or by practice setting.

Occupational Employment Survey

The OES is a 3-year sample survey of over one million non-farm businesses throughout the U.S., with one-third of the sample surveyed once during the 3-year cycle (http://www.bls.gov/oes/). The data count jobs and ultimately produce estimates of the number of current jobs as well as wages and salaries for both full- and part-time employees by industry and occupation using the NAICS and SOC, respectively

OES data are available at the national, state, MSA, and non-MSA levels, but are not generally available at county and subcounty levels. OES data are also available at multiple industry and occupational levels. For example, an RN job can be counted for a specific type of provider office, such as offices of physicians except mental health specialists, and then aggregated to higher levels, including offices of physicians, ambulatory health care services, and health care and social assistance.

Similarly, RN jobs have their own SOC code, and can be included with other health professionals and aggregated to the level of "health diagnosing and treating practitioners" and then to "health care practitioners and technical occupations." Under the 2000 SOC coding scheme, "RN job" was a standalone occupation, but under the revised 2010 coding scheme, nurse anesthetist, nurse midwife, and nurse practitioner jobs are now reported separately from other RNs.

While the OES can be used to count nursing jobs at the various geographic, industry, and occupation levels, as described above, it cannot be used to count individual RNs. For example, one RN working two jobs would be counted as two jobs in the OES data, regardless of the number of hours at each of the positions. Additionally, since OES surveys employers about the number of their employees, jobs for individuals who are self-employed are not counted; consequently, the number of private duty RNs or those conducting private consulting would not be counted using the OES. There is also no demographic (age, gender, race/ethnicity) or practice (job title, hours worked) information, thus limiting the usefulness of these data to describe characteristics of the RN workforce.

Area Resource File

The Area Resource File (ARF) is a county-level dataset compiled by the HRSA from a variety of sources, and includes demographic, geographic, economic, and health care data (http://bhpr.hrsa.gov/healthworkforce/data/arf.htm). Data sources include professional and trade associations (e.g., the American Medical Association, the American Hospital Association [AHA]) and government agencies (e.g., the Bureau of Labor Statistics, the Census Bureau, the Centers for Medicare and Medicaid Services).

The ARF includes information on government classifications of counties (e.g., rural-urban continuum codes, status as a persistent poverty county, designation as a health profession shortage area), and data on health professionals, health facilities, health care utilization, health care expenditures, populations (including demographic and economic characteristics), and vital statistics. Although the ARF is updated annually, the source data are frequently often 2 or

3 years old when the ARF is released. Each release of the ARF contains variables from previous years, allowing researchers to conduct trend analysis.

The nursing workforce analyses that can be conducted using the ARF alone are limited in scope, because the only variables that explicitly pertain to RNs are the number of RNs living in each county at the time of the last decennial census, and the number of full-time and part-time RNs employed in hospitals in the county. Nonetheless, the ARF is a valuable source of data, and when used in conjunction with other sources of nursing data enables researchers to incorporate contextual variables into their analyses.

OTHER NATIONAL DATASETS

There are other datasets that collect nursing-related data that were not reviewed in detail in this study. Each of these datasets may be useful to researchers in understanding some very specific nursing issues such as education or licensing exam pass rates. These data sources are briefly described below.

Integrated Postsecondary Education Data System

The Integrated Postsecondary Education Data System (IPEDS) is an annual survey of post-secondary educational institutions that collects data on enrollments, graduations, faculty, staff, and finances (http://nces.ed.gov/ipeds/datacenter/). Enrollments are collected at the school level rather than at the program level, and graduations are categorized by race and ethnicity, gender, and program. Educational institutions that confer 2- and 4-year nursing degrees report their RN degrees separately by the different programs. Likewise, educational institutions with 4-year and master's-level degrees report them separately. While these data are useful in describing the graduates of nursing education programs, especially by race and ethnicity, there is no information about the career paths of the new graduates. IPEDS is useful for tracking total graduation trends over time, such as the racial/ethnicity diversity of graduates, but with the caveat that those numbers may not accurately represent the number of RNs who ultimately enter the nursing workforce.

National League for Nursing

The National League for Nursing (NLN) conducts an annual survey of nursing programs, collecting data on the number of applications, admissions, and graduations; the percent of the students in the nursing programs who are racial/ethnic minorities; and age distribution of the students in the nursing program (http://www.nln.org/). Data are collected on licensed practical/vocational nurses (LP/VNs) and all levels of registered nursing education, from diploma and associate level degrees to the doctorate level. These data are useful in understanding trends in the nursing education pipeline, but as with the IPEDS data, do not provide any information on career paths of graduates.

National Council of State Boards of Nursing

The National Council of State Boards of Nursing (NCSBN) publishes data on the number of individuals (both RNs and LP/VNs) who pass the National Council Licensure Examination (NCLEX) (https://www.ncsbn.org/index.htmm). These data are available on a quarterly basis (January–March, April–June, etc.) and include data on pass rates for first time candidates as well as repeat candidates for both U.S.-educated and internationally educated nurses. These data may be a better proxy for estimating the number of RNs entering practice than IPEDS or NLN data because individuals who pass the NCLEX are most likely to practice or plan to enter practice, though there may be a time delays between when the test was taken and when an individual actually begins practicing.

American Hospital Association

The AHA conducts an annual survey of hospitals that includes limited information about RNs who work in hospitals (http://www.aha.org/). RN-specific data collected include the number of RNs who work full time (35 hours a week or more), the number of RNs who work part time, and total RN FTEs. Additionally, the survey collects information about the hiring of foreign-educated RNs, including their countries or continents of training. While AHA data allow for some analysis of the number of RNs working in hospitals, basic demographic information on hospital RNs, such as age, gender, or race/ethnicity, is not available.

LIMITATIONS OF NATIONAL DATASETS

Data Considerations

It is clear that the national data sources described above do not provide data in a consistent manner. For example, some sources of data provide information on where RNs live rather than where they work. In some communities, this is not an issue, but in others (particularly major metropolitan areas where health care tends to be provided in the central city, but many RNs may live in the suburbs), using location of residence as a proxy for location of employment may overestimate or underestimate RN supply.

The most common data available to inform the measurement of RN shortages are supply data, that is, how many RNs or RN jobs exist within a given geography. Using the number of RNs in a given area, researchers calculate the ratio of active RNs to the population to evaluate whether a given state, MSA, or county has a shortage of RNs based on a standard, usually the national or state ratio of RNs-to-population. While supply ratios may be appropriate for providers such as physicians who can set up private practice, they are of limited use when considering RN shortages since typically, RNs must be employed by health care providers (e.g., hospitals, private physician practices, and home care agencies). Some of the most disadvantaged (i.e., persistently poor) counties in the United States have a great need for health care services, but, however, may have almost no demand for RNs because of a lack of a health care providers. Both supply and demand data are necessary to truly measure whether a shortage of RNs exists.

RN data can be used to measure jobs (such as government employment data) or individuals. Some data sources provide FTEs. It is critical that the researcher using RN data from two or more different sources ensures that the data are presented in the same metric. Another complication of RN data is that it may or may not include advanced practice nurses (APNs), such as nurse practitioners or certified nurse midwives. Thus, APNs must either be removed from an analysis of RNs or analyzed separately.

Additionally, while the national sources of nursing data are updated on a regular basis, thus allowing the examination of trends, none of them are longitudinal (i.e., they do not track the same nurses over time). Therefore, there is great reliance on retrospective data to determine when and why key transitions in an RN's work life occurred.

Finally, the questions of sampling and response rate must be addressed and understood. Is the data being collected a sample or the entire population of RNs in a given geographic area? Large datasets that are samples of the RN population may be less reliable as different levels of analysis are undertaken (e.g., race/ethnicity by setting by practice specialty, especially at a state level), than smaller, population-based datasets. Additionally, population-based surveys with low response rates may be less reliable than a sample survey with a high response rate. Ultimately, the researcher must decide which survey and sampling truly represent the RN population being studied.

STATE DATA ON RNs

Nursing shortages tend to be specific to particular localities, and national data, even used at a state level, may not be adequate to document the supply of and demand for RNs. Even in the face of the most severe national RN shortages, some communities will have enough RNs to meet patient care needs, and even when RNs are plentiful, there are communities that will have difficulty meeting their need for RNs. While national data are a useful barometer for tracking trends over time, the presence and severity of RN shortages are best determined at the MSA or county level, and these geographies are more often found in state-level data-sets such as state licensure data, additional data collected at the time of license renewal, or other state-level data collection efforts.

State Licensure Data

States are responsible for licensing RNs and each state has its own rules for licen-sure and, consequently, the data collected on RNs at licensure is not standard-ized across states. Some states collect only the data essential for licensure or license renewal, such as name, address, RN education, NCLEX exam score (if initial licensure), information on legal offenses, continuing education credits if required, and whether the individual holds RN licenses from other states.

State licensure data generally allow for substate analysis, although in many states that may be limited to counts by county or zip code. The accuracy of these counts may be questionable, as described more fully below. Additionally, many states have very restrictive policies on how state licensure data may be used, making the data less accessible to researchers.

Addresses provided by the RNs for licensure represent either their work address or their home address, and state licensing boards may not know which it is. Additionally, many RNs maintain an active license but may be employed in occupations outside of nursing. Further, some states do not regularly update information on RNs who do not renew their licenses. Counts of RNs based on licensure data at the state, county, or zip code levels are, consequently, unreliable at best and generally tend to be an overestimate the potential supply of active RNs in a state or community. Licensure data without additional detail cannot be used to describe such aspects as basic demographics, practice settings, hours worked, or a second practice location.

There is great variability among states on the amount of additional infor-mation above what is necessary for RN licensure renewal. For example, New York includes an optional two-page survey in its re-registration materials. In addition to the basic demographic questions, the survey has questions about practice setting, employment status, job title, the zip code of the primary and, if applicable, secondary work location(s), shifts worked, hours worked, job satis-faction, and future plans. Texas includes questions on the license renewal form about employment status, primary practice setting, primary practice position, primary specialty, highest degree, and primary employment zip code.

While some states, using additional questions or separate surveys as described above, may capture more indepth information on RN demographic and practice characteristics at re-licensure, lack of continuity of the data collected across the different states makes it impossible to conduct cross-state analysis.

Additionally, basic information on newly licensed RNs may be missed if data are only collected as part of the licensure renewal process.

The Forum of State Nursing Workforce Centers has identified minimum datasets for assessing a state's nursing workforce. The minimum dataset recommendations were based on a review of scientific literature and a survey of states to determine the most significant variables for measuring supply, demand, and education. More information on these minimum datasets is available from the Forum of State Nursing Workforce Centers at: http://www.nursingworkforcecenters.org/minimumdatasets.aspx.

Other State Data

Other RN data may be available from surveys conducted within a state using addresses from licensure data or other state-level datasets such as those provided by state nursing associations. Mailing lists obtained from membership organizations may be limited to active members, thus potentially creating a sample bias. The size, scope, and frequencies of RNs surveys may be limited by financial considerations or interest in particular nursing issues. Additionally, surveys developed for one nursing issue, such as job satisfaction, may be less useful for analysis on other nursing issues such as retirement or education.

RNs IN NEW YORK: THREE DIFFERENT VIEWS

Similar data variables can produce very different results depending on the data sources that are used and can lead to different conclusions about the RN workforce. To best illustrate this, race/ethnicity and practice setting for New York RNs were estimated using 2006–2008 ACS, the 2008 NSSRN, and the 2007–2010 New York RN Re-licensure Survey. The CPS was excluded from this analysis due to the small number of New York RNs in the 2007 sample.

RNs actively working in New York (regardless of where they lived) were selected from each of the three datasets and then frequencies were run on race/ethnicity (Table 3.1) and practice setting (Table 3.2). There was variability in the estimates of individuals who were non-Hispanic White across the three datasets. For example, the NSSRN estimated 75% of New York RNs were non-Hispanic White, while the ACS showed 64% of New York RNs to be non-Hispanic White, and New York's RN Re-licensure Survey indicated 70% of the RN population was non-Hispanic White. In contrast, the ACS estimates showed higher percentages of individuals who were Asian/Pacific Islander, non-Hispanic (13%), Black/African American, non-Hispanic (18%), and Hispanic/Latino (4%) than either the 2008 NSSRN (11%, 10%, and 3%, respectively) or the New York RN Re-licensure Survey (10%, 10%, and 4%, respectively).

TABLE 3.1
Distribution of New York RNs by Race/Ethnicity

	2006–2008 ACS Estimates (%)	2008 NSSRN (%)	2007–2010 NY RN Re-licensure Survey (%)
Asian/Pacific Islander, non-Hispanic	12.5	10.9	9.8
Black/African American, non-Hispanic	18.1	10.0	9.7
Hispanic/Latino	4.4	3.1	3.8
White, non-Hispanic	63.7	74.9	69.8
Other/multiracial	1.3	1.1	6.8

Sources: New York Center for Health Workforce Studies, RN Re-licensure Survey, 2007–2010; U.S. Census Bureau, 2006–2008 ACS Estimates; U.S. Department of Health and Human Services, Health Resources and Services Administration, 2010.

TABLE 3.2
Distribution of New York RNs by Practice Setting

	2006–2008 ACS Estimates (%)	2008 NSSRN (%)	2007–2010 NY RN Re-licensure Survey (%)
Hospitals	63.6	59.2	47.4
Long-term care	8.5	6.1	11.5
Home health care	4.5	7.3	6.5
Ambulatory care	7.0	10.4	14.4
Other/unknown	16.4	17.0	20.2

Sources: New York Center for Health Workforce Studies, RN Re-licensure Survey; Bureau of Census, 2006–2008 ACS Estimates; U.S. Department of Health and Human Services, Health Resources and Services Administration, 2010; New York Center for Health Workforce Studies, RN Re-licensure Survey.

The differences in practice setting were more pronounced, as shown in Table 3.2, with 64% of RNs in the ACS estimates practicing in hospitals —greater than the percent from the 2008 NSSRN (59%) or the New York RN Re-licensure Survey (47%). In contrast, the New York RN Re-licensure Survey estimated a higher percent of RNs in long-term care (12%) and ambulatory care (14%) than either the ACS (9% and 7%, respectively) or the 2008 NSSRN (6% and 10%, respectively), and a slightly greater percent for RNs in home health care (6%) than the ACS (5%), but less than the 2008 NSSRN (7%).

What causes these differences in results between the datasets may be a combination of factors, such as sampling methodology, sample size, survey question construction (available choices for the survey questions), and response bias. As indicated earlier in this study, the NSSRN undersamples larger, more metropolitan states. It is possible that this sampling method undercounts RNs working in cities in New York which have more hospitals and more RNs who are people of color. There were slightly more than 1,200 RNs from New York in the 2008 NSSRN sample (HRSA, 2010).

Based on the limitations on the NSSRN, one might conclude that a population sample, such as the New York RN Re-licensure Survey would provide a better estimate of RNs by race/ethnicity and by practice setting for New York. That may not be the case, however. The number of RNs reporting working in hospitals and reporting themselves as a racial/ethnic minority is lower than either the ACS or the 2008 NSSRN. One possible conclusion is that there may be a response bias in the New York RN Re-licensure Survey data, with RNs working in larger cities not responding to the survey at the same level as RNs working in smaller cities or in rural communities. The overall response rate for the 2007–2010 New York RN Re-licensure Survey was approximately 40%.

Survey question construction may also influence individual question responses and thus results. For example, when identifying practice settings, the ASC uses the NAICS codes for practice setting, identifying ambulatory practice settings in detail, including offices of physicians, offices of dentists, offices of other health practitioners (chiropractors, podiatrists, etc.), and breaks out outpatient clinics into a number of categories. The 2008 NSSRN also has a number of practice settings under the main categories of "hospital" and "ambulatory care setting, not located in hospitals." The hospital category includes outpatient owned by and/or located at the hospital. In contrast, the New York RN Re-licensure Survey aggregates all the outpatient settings together and includes two separate categories for hospitals, acute care inpatient and emergency room. The choices for identifying practice setting, as well as how data may be reported, in the case of the 2008 NSSRN, may affect the variation in practice setting information for New York RNs.

CONCLUSION

This study described the national data sources available to nursing workforce researchers to study the supply and distribution of the RN workforce and evaluated each source's strengths and limitations. This study also explored the potential for using state-level data for nursing workforce research.

Future RN shortages are likely and, in the long-term, shortages will be less likely than in the past to be resolved through market response (e.g., more entrants into nursing in response to widely publicized shortages). A national shortage of about 6% was believed to exist as early as 2000. By the year 2020, the supply of RNs nationally is projected to fall 36% below predicted requirements (HRSA, 2004).

Appropriate tracking of the size and characteristics of the RN workforce is critical to determine the supply and distribution of RNs. Lack of relevant and timely data about the nursing workforce is a significant barrier to identifying where nursing shortages exist, where they are most severe, and determining the factors that contribute to them. This lack of understanding impedes the development of health workforce programs and policies to mitigate shortages and the ability to evaluate these programs for effectiveness.

ACKNOWLEDGMENT

Contributions from Dayna Maniccia and Tracey Continelli at the Center for Health Workforce Studies and from Stephanie Fry and Vasudha Narayanan of Westat are gratefully acknowledged.

REFERENCES

Buerhaus, P. (2008). Current and future state of the U.S. nursing workforce. *JAMA: The Journal of the American Medical Association, 300*(20), 2422–2424.

Cleary, B. L., McBride, A. B., McClure, M. L., & Reinhard, S. C. (2009). Expanding the capacity of nursing education. *Health Affairs, 28*(4), w634–w645.

Kuehn, B. (2007). No end in sight to nursing shortage; Bottleneck at nursing schools a key factor. *JAMA: The Journal of the American Medical Association, 298*(14), 1623–1625.

Moore, J. (2008). Health workforce research: What are the issues? In D. Holmes (Ed.), *From education to regulation: Dynamic challenges for the health workforce* (pp. 85–100). Washington, DC: Association of Academic Health Centers.

New York State Education Department. (2003). *Registered nurses in New York State, 2002. Volume 1: Demographic, educational, and workforce characteristics.* Albany, NY: NYSED, Office of Professions.

U.S. Department of Health and Human Services, Bureau of Health Professions, National Center for Health Workforce Analysis Reports (HRSA). (2004). *What is behind HRSA's projected supply, demand, and shortage of registered nurses?*

U.S. Department of Health and Human Services, Bureau of Health Professions, National Center for Health Workforce Analysis Reports (HRSA). (2010). *The Registered Nurse Population. Initial Findings from the 2008 National Sample Survey of Registered Nurses.*

CHAPTER 4

State Policy and Research Initiatives Focused on Improving Nursing Workforce

An Integrative Literature Review

Alexia Green, Aileen Kishi, and M. Christina R. Esperat

ABSTRACT

The purpose of this chapter is to examine to and synthesize nursing workforce research and policy initiatives at the state level. An integrative literature review was systematically conducted using Ganong's Stages of an Integrative Research Review (1987). Searches were limited to English-language publications in the years from 2000 to 2010 which focused on workforce issues in the United States. A total of 155 published articles were included in this review. Overall, the literature indicated that significant research is examining nursing workforce issues and that states are actively engaged in policy initiatives to address nursing workforce issues, particularly those related to a shortage of nurses and faculty. The findings also indicated a major disconnect between nursing workforce research and patient outcomes research. Recommendations include connecting research and policy links between nursing workforce research and patient outcomes research and creating clear correlations to system-level determinants of quality. Additional implications for further research are provided which include the important role of nurse researchers in connecting nursing care and nurse staffing to processes and outcome measures, which demonstrate the financial impact upon health care.

© 2011 Springer Publishing Company
DOI: 10.1891/0739-6686.28.63

Over the past decade a global and national nursing shortage has emerged which is multifaceted and complex. As a result of this shortage, which is projected to worsen over the next 15–20 years (Cleary et al., 2005), the nursing workforce is being examined through a variety of lens, including policy makers attempting to devise effective strategies to abate or stem impacts upon patient populations. Global, national and state perspectives of the shortage have emerged with accompanying implementation of a cadre of policy interventions and strategies to assure an adequate, competent and effective nursing workforce. The purpose of this integrative literature review is to examine and synthesize nursing workforce research and policy initiatives at the state level.

BACKGROUND

Nursing workforce shortages have emerged cyclically across the United States over the past 150 years. As the U.S. population has grown, so has the need for additional nurses and other cadres of health care professionals. Most recently, national nursing workforce research agendas have focused on a variety of topics including but not limited to the size and composition of the nursing workforce (Buerhaus, 2000, 2008; Buerhaus, Staiger, & Auerbach, 2000; Buerhaus, Staiger, & Auerbach, 2009), the relationship between work-environments and shortages (Aiken et al., 2001; Brewer, Kovner, Greene, & Cheng, 2009), the quality of the nursing workforce (Aiken et al., 2001), staffing and outcomes (Clarke & Donaldson, 2008), and economics and nursing practice (Aiken, 2008). Bleich and Hewlett (2004) described the nursing shortage as "the perfect storm" identifying four areas where national efforts were being focused: supply and demand; work-environment; new partnerships and public/private ventures; and patient-centered and essential patient-safe care. Workforce regulation has also been addressed by a variety of national entities and taskforces, including the Pew Commission's Taskforce on Health Care Workforce Regulation (Parkman, 1997). Most recently, Donelan, Buerhaus, DesRoches, and Burke (2010) conducted a national survey of thought leaders about the nursing workforce, with the majority agreeing that the quality and safety of the U.S. health care system is dependent upon a highly educated nursing workforce of sufficient quantity and quality. All of these researchers stressed the need to influence policy and to increase policy attention to the many issues that face the nursing workforce over the coming decades.

An overview shows that national research and policy initiatives have focused on a variety of concepts, variables and strategies at the national level. The authors' own interest and involvement in research and policy initiatives emanates from their work within their home state, and the state nursing workforce center, resulting in their direct involvement in both processes focused on improving responses to the nursing shortage. An integrated review of research and policy initiatives framed at the state level and utilizing a defined conceptual model may help to add clarity to this body of knowledge. More importantly, the authors are hopeful that this review might help to inform state policy decisions, in the future, related to nursing workforce.

PURPOSE

Although national strategies to address the nursing shortage continue to emerge, it is often at the state level where practice and education are regulated and legislated. A national agenda alone cannot fully address the complexity of the nursing shortage and assure a competent and quality nursing workforce. Careful consideration of nursing workforce research and recommendations focused on state level interventions are necessary as a complement to federal policies and interventions. The purpose of this integrative literature review is to organize and examine the body of literature focused on research and policy addressing state nursing workforce issues and initiatives. Specifically this chapter has five purposes:

1. To review research on state nursing workforce issues and initiatives, exploring various foci of research;
2. To explore methodologies and processes being employed in research focusing on state nursing workforce issues, creating recommendations for improvement;
3. To examine state nursing workforce policy initiatives reported in the literature, exploring if such initiatives were supported by research;
4. To briefly explore the role and impact of state nursing workforce centers on nursing workforce research and policy;
5. To create recommendations to advance an agenda for future research and policy initiatives at the state level.

CONCEPTUAL FRAMEWORK

The authors utilized the framework described by L. H. Ganong (1987), declaring that integrative reviews are a valuable part of the process of creating and organizing a body of literature and yet should be held to standards similar to primary research. The authors found the framework—Ganong's Stages of an Integrative Research Review—valuable in organizing and conducting this review. Table 4.1 summarizes Ganong's methodology.

Furthermore, Ganong (1987) recommends that in order for an integrative literature review to make a meaningful contribution it should: "(a) use methods

TABLE 4.1
Ganong's Methodology for an Integrative Literature Review

- Develop purpose and research questions
- Establish inclusion and exclusion criteria (may be changed as review progresses)
- Search literature using appropriate search engines
- Design data collection tool
- Identify rules of inference for data analysis and interpretation
- Revise data collection tool as necessary
- Conduct literature review utilizing data collection tool
- Analyze data in a systematic way
- Discuss and interpret data
- Synthesize findings into manuscript for dissemination

Source: Adapted from Ganong (1987).

to ensure accurate, objective, and thorough analyses; (b) consider theory as well as the results, methods, subjects, and variables of the studies; (c) provide the reader with information about the studies reviewed...; and (d) inform rather than overwhelm the reader" (p. 1). Ganong (1987) proceeds to state that the reviewers should include enough information about the studies reviewed for readers to examine the evidence and draw their own conclusions. The authors attempted to meet Ganong's standards in this integrative review of research and policy focusing on state nursing workforce issues and initiatives.

METHODOLOGY
Hope (2004) and team organized a round table focused on the national nursing workforce, identifying gaps in current research, and suggesting specific areas for further research. Discussions focused on barriers to good research, including utilization of a sound methodology. The methodology followed for this review, as recommended by Ganong's framework (1987), included: (a) formulation of the purpose of the review and development of questions to be answered by the review; (b) establishment of tentative criteria for inclusion of studies in the review; (c) conduction of the literature search including sampling decisions (such as elimination of manuscripts which did not clearly emerge from problem identification at the state or multistate level); (d) development of a tool for reviewing the studies; (e) identification of rules of inference including those related to

classification as "research," "research and policy," or "policy" and interpretation within this classification, (f) reading the studies using the tool to gather data; (g) analysis of data in a systematic fashion; (h) discussing and interpreting data; and finally, (i) reporting the review as clearly and completely as possible.

Sample

Using the keywords of nursing workforce research, nursing workforce policy, workforce legislation, retention of nurses, and work-environment for nurses, the following search engines were used: Cumulative Index of Nursing and Allied Health Literature (CINAHL), Google, Google Scholar, PubMed, Medscape, and the National Forum of State Nursing Workforce Centers' website that provided links to all of the state nursing workforce centers in the United States. We collected 265 articles, publications and reports. One hundred fifty-five (n = 155) were selected for review using the inclusion criteria.

The sample consisted of manuscripts published from January 2000, through August 2010. As recommended by Ganong, the authors established tentative inclusion and exclusion criteria. Literature included for review was that which focused on U.S. state nursing workforce research or policy initiatives. A requirement for inclusion related to literature with a multistate perspective was that the manuscript must have identified the number of states included or named the specific states. One manuscript included up to 50 states, but most multistate manuscripts involved five to six states. Excluded were articles that specifically focused on national or international nursing workforce.

Measures

Sparbel and Anderson (2000a, 2000b) followed Ganong's methodological recommendations in their integrated literature review of continuity of care, developing a review tool framed upon Ganong's Stages of an integrative research review. The authors further modified this tool (Table 4.2) to accommodate the purposes of this study, which included incorporation of policy indicators as the researchers assumed that most nursing workforce studies would be accompanied by policy recommendations. The tool required the authors to consider whether literature being reviewed was solely research, research with policy recommendations or policy focused without a research foundation.

The authors, all three doctoral prepared nurse researchers, independently reviewed articles for adherence to inclusion and exclusion criteria. Those articles selected for inclusion were further reviewed using the data collection tool designed for this literature review. Each manuscript was treated as a single datum. The manuscripts were then further divided into three groups or classifications: research, research and policy, or policy only. A qualitative descriptive approach

TABLE 4.2

Data Collection Tool

State Workforce Literature Review Tool	
Parameters	Findings
1. Researcher/author/s	
2. Article/report title	
3. Year of study/report	
4. State of origin	
5. Research or policy focus	
A. If policy—Who is target audience?	
B. On what are the policy recommendations made?	
6. Workforce focus	
7. Purpose of study	
8. Conceptual model type (describe)	
9. Research question/hypothesis	
10. Variables examined/included	
11. Methodology described type	Yes No
12. Sampling methodology	
13. Instruments/tools used	
14. Sample size	
15. Validity (addressed) comments	
16. Reliability (addressed) comments	Yes No
17. Methodological limitations	
18. Factors identified affecting workforce	Yes No
19. Study conclusions/recommendations	
20. Do the interpretations of results include	
A. Suggestions for further research?	
B. Recommendations for policy?	
21. Other comments/notes	
22. Reviewer	

was then used to synthesize the literature findings, identifying common themes and content.

Limitations

One of the most notable limitations of this study relates to the difficulty often encountered in determining the conclusions drawn from the research or policy initiatives. Parameters were not consistently reported by all authors in the same way or format. Often lacking was a clear statement of a conceptual framework or model and of research methodologies. In particular, reliability and validity were often not addressed in the literature being reviewed.

When developing the review tool, the authors decided to classify the reviewed literature into one of three categories: research, research and policy or policy. This classification proved to be more difficult than first envisioned. To be considered "research," the literature being examined must have included a description of three or more of the following research components: conceptual model, research questions or hypothesis, variables being examined, a description of the methodology, sampling methodology, instruments/tools used, validity, reliability, methodological limitations and study conclusions and recommendations. Literature that was found to contain three or more of the above research components and a policy framework and/or policy recommendations were classified as "research and policy."

To be classified as "policy," the literature contained two or less of the research components described above yet provided strategies and/or recommendations on addressing a state nursing workforce issue/s. Because state nursing workforce initiatives are often grounded in research findings (primary or secondary), most nursing workforce researchers have an assumed intent to impact policy decisions with the findings and recommendations. However, there were numerous publications with policy recommendations that were not substantiated with research findings.

A group of noted workforce researchers (Hope, 2004) elaborated on strengthens and barriers to good nursing workforce research, including the "usefulness" of current research to increase the visibility of the problems in the work-environment and nursing workforce, suggesting that researchers have done a good job in this arena. However, these same national leaders (Hope, 2004) stated that few research initiatives have done a thorough job in assisting the profession and policy makers in determining interventions that need to occur. The authors encountered similar findings in conducting this integrative literature review as expressed by Hope (2004) in that few interventions studies were identified. Not surprisingly, most of the policy manuscripts did include policy recommendations; however, these recommendations were not necessarily grounded or based upon research.

FINDINGS AND DISCUSSION

Categorization, Characteristics, and Foci of the Literature

The literature review yielded 265 citations. Using sample inclusion criteria, 155 were reviewed and 54 were selected. The findings will be presented in the categories (groupings) related to either "research," "research and policy" or "policy." Of the 54 publications selected for in depth review, 9 (16%) were classified as "research" and 18 (33%) focused only on "policy." Most of the literature reviewed (n = 27, 50%) was classified as "research and policy" meaning research and policy were interfaced with research findings usually informing policy recommendations. In addition, the authors will explore various foci of the literature, thus addressing "purpose one" which was "to review research on state nursing workforce issues and initiatives, exploring various foci of the literature." Table 4.3 summarizes these foci including: (a) workforce planning, (b) nursing education, (c) retention—work environment, (d) supply and demand, (e) workforce centers—history/initiatives, (f) long-term care workforce, (g) public health workforce, (h) aging workforce, and (i) workforce legislation.

TABLE 4.3
Summary Table of Literature Foci

Foci of Literature	Reviewed (n)
Workforce planning	18
Nursing education	11
Retention—Work environment	6
Supply and demand	6
Workforce centers/history/initiatives	4
Long-term care workforce	3
Public health workforce	2
Aging workforce	2
Workforce legislation	2
Total literature reviewed	n = 54

Research Literature

A total of nine articles (n = 9, 16%) were classified by the review criteria as research, meaning the literature being examined included a description of three or more of the following research components: conceptual model, research questions or hypothesis, variables being examined, a description of the methodology, sampling methodology, instruments/tools used, validity, reliability, methodological cal limitations and study conclusions and recommendations.

All nine ($n = 9$) of the research articles clearly stated a purpose and related the importance to a particular sector or foci related to or impacting the nursing workforce (Table 4.4). Further examination and categorization of foci of these nine research studies revealed that three ($n = 3$) of the research studies focused on retention and the nurse work-environment, two ($n = 2$) focused on the public health nurse workforce, two ($n = 2$) on nursing education, one ($n = 1$) on workforce planning and one ($n = 1$) on supply and demand.

A total of six ($n = 6$) of the research studies utilized a conceptual model or framework. Five ($n = 5$) of the research studies (Andrews & Wan, 2009; Brewer, Kovner, Greene, et al., 2009; Cramer, Nienaber, Helget, & Agrawal, 2006; Kalb et al., 2006; Kotzer & Arellana, 2008) clearly identified the use of a conceptual framework, while a sixth study (Cox, Anderson, Teasley, Sexton, & Carroll, 2005) discussed a well known conceptual model (Forces of Magnetism) but failed to clearly state its utilization as a framework for the study. All nine of the research studies described a methodology, with the most common being survey methodology ($n = 7$), while one research team used a cross-sectional data analysis ($n = 1$), and another focused on a pilot methodology ($n = 1$) to test an evaluation tool. Four of the research articles ($n = 4$) clearly addressed validity and reliability, while one study ($n = 1$) addressed only validity. Three failed to address both validity and reliability. All seven of the research studies appeared to have robust sample sizes and response rates.

Retention and improving the work-environment ($n = 3$) were the most prevalent area of focus of the research manuscripts reviewed. Andrews and Wan's (2009) research evaluated the causal relationships between job strain, the practice environment and the use of coping skills. Their purpose included the desire to predict factors that resulted in a risk for the voluntary turnover of nurses and to identify potential intervention strategies. Findings indicated that while a nurse's physical health contributes significantly to the overall experience of job strain, mental health stressors were the most important influence upon propensity to leave. The authors discussed the importance of these findings in relation to the large number of nurses reported to be leaving the workforce and offered strategies for nurse administrators and managers to improve the mental health of the nursing workforce. Cox et al. (2005) focused on perceptions of nurses employed in states with and without mandatory staffing ratios and/or mandatory staffing plans. Surveying nurses in 10 states, Cox and team provided preliminary evidence that mandatory staffing plan legislation may be linked with the most positive nurse work-environment perceptions when compared with implementation of mandatory staffing ratios or no workforce regulation. The researchers

TABLE 4.4

Characteristics of State Nursing Workforce Research Literature (n = 9)

Author(s) (Year) State(s)	Workforce Focus/Purpose	Conceptual Model	Methodology (Validity) [Reliability] Sample Size	Primary Findings/ Policy Recommendations
Andrews & Wan (2009) Multistate	Retention—Workforce environment/staff RNs. To evaluate the causal relationships between job strain, the practice environment and the use of coping skills to predict risk of voluntary turnover.	Yes Occurrence of job strain	Exploratory cross-sectional survey (Yes) {Yes} N = 1235 RNs n = 308 RNs	Mental health stressors influence upon propensity to leave job. Hypothesized direct relationship between professional practice and propensity to leave significant (–0.58) using SEM. Suggest attention to role that mental health plays in decision making process and coping skills of individual staff nurses.
Bartee, Winnail, Olsen, Diaz, & Blevens (2003) WA	Public health workforce/RN competencies. To determine perceived proficiency on Public Health Core Competencies. Includes RNs.	No	Survey (Yes) {Yes} N = 696 N = 445	Strong communication competencies. Low in 7 other domains especially financial planning/ management skills, policy development, and program planning. Recommends discipline specific training.
Brewer et al. (2009) 35 States	Nursing Education/ baccalaureate educated RNs (BSN). To describe the differences between traditional BSN and second degree BSN graduates.	Yes Turnover model	Cross-sectional survey (Yes) {Yes} n = 3,391 RNs	Suggest significant differences between traditional and second degree baccalaureate graduates. Second degree performed higher in planning, evaluation, interpersonal relations, and communication. However, second degree grads have less workgroup cohesion (p = .001) and greater turnover.

Cox, Anderson, Teasley, Sexton, & Carroll (2005) 10 states	Retention—Workforce environment/nurses (does not specify type). Perceptions of work environment related to staffing ratios.	Not stated but appears to be "Forces of Magnetism"	Survey (No) [No] $N = 4000$ nurses n = not stated	Means and percentages were derived. Variations in state-specific nurse work environment perceptions may exist. Variation may be dependent upon adopted mandatory staffing ratios/plans. Recommends that states give careful consideration to potential trade-offs of alternative types of legislation, with first consideration being given to adoption of mandatory staffing plans.
Cramer, Nienaber, Helget, & Agrawal (2006) NE	Supply and demand/RN workforce. To determine trends in RN shortages between urban and rural areas.	Yes Predictive model to determine need for nursing workforce	Cross-sectional data analysis (Yes) [Yes] $N = 66$ counties	Rural areas of state consistently exhibited significantly greater RN shortages than did urban areas ($p = .013$). Suggest the full extent of rural RN shortage seriously underestimated. Recommends federal designations similar to that for physicians to entice RNs to rural areas.
Foxall, Megel, Grigsby, & Billings (2006) NE	Nursing education/nursing faculty (NF). Explore conditions and situations which would entice faculty to continue working beyond intended retirement date.	No	Survey (No) [No] $N = 270$ NF $n = 56$ NF	Percentages of responses were reported. Faculty might be enticed to work past retirement age if certain incentives are offered: flexible schedule, no clinical teaching or reduced workload, and higher salaries and additional benefits.
Kalb et al. (2006) WA	Public health workforce/ public health nurses (PHN). To integrate PHN competencies into a comprehensive performance review instrument for nurses at an urban PH department.	Yes Domains of PH nurse competencies	Pilot testing (No) [No] $n = 50$ PHN	No psychometric properties were reported. Supervisors found tool easy to use and reported tool facilitated communication between employee and supervisor. Tool proved efficient for performance appraisal. Use of tool reinforces population-based practice and translates into improvement of population health.

(Continued)

TABLE 4.4

Characteristics of State Nursing Workforce Research Literature (n = 9) *(Continued)*

Author(s) (Year) State(s)	Workforce Focus/Purpose	Conceptual Model	Methodology (Validity) {Reliability} Sample Size	Primary Findings/ Policy Recommendations
Kotzer & Arellana (2008) Colorado	Retention—Workforce environment/staff nurses (SN). To describe and compare SN's perceptions of their real and ideal work environment in a tertiary pediatric facility. To provide administrators with research evidence for identifying areas for improvement.	Yes Kanter's theory of organizational empowerment	Descriptive survey (Yes) {Yes} N = 385 SN n = 157 SN	Perceptions of real (R) and ideal (I) work settings were compared. Statistically significant findings were derived from the instrument used (p = .001). Despite moderate work pressure, staff affirmed a highly positive work environment on their units. Understanding dimensions of the nurse's work environment needing improvement and involving staff in making and evaluating change supports an evidence-based environment to attract and retain qualified staff.
Seago, Spetz, Coffman, Rosenoff, & O'Neil (2003) CA	Workforce planning/RN and LVN. To cescribe current RN and LVN staffing levels in medical-surgical nursing units in CA acute care hospitals and identify impact of new mandatory staffing regulations.	No	Cross-sectional survey (No) {No} N = 410 acute care hospitals N = 115	Mean characteristics of rural vs. non-rural hospitals were analyzed, statistically significant (p = .001) differences were found. Projected that new mandatory staffing regulations would impact ability to adequately staff in the state of California due to insufficient size of workforce. Rural hospitals would have most difficulty in meeting mandatory ratios, taking longer to recruit sufficient staff.

suggest that further analysis comparing the relative benefits and costs of workforce regulation is needed. Adding to the research evidence on work-environment were Kotzer and Arellana (2008), examining staff nurses' perceptions of their real and ideal work-environment in a tertiary pediatric facility. The researchers found that a consistent pattern was seen across all units with reported high levels of involvement, peer cohesion, task orientation and managerial control. Significant differences were reported between real and ideal work-environments suggesting that staff were able to identify areas for improvement. These researchers recommended that administrators utilize standards for establishing and sustaining healthy work-environments, such as those defined by the American Association of Critical Care Nurses in 2005.

The public health workforce was the foci of two research articles ($n = 2$). Bartee and team addressed competencies of the public health workforce, including registered nurses (RNs), in a rural frontier state (Bartee, Winnail, Olsen, Diaz, & Blevens, 2003). Interestingly, their findings indicated that all public health workforce members surveyed lacked sufficient expertise in program planning skills and policy development. This finding seems to have particular implications for nursing as implementation of health care reform emerges over the next 5–10 years. Kalb et al. (2006) specifically examined the public health nursing workforce in their research focused on piloting a competency based performance evaluation instrument. Both of these research articles stressed the correlation between a strong and effective public health workforce and population health.

Two research articles focused on nursing education—one focusing on nursing faculty and the other on differences between two types of baccalaureate-educated graduates. Brewer and team conducted a very interesting study examining the differences between traditional baccalaureate nursing graduates and those who held a baccalaureate in another field and graduated from a second-degree baccalaureate nursing program (Brewer, Kovner, Poornima, et al., 2009). Interestingly, Brewer and team documented differences between the two types of graduates that have implications for workforce productivity. The demographics between the two groups were strikingly different, with second-degree graduates being older, more likely to be Asian (double the proportion of traditional graduates) and male (triple the proportion of traditional graduates). The second-degree graduates also reported more family-work conflict, yet were optimistically inclined as a group. Second-degree graduates were more likely to remain in their first job past 1 year, and earned a higher salary. An important finding for employers of second-degree graduates was that they experienced less workgroup cohesion than traditional graduates did. Foxall, Megel, Grigsby, and Billings (2009) explored conditions impacting an aging nursing faculty workforce and found that aging faculty might be enticed to work past retirement age if certain incentives were provided. Of particular interest to aging faculty were flexible teaching schedules, limited or no clinical teaching, reduced workload. Aging faculty also reported that higher salaries and additional employee benefits might entice them to remain in the workforce longer (Foxall et al., 2009).

The final two research studies in this section focused on supply and demand ($n = 1$) and workforce planning ($n = 1$). Cramer et al. (2006) focused on supply and demand, utilizing a cross-sectional analysis examining differences in the nursing shortage between rural and urban areas of Nebraska and suggested that the rural shortage of nurses was greatly underestimated, recommending federal designations similar to those used for physicians to recruit nurses to rural areas of the state. Seago and team's research question focused on the impact of mandatory staffing laws passed in California, asking how those laws would impact the capacity to staff in rural versus urban hospitals (Seago, Spetz, Coffman, Rosenoff, & O'Neil, 2003). The findings suggested that it would be difficult for rural hospitals to meet the mandatory staffing mandates and require significantly longer periods of time to recruit nurses to rural areas of the state.

Research and Policy Literature

Dickson and Flynn (2009) in discussing the research to policy connection identified the convergence of three streams: problem, politics, and policy. The literature classified as "research and policy" (Table 4.5) were found to contain two or more of Dickson and Flynn's converging streams and many contained all three. One-half of the literature reviewed ($n = 27$, 50%) was classified as both "research and policy," containing three or more of the required research components and a policy framework and/or clearly stated policy recommendations. The researchers further classified or grouped the "research and policy" literature into areas of emphasis or foci for purposes of discussion.

Research and policy literature focused on workforce planning ($n = 10$) and supply and demand ($n = 5$) comprised the largest categories. Interestingly, many of these researchers utilized national data sets and extrapolated state workforce data for use in workforce planning. Brewer, Feeley, and Servoss (2003) used the national sample survey of RNs to illustrate to other nursing workforce professionals and scholars the value of using a state-level or regional subset of the data to inform state workforce planning. Courtney (2005) visualized nursing workforce distribution via federally designated Health Profession Shortage Areas (HPSAs) in Missouri using geographic information systems. Lin and team used primary metropolitan statistical areas as the principal data unit to examine the California workforce, finding that the state will face major challenges over the next 15 years in meeting workforce demand (Lin, Juraschek, Xu, Jones, & Turek, 2008). Recommendations were made which included policy initiatives to

TABLE 4.5

Characteristics of State Nursing Workforce Research and Policy Literature (n = 27)

Author(s) (Year) State(s)	Workforce Focus/Purpose	Conceptual Model/Policy Framework	Methodology (Validity) [Reliability] Sample Size	Primary Findings/Policy Recommendations
Bargagliotti (2009) Multistate (50)	Nursing education—Supply. Funding for RN education	No Coalition building	Secondary data analysis/comparative analysis (No) [No]	Using 2004 National Sample Survey and 2004 National Council of State Boards statistics predictions of RN replacement (RNRRS) rates were calculated. Stepwise regression analysis found that percentage of state budget fiscal year 2004 used for higher education ($p = .000$) and percentage of LVNs in 2004 ($p = .000$) predicted 2004 RNRRs in states studied. Descriptive statistics. One of three new US nurse graduates comes from only 6 states: CA, NY, TX, FL, OH, IL. Three of these states had state budget deficits. CA is highest producer of RNs but has lowest density per population. Recommends monitoring of RN replacement rate versus just monitoring number of graduates. Monitoring replacement rate will be especially important in future due to retirements. Suggest correlation in minimal increases in funding to big changes in RN replacement. Recommends to state nurses associations to pursue "friend raising" with state governors and staff.

(Continued)

TABLE 4.5

Characteristics of State Nursing Workforce Research and Policy Literature (n = 27)   *(Continued)*

Author(s) (Year) State(s)	Workforce Focus/Purpose	Conceptual Model/Policy Framework	Methodology (Validity) [Reliability] Sample Size	Primary Findings/Policy Recommendations
Brannon, Kemper, & Barry (2009) NC	LTC Workforce/LTC direct care workforce. Evaluation of Better Jobs Better Care Initiative	Complex adaptive systems coalition building	Single-case study/evaluation (No) [No]	Qualitative data from project work plans and progress reports as well as notes from interviews with key stakeholders and observation of meetings were coded into a simple rubric consisting of characteristics of complex adaptive systems. Found leaders who view coalitions as systems are likely to allow developments to evolve rather than attempt to plan every detail thus having greater success. Do just enough and just-in time planning, build good enough vision, practice covert leadership, develop relationships for sustainability, respect role of process.
Brewer & Kovner (2009) Multistate	Retention—Workforce environment/RN staff nurses. Predictors of RN staff nurse satisfaction.	Price model	Descriptive/ survey (Yes) [Yes] N = 1.2 million hospital staff RNs in U.S.	The following predictors were positively related to hospital staff RNs' work satisfaction: fair rewarding of staff, group cohesion, supervisor support + relationship; and work/family conflict, organizational constraint, quantitative workload –relationship were negatively related to satisfaction (p values ranged from .000 to .024). Working conditions accounted for 51% variance in job

			$n = 533$ hospital staff RNs from 29 states	satisfaction, and more than 37.8% of the variance in satisfaction was explained by various work attitude scales. Income and benefits were not related to satisfaction but important in staying in their job; up to 63% reported work related injuries; change in supervisors is a common experience for staff RNs; staff RNs work more hours than scheduled to work (average of 100 hrs more for FT nurses); 51% plan to leave the organization or change their position within a year. Recommended policies that relate directly to keeping nurses safe from injuries, providing competent and stable managers, implementing fairness in salaries and tying work rewards to work efforts.
Brewer, Thomas, & Servoss (2003) NY	Workforce planning/RN workforce. To illustrate to other nursing workforce professionals and scholars the value of using a state-level or regional subset of a national data set to inform and complement understanding of factors affecting RN supply	Demonstration project	Secondary data analysis and geocoding	Recommendation to use secondary data analysis and geocoding of national data set may be worthwhile to state to "home in on" specific issues for the state, using this data to develop policy strategies to correct identified problems. Methodology also allows for examination of regional differences. NSSRN data set are useful for policy planning for state policy makers.

(*Continued*)

TABLE 4.5

Characteristics of State Nursing Workforce Research and Policy Literature (n = 27) *(Continued)*

Author(s) (Year) State(s)	Workforce Focus/Purpose	Conceptual Model/Policy Framework	Methodology (Validity) [Reliability] Sample Size	Primary Findings/Policy Recommendations
Cleary, Bevill, Lacey, & Nooney (2009) NC	Nursing education/ nursing faculty. To identify supply and demand needs for nursing faculty in NC via analysis of RN licensing data and calculation of nurse faculty supply and demand estimates.	Supply and demand model	Descriptive, longitudinal analysis (No) [No] N = 9,380 RNs	Means and percentages were reported. The vast majority of RNs from the 1983/84 and 1993/94 cohorts who pursued graduate education by 2003 to become prepared at or above the master's level originally had entered nursing with a BSN. Policy recommendations: obtaining additional financial resources in baccalaureate and higher degree nursing programs to increase the educational mobility of nurses, offer opportunity for ADN nurses to pursue directly a master's degree, continue developing partnerships between community colleges and 4-year colleges and universities, further develop partnerships between nursing education and nursing service, further develop use of clinical simulation to augment clinical instruction.
Courtney (2005) MO	Workforce planning/ RN workforce. Nursing workforce distribution related to HPSAs	No	Outcomes evaluation via geographic information systems (GIS)	Used GIS data visualization and statistical techniques which did not demonstrate an expected trend of decreasing group differences between HPSA and non-HPSA designated counties over time. Between 1993 and 1999, the loss in nurse to

| | | Visualization (No) [Yes] N/A | population ratios in HPSA counties was significant ($p < .001$); however, between 1999 and 2001, the growth in nurse to population ratio changes in HPSA counties was significant ($p = .001$). Goal of recruiting RNs to underserved areas (HPSAs) was not achieved by state policy initiative. Policy definitions of underserved areas may not be effective in defining areas of nursing shortages and the existing policy may not be achieved by the stated goals. |
| Dickson & Flynn (2009) NJ | Supply and demand/RN workforce. To project supply and demand for RNs to meet state needs. | Supply and demand model | Descriptive survey (no) [no] $N = 44,000$ RNs $n = 24,406$ RNs | Frequencies and percentages were reported. 24% of NJ RNs were dissatisfied with their job, 12% plan to resign from their facility within a year, over 9,800 nurses reported the following as problem areas: high patient-to-RN ratios and heavy workloads, unsupportive nurse managers, inflexible work schedules, unsupportive work environments, high rates of occupational injuries, and high levels of occupational burnout. Descriptive survey of 50% of all RNs licensed in NJ, update on NJ supply and demand calculations, and review of published research. Among the 5 evidence-based supply recommendations, 3 focused on improvements in the workplace to retain experienced nurses and 2 on increasing educational capacity to increase the long-run supply of nurses. |

(Continued)

TABLE 4.5

Characteristics of State Nursing Workforce Research and Policy Literature (n = 27)   (Continued)

Author(s) (Year) State(s)	Workforce Focus/Purpose	Conceptual Model/Policy Framework	Methodology (Validity) {Reliability} Sample Size	Primary Findings/Policy Recommendations
Florida Center for Nursing (2010) FL	Supply and demand/ LPNs and RNs. To provide an update on the demand for nurses by employers in 6 settings: hospitals, psychiatric hospitals, home health agencies, skilled long-term care facilities, public health departments, hospices.	Supply and demand model	Descriptive survey (Yes) {Yes} in a separate technical manual $N = 1,904$ employers $n = 597$ employers	Frequencies, means, vacancy and turnover rates, and growth percentages were reported. Employers reported higher than expected vacancies, turnover, and projected growth in nursing positions. The recession had eased the nursing shortage in several ways: more nurses returned to work, nurses were working more hours, turnover had decreased, and employers had cut vacant positions. Increasing the number of new nurses alone will not satisfy the health care system's need for experienced nurses with specialized skills. Policies are needed to retain the older, experienced nurses taking into consideration the physical demands of nursing work (e.g., work schedules, patient loads, physical demands) and how to draw from the strengths of a multigenerational workforce.
Flynn (2009) Multistate	Retention—Workforce environment. Home health staf RNs. To identify relationships	Job satisfaction and retention of nurses in the work place	Descriptive correlational design (No)	Correlation coefficients, analysis of variance, and logistic regression were used to analyze data. 30% of the sample indicated they were dissatisfied with their job, 26% reported plans to leave their job

that workload, quality of
care and job satisfaction
have on retention.

{No}
N = 325
n = 137
from 38 states

within 12 months. No significant relationships
between demographic characteristics and job
satisfaction. High ratings of nurse assessed quality
of care were associated with higher level of job
satisfaction ($r = .355$, $p = .000$); patients' lack of
preparation for discharge was associated with
lower job satisfaction ($r = -.253$, $p = .003$). Nurses
who reported that patients' visit frequencies were
appropriate to their skilled nursing needs were
3 times more satisfied with their jobs than those who
felt their patients received fewer visits than needed
($OR = 294$ [1.25, 6.94], $p = .013$). Three measures
of workload were associated with a higher frequency
of patients' lack of preparedness for discharge.
These findings indicated that workload may have
an indirect effect on job satisfaction by negativey
influencing quality-care processes. 2 of the 3 quality-
care indicators and 2 of 3 workload indicators were
significantly associated with intent to leave the job.
Results indicated that the higher the ratings of quality
of care, the lower the odds on nurses' intent to leave.
Need for policies related to organizational processes
and structures that support nursing practice and,
thereby, enhance quality of patient care, which are
important in improving job satisfaction and retention
of staff nurses in home health.

(Continued)

TABLE 4.5

Characteristics of State Nursing Workforce Research and Policy Literature (n = 27) (Continued)

Author(s) (Year) State(s)	Workforce Focus/Purpose	Conceptual Model/Policy Framework	Methodology (Validity) {Reliability} Sample Size	Primary Findings/Policy Recommendations
Kemper, Brannon, Barry, Stott, & Heier (2008) IA, NC, CA, OR, PA, and VT	LTC Workforce/LTC direct care workforce. Evaluation of Better Jobs Better Care Initiative	No Demonstration Project	Evaluation (No) {No}	Analysis of qualitative data from project work plans and progress reports, and notes from telephone and in person interviews with project staff, coalition stakeholders, and state policy experts. Data were abstracted, categorized and summarized. No psychometric properties were reported. Each state varied in methodologies used to advocate for LTC direct care workers. Found insufficient demonstration resources, strong stable project leadership and coalitions of key stakeholders, neutral lead agency, clear goals, effective processes, favorable state histories and contexts. Policy change is difficult to improve direct care jobs.
Lin, Juraschek, Xu, Jones, & Turek (2008) CA	Workforce Planning/RN workforce forecasting	Shortage Projection Model	Supply and Demand Modeling (NA) {NA}	Using Primary Metropolitan Statistical Area/ Metropolitan Statistical Area as the principal data unit, the report projects severe shortages in RN workforce by 2020. 22 of 24 PMSA/MSA will have severe ratios; population growth and aging will be the most important factors in these ratio changes. California has lowest RN ratio in US and RN forecasting model

				shows that over the next 15 years, the majority of P/MSAs will have increasing RN shortages. Recommends policy initiatives to curtail shortage.
Lundeen, Kaufmann, & Krause (2007) WI	Nursing Education/ Nurse faculty. Nurse faculty shortage and restrictions on faculty qualifications to teach	No	Survey (No) {No} $N = 39$ nursing programs $n = 32$ nursing programs	Means and percentages reported. Surveyed WI nursing schools on a variety of variables. Found a shortage of faculty existed, evidence of unmet demand for potential nursing students, insufficient clinical training sites, non-competitive faculty salaries and other factors negatively impacting nursing education capacity in state. Recommended increased financial support and other incentives for nursing graduate students to become faculty, competitive nursing faculty salaries, collection of supply/demand data, strategies to promote faculty satisfaction and effectiveness, and expansion of the existing board of nursing faculty exception program.
McHaney & Varner (2006) AL	Aging workforce/RNs. Awareness of and plans to address aging RN workforce by nurse administrators in hospitals and nursing homes	No	Survey (Yes) Face validity only {No} $N = 129$ hospitals $N = 42$ hospitals $N = 227$ nursing homes $N = 63$ nursing homes	Means and percentages were derived. Lack of policies to assist retention of aging RNs. Limited action by administrators to address aging workforce. Need for flexible work schedules, weekend-only work opportunities, flexible shifts, policies which support retention.

(Continued)

TABLE 4.5

Characteristics of State Nursing Workforce Research and Policy Literature (n = 27)   (Continued)

Author(s) (Year) State(s)	Workforce Focus/Purpose	Conceptual Model/Policy Framework	Methodology (Validity) [Reliability] Sample Size	Primary Findings/Policy Recommendations
Michigan Center for Nursing (2009) MI	Workforce planning/ workforce profile of RNs and LFNs	No State workforce center	Descriptive/ secondary data analysis (No) [No]	Means and percentages were derived. Profile of Michigan nursing workforce for use by state and Michigan Center for Nursing to develop strategic plan to address nursing shortage. Describes characteristics of active RNs and LPNs, education, work settings, number of nursing programs and students. Use HRSA data to project shortage in Michigan and makes policy recommendations.
North Carolina Institute of Medicine (2007) NC	Workforce planning/ state nursing workforce plan assessed for progress	No	Assessment (NA) [NA] N/A	Means and percentages reported. Original plan (2004) contained 74 recommendations. 2007 assessment indicated that 13 (18%) fully implemented; 52 (71%) partially implemented, 8 (11%) no implemented or no progress made. Comprehensive data included supporting policy recommendations. Original plan made recommendations in eight areas—all areas improved. Continue trajectory/plan.

Palumbo, McIntosh, Rambur, & Naud (2009) VT	Aging workforce/RNs. Retention of older experienced nurses in the workforce.	Retention model	Descriptive survey (Yes) {Yes} n = 583 RNs	Means and percentages reported. Challenges of managing a nursing workforce with the majority of nurses over 45 years of age are now necessitating attention to policies for recruitment and retention of older nurses, particularly in rural areas. Nurses in this study are willing to work longer if the organization creates a responsive work environment, managers are able to promote intergenerational understanding and teamwork, and address certain HR practices that would affect a nurse's attention to remain in the organization. Recommendations for improving recruitment and retention of older nurses were made in relation to staffing, development, work design, feedback/recognition, compensation, and culture.
Pennsylvania Department of Health Professions Study Group (2004) PA	Workforce planning/ RNs and LPNs	Nurse supply and demand model	Multiple surveys, Facilitated discussion, Secondary data analysis (No) {No} Multiple Groups	Means and percentages were reported. Flexibility in the education process, enhancement of retention strategies, increase supply of nurses, improve workplace, conduct additional research on supply and demand, development of targets based on the Nurse Retention Assessment Index of counties at risk of experiencing nurse shortage, flexibility by employers to assure retention of nurses.

(Continued)

87

TABLE 4.5

Characteristics of State Nursing Workforce Research and Policy Literature (n = 27)   (Continued)

Author(s) (Year) State(s)	Workforce Focus/Purpose	Conceptual Model/Policy Framework	Methodology (Validity) [Reliability] Sample Size	Primary Findings/Policy Recommendations
Roth (2008) NC	Retention–work environment/Newly licensed RNs. To identify factors contributing to safe practice and critical areas of need for focused competence and confidence development of newly licensed RNs and to create intervention activities to enhance competence and confidence development.	Development of a transition to practice model for newly licensed RNs	Longitudinal design (Yes) [Yes]—stated it was done but did not describe n = 512 new nurse-preceptor dyads (1,024 individuals) in 29 hospitals in North Carolina	Description of Phase I of a collaborative project and the research that will be conducted. Findings were not reported at the time of this publication. Author does indicate that data will describe competence and confidence development of new graduates practicing in acute care hospitals. Longitudinal data about practice errors and risk for practice breakdown in the first 6 months of employment will also be collected. The goal of this evidence-based project is to determine if the evidence supports enacting legislation requiring statewide implementation of a formal transition experience for all newly licensed nurses in N.C
Rudel & Moulton (2009) ND	Workforce planning. High school students. To provide evidence base for development of recruitment strategies to encourage high school students to	No	Stratified Survey (No) [No] n = 571 students representing 25 high schools	Frequencies and percentages were reported. Provided an evidence base for a state to develop: action steps to introduce health care careers, including nursing, to elementary and high school students; a curriculum plan and workshop to engage parents; and a program that uses health care employers and other resources to market

	consider a career in nursing.		career opportunities, increase student experiences, and increase resources for career counselors and teachers to use.
Simon & Hoffman (2004) ID, MO, MT, NJ, OH, VA	Workforce planning/ Nursing as prototype. Development of a conceptual framework and action plan for the next generation workforce system.	Shared vision for transformation	Multimethod: national focus groups, environmental scans, regional forums, policy academy (No) {No}	Two-phase project: research phase to develop conceptual framework; second phase developed policy academies. Framework developed includes focus on connecting workforce development to economic needs; building stronger education pipeline; expanding lifelong learning opportunities; enhancing worker's ability to manage careers; strengthen employment retention and career advancement; strengthen governance and accountability in workforce system. Nursing was used as prototype for development of policy academies.
Spetz (2009) CA	Workforce planning/RN workforce forecasting	Forecasting model	Forecasting (No) {No}	Used forecasting model for long term supply and demand, based on inflow and outflow of RNs and numbers from national data base. In the long term the forecast predicts that demand will continue to increase pushing CA to the 25th percentile by 2016 and national RN average FTEs per population by 2025. Forecast need for more nurses to meet CA workforce needs. Multiple factors identified which affect forecasting including: migration, immigration, supply, movement from active to inactive license status, demand for nurses. Recommends increasing graduates from schools and increase FNG migration/immigration.

(Continued)

TABLE 4.5

Characteristics of State Nursing Workforce Research and Policy Literature (n = 27)   (Continued)

Author(s) (Year) State(s)	Workforce Focus/Purpose	Conceptual Model/Policy Framework	Methodology (Validity) {Reliability} Sample Size	Primary Findings/Policy Recommendations
State of Illinois Department of Financial and Professional Regulation (2007) IL	Workforce planning/ RNs, LVNs, APNs. Nursing shortage, nurse work experience of RNs, LVNs, APNs	No	Survey (Yes) {Yes} N = 22,889 n = 9,028	Means, frequencies and percentages were derived. Purpose was to gather supply data, better understand the nurse work experience and identify areas of health care policy and planning that may resolve shortage. Findings indicate need to recruit more nurses, need for retention strategies across all work settings and types of nurses, need to address dissatisfiers (salary/workload). Develop campaign to improve image of nursing and nursing education.
Tate & Moody (2005) LA	Nursing education/ nursing students—need for criminal background checks	No Regulatory	Case study/ survey (No) {No}	Percentages reported. Louisiana only state not requiring criminal background checks on nursing students on admission to nursing school and at licensure. Recommended change of regulatory policy to protect public.
Texas Center for Nursing Workforce Studies (2006a) TX	Supply and demand/RN workforce. To develop supply and demand projections for RNs and nurse graduates in Texas.	HRSA Supply and Demand Model	Longitudinal analysis and statistical calculations (NA) {NA} Nursing	Supply and demand projections for RNs and new RN graduates were calculated from 2005 to 2020. Cost for increasing the number of new graduates to meet targeted goals was also calculated. Model assisted state workforce center to create state supply and demand model for use in policy decisions.

			education data from all RN nursing programs and RN licensing data over a 5-year period and calculation of annual costs to increase targeted enrollments and graduates over a 6-year period	Policy recommendations presented to the TX Legislature included: funding amount needed to meet projected target number of graduates along with recommendations on how new funds could be used to provide financial incentives to professional nursing programs who increase the number of graduates, provide additional financial aid for both undergraduate and graduate nursing students, increase nurse faculty salaries, and continue to allocate dedicated tobacco fund earnings for innovative nursing education projects and research.
Texas Center for Nursing Workforce Studies (2008a) TX	LTC nursing workforce. To project supply and demand for nurses in long term care (LTC) facilities.	Nurse supply and demand model	Descriptive survey. (Yes) (Yes) $N = 1,158$ LTC facilities $n = 473$ LTC facilities	Frequencies, means, and vacancy and turnover rates were reported. Examined length of tenure, reasons for turnover and salaries of directors of nursing; turnover and vacancy rates of licensed and unlicensed nursing staff; staff compensation and benefits, and implementation of safe patient handling legislation in LTC. Policy recommendations were made on funding and reimbursement and training standards required for certified nurse aide to state agency that regulates LTC facilities. Policy recommendations were made to LTC facilities on compensation and benefits, work place environment, staff training and career development, and partnerships with other organizations and institutions.

(Continued)

TABLE 4.5

Characteristics of State Nursing Workforce Research and Policy Literature (n = 27)   *(Continued)*

Author(s) (Year) State(s)	Workforce Focus/Purpose	Conceptual Model/Policy Framework	Methodology (Validity) [Reliability] Sample Size	Primary Findings/Policy Recommendations
Texas Center for Nursing Workforce Studies (2008b) TX	Supply and demand/ nurse workforce. Examined supply and demand for nurses in hospital in-patient facilities.	Nurse supply and demand model	Descriptive survey. (Yes) (Yes) N = 542 licensed in-patient hospitals n = 289 licensed in-patient hospitals	Frequencies, means, vacancy and turnover rates, and growth percentages were reported. Surveyed vacancy and turnover rates for licensed and unlicensed nurses, methods and cost for interim staffing of RNs, plans for expansion and projected need for RNs and LVNs in the next 3 years, assessment of the nursing shortage in clinical specialty areas and impact hospitals are experiencing in RN shortage. Policy recommendations encouraging partnerships between hospitals and academic institutions and nursing programs, retention of older experienced nurses, development of an effective transition program for new graduates, and strategies that improve the work environment and contribute to the recruitment and retention of nurses in the work setting.
University System of Georgia Board of Regents (2009) GA	Supply and demand/ RN workforce.	HRSA workforce model Policy brief	Secondary data analysis (No) [No] N/A	Means and percentages reported. Utilized a final report from a task force on health professions education and analysis of HRSA data. Extensive data and appendices describing RN workforce in GA. Recommendations include: GA must expand its production of new nurses and perform better surveillance of existing nursing workforce.

curtail the predicted worsening of the California workforce shortage. The Health Resources Service Administration's (HRSA) Supply and Demand Model was used by the Texas Center for Nursing Workforce Studies (2006a, 2008b) to develop a state supply and demand model which generated projections which were used to inform policy makers and drive legislative agendas. Many of the nursing workforce research and policy initiatives emerged from state nursing workforce centers, including the North Carolina Center for Nursing (Cleary, Bevill, Lacey, & Nooney, 2009) and the Florida Center for Nursing (2010), and other state entities—University of Georgia Center for Health Workforce Planning & Analysis (University System of Georgia Board of Regents, 2009); the Center for Health Professions at University of California San Francisco (Spetz, 2009), and the Pennsylvania Department of Health Professions Study Group (2004).

In Courtney's work (2005) focused on nursing workforce distribution using geographic information systems, which included HPSAs, the findings converged with policy recommendations suggesting that the current methodology of recruiting workforce RNs to underserved Missouri areas was not effective. Courtney recommended that federal policies for recruitment of nurses to rural areas be redesigned, employing strategies similar to those used for physician recruitment. The National Governor's Association Center for Best Practices, engaged three university policy centers (University of Washington, Rutgers, and University of Texas) to develop the next generation workforce system (Simon & Hoffman, 2004). These researchers used nursing workforce as a case example connecting workforce development to economic need in six states. The Michigan Center for Nursing (2009) profiled the state nursing workforce (RNs and licensed practice nurses [LPNs]) for use in developing a strategic plan to address the state nursing shortage. This work was contracted to a public policy research firm that worked with the Michigan Health Council to link or converge the report to ramifications of recently passed health care reform legislation. The North Carolina Institute of Medicine (2007) collaborated with a task force composed of multiple advocacy groups focused on the nursing workforce to produce a report that included specific recommendations to a variety of entities including trade and professional organizations, nurse leaders, regulatory boards, health care employers, Area Health Education Centers (AHECs), educational systems, and legislators. These recommendations clearly modeled the convergence of research, policy and legislative streams. The State of Illinois Department of Financial and Professional Regulation (2007) contracted with the National Research Corporation to produce the report entitled "The 2007 Illinois Nursing Workforce Survey Report" which included data to better understand the LPN, RN, and advanced practice nurse (APN) work experience and identify areas of health care policy and planning that may resolve the nursing shortage impacting the state; and finally, two independent researchers, Rudel and Moulton (2009) examined high schools students' perceptions of nursing as a career and made policy recommendations for workforce planning in North Dakota.

Multiple policy and research literature focused on nursing education capacity and/or on the nursing faculty shortage (n = 3). A very interesting study by Bargagliotti (2009) focused on the three converging streams of research, policy and legislation, by examining how the percentage of state funding (50 states) to higher education and other RN workforce variables may be related to RN replacement rates in states. One of the most striking findings is that one in three new US nurses graduates come from only six states: California, New York, Texas, Florida, Ohio, and Illinois. Bargagliotti further linked these findings to the fact that three of the above states had budget deficits at the time and suggested that RN replacement rates will need to be monitored very carefully in the future in relation to the economy and projected retirement of large numbers of nursing faculty. Very clear policy recommendations are made by Bargagliotti, including advice to state nurses associations to "friend raise" with state governors and policy staff. The Wisconsin Nurse Faculty Shortage Task Force through the Wisconsin Center for Nursing examined issues around the perceived nurse faculty shortage and then examined restrictions imposed on faculty qualifications to teach (Lundeen, Kaufmann, & Krause, 2007). Recommendations emanating from the Wisconsin study were directed at the state's nursing regulatory agency, encouraging the adoption of an "exception program" for nurse educators. In another policy and research study, Tate and Moody (2005) examined the streams of nursing education and regulation via exploration of state requirements of criminal background checks for nursing students. Supply and demand for nursing faculty were also examined by Cleary, Bevill, et al. (2009) with a study emanating from the North Carolina Nursing Workforce Center.

Long-term care workforce supply and demand (n = 3) was also examined by three teams of researchers. Two focused on "Better Jobs, Better Care" (BJBC) demonstration projects funded by the Robert Wood Johnson Foundation and the Atlantic Philanthropies that sought to create changes in policy and practice to improve the recruitment and retention of direct care workers (non-licensed) in both nursing homes and home and community-based settings. Although these two studies focused on non-licensed caregivers versus licensed nurses, the findings have significant implications for nursing workforce coalitions and thus were included in the literature review. Kemper and team analyzed five BJBC projects and presented the lessons learnt, including the recognition that workforce policy and management practice change is difficult and requires time (Kemper, Brannon, Barry, Stott, & Heier, 2008). A similar BJBC analysis was conducted as a case-study by Brannon, Kemper, and Barry (2009) in North Carolina, pro-viding insights into a single case, finding that leaders who view coalitions as systems are likely to allow developments to evolve rather than attempt to plan every detail (Brannon et al., 2009). Building upon the model of complex adaptive systems used by Brannon et al. (2009), this study and its finding certainly has implications for the numerous state workforce coalitions that have formed to address the nursing shortage. And lastly related to long-term care, the Texas Center for Nursing Workforce Studies (2008a) conducted a supply and demand study focused on nursing workforce (including licensed and non-licensed care-givers), converging the research and policy streams via several recommendations to both long-term care employers and state policy makers.

Of the research and policy literature were three studies classified by the authors as focus on retention, including one very interesting study focusing on newly licensed RNs (Roth, 2008) to identify factors contributing to safe practice during the first 6 months of employment. The issue of transition into practice has long been a topic of debate in nursing since new graduates were transitioned from becoming "graduate nurses" to directly entering the workforce as RNs upon licensure. Roth was unable to report findings in this initial publication, but indicates that outcomes data will describe the competence and confidence development of new graduates practicing in acute care settings. Roth indicates that the findings of this research may drive enactment of legislation to address transition of new graduates into practice, converging the streams of problem (inexperienced new graduates) with policy. Brewer and Kovner (2009) focused on RN staff nurse satisfaction, while Flynn (2009) examined home health staff RNs satisfaction. Both merged the research findings with policy recommenda-tions directed to employers related to improving nurse satisfaction. Lastly, two studies were focused on the aging workforce both having sound methodologies and reaching similar conclusions and recommendations (McHaney & Varner, 2006; Palumbo, McIntosh, Rambur, & Naud, 2009).

Policy Literature

Eighteen (n = 18, 33%) of the reviewed literature were categorized as "policy" literature (Table 4.6). It is interesting to note that the convergence of the streams outlined by Dickson and Flynn (2009) relating to the research—policy con-nection which includes problem, politics and policy was most notable with the literature classified in this integrative literature review as "policy literature." In particular, the political component stands out in these manuscripts and provides important lessons, frameworks and pathways for others interested in improving the nursing workforce at the state level. Each of these manuscripts focused on state level nursing workforce initiatives and was included in hopes of fostering

TABLE 4.6

Characteristics of State Nursing Workforce Policy Literature (n = 18)

Author(s) (Year) State(s)	Workforce Focus/Purpose	Policy Framework	Policy Approach	Primary Findings/Policy Recommendations
Cleary et al. (2005) FL, NC, CA, IA, MS, NJ	Nursing workforce centers/state workforce centers review of long-range strategic initiatives in 5 states	Call to action	Case studies	Summarizes progress in establishing a national network of state nursing centers for sharing of workforce data, new education models workplace and policy initiatives. Encourages similar initiatives across country and support for nursing workforce centers.
Cleary (2001) NC	Nursing workforce centers/describes the creation and implementation of the NC Center for Nursing, including the Center's enabling legislation	Nursing workforce center	Legislative	Recommends other states create nursing workforce centers to a) provide objective information to health care providers, policy makers, and stakeholders; b) develop a strategic planning mechanism for nursing resources; c) promote recruitment and retention by recognizing and rewarding excellence/recognition of nursing colleagues.
Cleary, Hofler, & Seamon (2005) NC	Nursing workforce centers/describes an 18 month policy fellowship for nurses in NC.	Leadership development	Health policy fellowship	Purpose of fellowship is to train and educate NC nurses regarding state health policy. Reported as state policy fellowship for nurses in the nation.
Green et al. (2004) TX	Workforce planning/describes the strategic planning process for development and passage of legislation to address nursing shortage, the content of the legislation, and provides a 2-year	Strategic leadership	Legislation	2001 legislation, with accompanying multimillion dollar funding, proved to be a success as an initial step to address the nursing shortage within the state, particularly the dramatic growth funding and the Nursing Innovation Grant Program. There has been a significant increase in awareness of the

	summary of the impact of the legislation on the Texas nursing education infrastructure.		nursing shortage in Texas. Enrollments increased by 18.9% as a result of legislation.
Green et al. (2006) TX	Nursing education/RN workforce. A statewide grant program was developed and implemented through legislative initiatives providing opportunities for schools of nursing to respond to the nursing shortage and need for innovation in nursing education.	Legislation Grant initiative	Shares some of the successes and challenges of implementing and evaluating a state wide grant program. Insights into the political and regulatory process are provided as a model for other states to consider. Examples of educational strategies that were successful in improving the recruitment and retention of students and faculty are discussed. Encourages other states to adopt similar strategy to infuse innovation into educational programs for rapid growth of nursing workforce.
Kaeding & Rambur (2004) VT	Nursing education/RN education. Examines a statewide merit-based scholarship program targeting academically excellent nursing students.	Leadership by foundation Scholarship program	A state-wide merit scholarship program reversed a decade-long decrease in enrollments in nursing schools. Academic indicators also increased (SAT and class rank). Proposes model for other states.
Kishi & Green (2008) TX	Workforce planning/RN workforce. Describes a statewide infrastructure for nursing workforce policy, including legislative and regulatory approaches.	Leadership in workforce development Strategic partnerships and planning, legislation, regulation	Statewide strategic partnerships are critical to success of nursing workforce planning. Success is dependent upon: (a) viewing issues from broad perspective; (b) leadership and vision; (c) expertise in developing strategic plans/policies; (d) ability to negotiate with diverse groups; (e) media, and marketing campaigns; (f) access to and ability to communicate with policy makers/legislators.

(Continued)

TABLE 4.6

Characteristics of State Nursing Workforce Policy Literature (n = 18)   (Continued)

Author(s) (Year) State(s)	Workforce Focus/Purpose	Policy Framework	Policy Approach	Primary Findings/Policy Recommendations
Kirschling, Harvey-McPherson, & Curley (2008) ME	Workforce planning/nursing workforce. Depicts a 6-year strategic effort to better understand the nursing workforce in Maine and describes efforts to persuade policy makers to invest in nursing education programs	Leadership in workforce development	State level strategic planning	Accurate and timely data are critical, need to educate state legislators, keep on message with legislators, must have universities/educational systems designate nursing has high priority before success in legislature, engage numerous stakeholders, having nurse legislator/s was key to success.
Loquist (2002) Multistate	Workforce planning/regulation. Directed to nursing administrators, describes the efforts of state boards of nursing to address nursing shortage.	Regulation	Partnerships	Encourages nurse administrators to work with state boards of nursing to embracing emerging innovations to address nursing shortage—working collaboratively to shape a preferred future to benefit profession and public.
McKay & Hewlett (2009) MS	Workforce centers/coalition building to support successful policy initiatives.	Workforce centers	Grassroots coalition	Identifies 10 strategies to impact coalition building to support nursing workforce development.
North Carolina Institute of Medicine (2004) NC	Workforce planning/recommendations from a taskforce on NC nursing workforce.	State workforce planning	Stakeholder task force	Recommendations included: need to focus on nursing faculty recruitment/retention; urges funding via legislature to increase production of RNs; encourages foundations to give to nursing students/schools; increase appropriations to schools; implement articulation across state; increase production of LPNs; work with AHECs to recruit to nursing profession.

Palumbo (2009) VT	Nursing education/use of a framework for research based problem solving, policy formation and legislative action to address faculty shortage.	John W. Kingdom's Theory used for policy development and legislation	Research based problem solving, strategic partnerships and coalition, policy development, legislation	Findings demonstrated how use of data, partnership coalitions, policy development, and recognition of windows of opportunity can lead to creation of a permanent funding for nurse faculty educational loan repayment in one state.
Sroczynski (2003) MA	Workforce planning/nursing workforce. Describes efforts in Massachusetts to address statewide nursing shortage and makes policy recommendations.	Leadership in workforce development	Strategic partnerships, planning, legislation	Strategies must be developed to address recruitment and retention. Create and strengthen partnership. Compress time to complete PhD, market the educator role. Develop mentor/preceptors roles in academic setting; find resources to maintain and expand lab facilities and other technologies; increase collaboration with stakeholders to generate funding and technology resources. Recommended specific legislative language to pending bills to incorporate faculty incentives. Recommended development of a statewide faculty initiative.
Tanner, Gubrud-Howe, & Shores (2008) OR	Nursing education/RN educatior. Describes a statewide coalition focused on increasing nursing education capacity.	Leadership in workforce development	Strategic partnerships and coalition, statewide planning and policy development	Describes development of the Oregon Consortium for Nursing Education, infrastructure development, creation of the shared curriculum, redesign of clinical education, faculty development, and plans for evaluation. Includes policy implications for development of nursing education systems, design and sharing of curricula, use of simulation as a component of clinical education, and delivery of clinical education.

(Continued)

TABLE 4.6

Characteristics of State Nursing Workforce Policy Literature (n = 18)   (Continued)

Author(s) (Year) State(s)	Workforce Focus/Purpose	Policy Framework	Policy Approach	Primary Findings/Policy Recommendations
Texas Center for Nursing Workforce Studies (2006b, 2010) TX	Workforce planning/RN workforce. Comprehensive statewide action plan/s to increase supply of RNs and nurse graduates to meet health care demands in Texas.	Leadership in workforce development	State workforce planning, strategic partnerships, legislation	Strategic plan based upon research and data obtained on recruitment and retention of nurses and supply and demand studies done in health care facilities. In addition to increasing the supply of new RN graduates, this evidence-based strategic plan included policy recommendations and strategies that focus on recruitment and retention of nurses and faculty in order to address the nursing shortage.
Texas Nurses Association (2006) TX	Workforce legislation/RN workforce. Description of policy recommendations for nursing workforce heading to legislature.	Leadership in workforce development	Professional association advocacy/ lobbying	Recommendations include: increase capacity in nursing education programs; provide financial incentives to ensure supply and sufficient faculty.
Texas Team Addressing Nursing Education Capacity (2008 and updated 2010) TX	Nursing education/RN education. Statewide nursing education capacity. Evidence and research based statewide strategic plan with focus on increasing educational capacity and the number of initial RN licensed graduates in Texas by targeted goals.	Leadership in nursing education capacity building	Strategic coalition/ partnerships Policy integration	Strategies and best practices used to increase the number of new graduates; evaluate progress in establishing individual and regional graduation targets; calculation of graduation rates; strategies for increasing diversity of nursing graduates; and use of regional academic partnerships and partnerships between and among health care consumers, health care systems, business communities and academic institutions. Illustrates the engagement, partnership and collaboration

of representatives from nursing education, health care and nursing organizations, state agencies, state legislature and governor's office as well as regional representatives in the ongoing development and implementation of statewide policies based upon data collected from studies done by TCNWS, the Texas Higher Education Coordinating Board, and the Board of Nursing.

Policy review

Compilation of state nursing legislation—addressing nursing education capacity—18 states had passed or pending legislation addressing capacity.

Legislation

Quinn (2008) Multistate

Workforce legislation/compilation and commentary on state-legislative bills passed or pending in 2008.

greater understanding of nursing workforce issues and comprehensive strategies and policy changes occurring across the United States. Many of these initiatives were data driven, although the actual research or evidence producing phase was not included in the publications.

Many authors focused on state workforce planning ($n = 7$; North Carolina, Maine, Massachusetts, Texas [3], and even one multistate project) related to health policy leadership and strategic planning, linking research generated data to support plan development and implementation. One extensive report addresses the North Carolina experience in strategic planning to address state workforce planning (North Carolina Institute of Medicine, 2004) and clearly links problem, policy and politics. Loquist (2002) addressed the role of state boards of nursing in responding to the nursing shortage by encouraging boards located in all states to recognize the role of innovation in nursing education. Nurse administrators in health care delivery systems were encouraged to embrace innovation as well. Kirschling, Harvey-McPherson, and Curley (2008) described the vital role of having accurate and timely data as critical to the planning process and to education of state legislators in Maine. Green et al. (2004) described a strategic planning process, which was supported by data generated from the state nursing workforce center, and resulted in passage of nursing workforce legislation to address the nursing shortage in Texas. Significant funds were appropriated by the Texas legislature, exceeding $14 million during a 2-year cycle, to schools of nursing to increase enrollments in response to the nursing shortage. The Texas Center for Nursing Workforce Studies (2006b, 2010) provides a comprehensive data driven statewide action plan to increase supply of RNs and nurse graduates to meet health care demands in Texas. Sroczynski (2003) describes the strategic planning process for workforce development in Massachusetts and provides comprehensive policy recommendations for consideration. Kishi and Green (2008) provided enlightening overviews of statewide strategies to address nursing workforce development through strategic planning and partnerships between professional associations, health care systems, foundations, regulatory agencies and legislatively established policy groups.

Statewide programs addressing nursing education initiatives were evident in five ($n = 5$) of the policy literature. Green et al. (2006) described how a statewide grant program developed and implemented through legislative initiatives, provided opportunities for schools of nursing to respond to the nursing shortage and need for innovation in nursing education. The cycle of research (data collection and analysis by the state nursing workforce center), policy development through the legislative process and the "politics" of lobbying to get the legislation passed are discussed in detail. Kaeding and Rambur (2004) discuss a similar initiative in Vermont to establish a statewide scholarship program and provide

outcome evidence linking the scholarship program to growth in nursing applicants and enrollments. Palumbo (2009) links evidence regarding a nurse faculty
shortage to a strategic initiative in Vermont creating a nurse faculty loan repayment
program, which was funded by the state legislature. The Texas Team Addressing
Nursing Education Capacity (2008, updated 2010) provided evidence of a statewide strategic plan developed in response to an American Association of Retired
Persons (AARP)/Center to Champion Nursing call to action. Multiple entities
were engaged including the Governor's Office, regulatory entities, professional
and hospital associations, schools of nursing, the workforce commission, and
AHECs. Lastly, in this category of nursing education, Tanner, Gubrud-Howe, and
Shores (2008) provide an important case-study review of the Oregon Consortium
for nursing education, which has been critically esteemed across the nation by
other educators attempting to address nursing education capacity. Changes in
state and educational policies clearly converged with problem of a nursing shortage in this Oregon initiative.

Workforce centers were the foci of four policy publications ($n = 4$). Cleary
(2001) describes the North Carolina Center for Nursing, including the political and legislative process resulting in its creation, and in a second manuscript
(Cleary et al., 2005) described efforts to establish a national network of state nursing centers encouraging other states to follow suit in order to effectively impact
policy changes at the state level. One last article by Cleary, Hofler, and Seamon
(2005) emerged from the North Carolina Center for Nursing and described the
creation and implementation of an 18-month policy fellowship for nurses in
North Carolina. It is interesting to note that the advent of state nursing workforce centers may have peaked in 2008, as many centers have been disbanded
as a result of depressed state economies, including the North Carolina Center
for Nursing, which was a leading center for many years. The full impact of the
dissolution of these centers will likely not be understood, but inarguably this
loss will have a negative impact upon nursing workforce advocacy and policy
decisions. McKay and Hewlett (2009) tell the story of effective coalition building
in Mississippi through the nursing workforce center, and how policy has been
positively impacted through advocacy.

The convergence of research, policy and politics was very evident in the
literature described above and two final publications ($n = 2$) most clearly made
the connection to politics through the legislative process. Those included a publication by the Texas Nurses Association (2006) which highlighted the trajectory
from planning to legislation to policy implementation addressing the nursing
shortage in Texas and another by Quinn (2008) which compiled state legislative
bills introduced and/or passed during 2007–2008, highlighting 18 states with
one or more legislative initiatives. Quinn proceeds to discuss the need for further

reform of health policy agendas at the state level to adequately address nursing workforce.

Role of Nursing Workforce Centers in Research and Policy

Milstead (2004) and Cleary and Rice (2005) discuss the role of nurses in acting as political entrepreneurs or strong messengers, providing evidence to facilitate the opening of windows of opportunity for policy change. Nursing workforce centers emerged in this literature review as key messengers for nursing in delivering data driven messages to policy makers. Seventeen ($n = 17$, 18%) of the 54 manuscripts review emanated from nursing workforce centers. Nursing workforce centers have joined individual researchers and others focused on highlighting the relevance of the nursing workforce to the public and to the attention of policy makers focused on improving health care systems in their states. Workforce centers appear to have resulted in a more knowledgeable set of key policy informants and have enhanced the number of research driven policies emerging from state legislatures.

Recommendations to Advance an Agenda for Future Research and Policy

State level nursing workforce research should be accompanied or complemented with patient outcomes research. Although the authors did not review patient outcomes research, this literature review found no mention or correlation of findings to patient outcomes research.

Mason, Leavitt, and Chaffee (2007) and Longest (2009) recommended better coordination of workforce research and patient outcomes research providing a clear correlation to systems-level determinates of quality. Together the knowledge gained from workforce research and patient outcomes research can deliver a powerful message to the public and to policy makers concerning issues of interest related to safety and quality of care. Outcomes research can assist the profession and policy makers in making the case for increased staffing levels and increased salaries for health care professionals. Equally important is the role of nurse researchers in connecting nursing care and nurse staffing to processes and outcome measures that demonstrate the financial impact upon the health care system. Conducting meta analyses of research that focuses on workforce and quality of care and outcomes of nursing care is also recommended.

Flynn's (2009) research reviewed in this study, suggest that there is a significant relationship between the quality of care perceived by home health nurses and the nurses' satisfaction with their jobs. In addition, Flynn points out that savings realized from reduced turnover and vacancies among the nursing staff could reduce cost to agencies and improve the quality of care delivered. Further research is needed and long overdue to determine the RNs' role in quality care delivery and carefully determining the economic savings of providing quality care, as well as the impact this has on enhancing nurse satisfaction and retention. Other than Flynn's research, the literature reviewed in this study made minimal connection between workforce and finance. This literature review reveals that most nursing research and policy planning has focused on outcomes impacting the profession, and not the public. To more effectively convey the importance of the nursing workforce related to public good and public policy, nurse researchers need to ask relevant questions. What are the consequences to patients and outcomes as a result of a nurse shortage? What are the economic and social costs of the nursing shortage on specific state policies—such as those related to public health? How does nursing education impact patient safety in hospitals, home health or long-term care?

Diers and Price (2007) discussed the challenge in disseminating research findings, to balance competing demands between complexity and simplicity in developing policy recommendations. Most of the literature reviewed by the authors in this study presented complex information, which would surely require major "reframing" before being presented to policy makers and/or the public. Diers and Price proceed to emphasize that the link between research and policy—policy research—hold the keys to the widespread adoption of effective nursing solutions that would benefit the public, most notably related to the safety and quality of care. Minimal connections were made to safety and quality in the literature reviewed.

Diers and Price proceeds in advising that nurse researchers must present sound evidence to effectively impact change. This literature review revealed that many nurse researchers and nursing workforce centers depend upon the HRSA to provide sound and reliable national nursing workforce supply and demand data for use at the state level. The authors recommend that HRSA continue to provide this data for use at the state level, to be used in workforce planning and policy generation.

This literature review identified the workplace of nurses as an area in great need of change through evidence-based policies. The current nursing shortage's impact upon acute care hospitals, where the majority of all nurses are employed, is highly important and was evident in this literature review. The literature review also revealed other problematic areas in non-hospital settings, including long-term care and public health. As states' populations age, the increased demand for nursing care continues to grow, just as the nursing workforce will be greatly diminished by massive retirements from the baby boom generation. Complicating an already complex problem is the much smaller potential pool of nurses available to fill the void between supply and demand of workers as the baby boomers retire and leave the workforce (Cleary & Rice, 2005). Further, this literature review indicates that policies focused on retaining experienced nurses in the health care workforce are an essential strategy toward reducing the projected shortage and providing experienced mentors for young and novice nurses. According to Dickson and Flynn (2009, p. 129):

> The severity of the current and projected nursing shortage requires serious thought in developing research-tested strategies for retaining experienced nurses in the workforce, while at the same time looking at the efficiencies of the work of nurses. The development of research-based retention policies, designed to create productive and healthy workplaces for nurses and their patients, are crucial to the overall health of the health care system.

Andrews and Wan (2009) provided clear evidence in their research of the role that mental health plays in decision making and coping skills of staff nurses and found a direct relationship between professional practice and propensity to leave the workforce. This finding correlates to national research findings related to the relationship of the work-environment with nurses' satisfactions with their work and link individual nurse characteristics to care delivery and in turn to patient outcomes (Brewer, Kovner, Greene, et al. 2009).

Two of the studies in this review addressed the aging nursing workforce (McHaney & Varner, 2006; Palumbo, McIntosh, Rambur, & Naud, 2009) reaffirming the fact that age matters in nurse burnout. Interestingly, these researchers found that the nurse under 30 reported the highest levels of burnout. To address these troubling and significant findings, policies should be developed that provide programs for new nurses to help ease the transition from the culture of nursing school to the culture of the workplace. The longitudinal study conducted by Roth (2008) provided beginning evidence for the potential need to develop policies requiring states to implement formal transition experiences for all newly licensed nurses. With further evidence, policies could be implemented which might deter the burnout rate of so many young nurses. Clearly, research and policies directed at understanding and intervening to assist nurses in navigating stressful work-environments should be undertaken to assure a quality workforce for tomorrow.

It is highly important that nurses make the research to policy connection. Research, in and by itself, is not sufficient to create the changes needed to improve the nursing workforce and health care delivery. The work of translating research into action is the most difficult to do. This literature review reveals that much work is being done and underway across the states to make this ultimate research to policy connection. As indicated in this review, many nurse researchers and nurse advocates are taking action to connect research and evidence to policy and legislative actions and outcomes. The literature classified by the authors as "policy" demonstrates the successes that some states have had in making this important connection. In fact, this is likely one of the most important findings emanating from this literature review. Many states have an effective cadre of nurse leaders capable of facilitating the research to policy connection and are having positive outcomes from those connections with passage of significant legislative initiatives aimed at improving state nursing workforces (Cleary, 2001; Green et al., 2004, 2006; Kaeding & Rambur, 2004; Kirschling, Harvey-McPherson, & Curley, 2008; Kishi & Green, 2008; Quinn, 2008). Equally important in the research to policy connection is "friend making" with state governors and policy makers as recommended by Bargagliotti (2009). Clearly some of the policy initiatives reported in this review indicate "friend raising" has been effective in positively building the nursing workforce. Another striking finding of this literature review is the relationship between "friend raising" and the formation of effective coalitions composed of a variety of stakeholders willing to tackle nursing workforce issues at the state level. Many of the authors in this literature review described the creation of coalitions and partnerships as key to their successful policy and legislative initiatives (Cleary et al., 2005; Green et al., 2004, 2006; Kaeding & Rambur, 2004; Kirschling, Harvey-McPherson, & Curley, 2008; Kishi & Green, 2008; Quinn, 2008; Tanner et al., 2008; Texas Nurses Association, 2006; Texas Team Addressing Nursing Education Capacity, 2008, updated 2010).

In considering the development of this literature review, the authors initially dialogued about including only those literatures that could be clearly described as "research." Further discussion on our part determined that it was indeed important to expand the review to include the literature described herein as "policy and research" and "policy." In order to establish a research to policy connection:

> ...the goal of research has to be expanded to include not only the generation of new knowledge, but also the 'translation' of that knowledge into constructive information that is (a) practical, (b) accessible, (c) actionable, (d) solution oriented, and (e) actively used by decision makers at clinical, organizational, or public policy levels. (Dickson & Flynn, 2009, p. 335)

Many policy makers have difficulty identifying the valuable information that is embedded in the complex, statistical reporting of research findings in peer-reviewed journals. Thus, the translation of research findings needs to be clear, concise, short, and compelling in order to capture the attention of policy makers and engage them in policy development and implementation (Dickson & Flynn, 2009). What the authors found by reviewing the literature classified as "policy" is that considerable "action" is occurring across states related to nursing workforce. Much of this action is being influenced by research and data—much of it emanating from state workforce centers and/or state related entities. However, the research or data gathering process that support these initiatives and decisions are not always clearly presented or included in the literature.

Shi and Singh (2008) discussed how funding sources could be excellent facilitators of the translation process. Organizations such as the Robert Wood Johnson Foundation, Northwest Health Foundation, Blue Cross and Blue Shield of Florida, the Moore Foundation and AARP's Center to Champion Nursing in America have played important roles in facilitating partnerships and creating opportunities for research and evidenced-based policies among researchers, nursing and workforce organizations with policy makers, legislators and project funders. There are also other people and organizations that can serve as invaluable translators and facilitators, including chief nursing officers, APNs, professional organizations, consumer groups, professional lobbyists, and community and business leaders. This literature review provided evidence of the importance of these relations to effectively impact policy. Mutual trust, reciprocity, and negotiation are key ingredients to sustaining successful partnerships between researchers as the producers of evidence and policy makers as the users of evidence (Cleary, Hofler, & Seamon 2005; Green et al., 2006; Green et al., 2004; Kirschling, Harvey-McPherson, & Curley, 2008; Texas Team Addressing Nursing Education Capacity, 2008, updated 2010).

One final thing to consider is that policy decisions are also influenced by personal and societal values, economics, politics, historical events, and the general mood of the public or organization (Longest, 2009). In order to effectively influence policy decisions, it is important that researchers and evaluators provide valid, rigorously produced, actionable and understandable evidence to the policy makers (Shi & Singh, 2008).

This literature review provides evidence that nurse researchers and nurse policy advocates have the opportunity to inform and influence clinical, organizational and public policy. Nursing's role in advocating for a strong nursing workforce must be grounded in evidence and be translated into effective public policies.

REFERENCES

Aiken, L. H. (2008). Economics of nursing. *Policy, Politics & Nursing Practice, 9*(2), 73–79.

Aiken, L. H., Clarke, S. P., Sloane, D. M., Sochalski, J. A., Busse, R., Clarke, H.,...Shamian, J. (2001). Nurses' reports on hospital care in five countries. *Health Affairs (Project Hope), 20*(3), 43–53.

Andrews, D. R., & Wan, T. T. (2009). The importance of mental health to the experience of job strain: An evidence-guided approach to improve retention. *Journal of Nursing Management, 17*(3), 340–351.

Bargagliotti, L. A. (2009). State funding for higher education and RN replacement rates by state: A case for nursing by the numbers in state legislatures. *Nursing Outlook, 57*(5), 274–280.

Bartee, R. T., Winnail, S. D., Olsen, S. E., Diaz, C., & Blevens, J. A. (2003). Assessing competencies of the public health workforce in a frontier state. *Journal of Community Health, 28*(6), 459–469.

Bleich, M. R., & Hewlett, P. O. (2004). Dissipating the perfect storm—Responses from nursing and the health care industry to protect the public's health. *Online Journal of Issues in Nursing, 9*(2), 5.

Brannon, S. D., Kemper, P., & Barry, T. (2009). North Carolina's direct care workforce development journey: The case of the North Carolina New Organizational Vision Award Partner Team. *Health Care Management Review, 34*(3), 284–293.

Brewer, C. S., Feeley, T. H., & Servoss, T. J. (2003). A statewide and regional analysis of New York State nurses using the 2000 National Sample Survey of Registered Nurses. *Nursing Outlook, 51*(5), 220–226.

Brewer, C. S., & Kovner, C. T. (2009). Working satisfaction among staff nurses in acute care hospitals. In G. L. Dickson & L. Flynn (Eds.), *Nursing policy research: Turning evidence-based research into health policy* (pp. 127–141). New York: Springer Publishing.

Brewer, C. S., Kovner, C. T., Greene, W., & Cheng, Y. (2009). Predictors of RNs' intent to work and work decisions 1 year later in a U.S. national sample. *International Journal of Nursing Studies, 46*(7), 940–956.

Brewer, C. S., Kovner, C. T., Poornima, S., Fairchild, S., Kim, H., & Djukic, M. (2009). A comparison of second-degree baccalaureate and traditional-baccalaureate new graduate RNs: Implications for the workforce. *Journal of Professional Nursing: Official Journal of the American Association of Colleges of Nursing, 25*(1), 5–14.

Buerhaus, P. (2000). A nursing shortage like none before. Interview by Carol Lindeman. *Creative Nursing, 6*(2), 4–7.

Buerhaus, P. I., Staiger, D. O., & Auerbach, D. I. (2000). Implications of an aging registered nurse workforce. *The Journal of the American Medical Association, 283*(22), 2948–2954.

Buerhaus, P. I. (2008). Current and future state of the US nursing workforce. *The Journal of the American Medical Association, 300*(20), 2422–2424.

Buerhaus, P. I., Staiger, D. O., & Auerbach, D. I. (2009). *The future of the nursing workforce in the United States: Data, trends, and implications.* Boston, MA: Jones and Bartlett.

Clarke, S. P., & Donaldson, N. E. (2008). Nurse staffing and patient care quality and safety. *Patient safety and quality—An evidence-based handbook for nurses.* Retrieved September 17, 2010, from http://www.ncbi.nlm.nih.gov/books/NBK2676/

Cleary, B., Bevill, J. W., Jr., Lacey, L. M., & Nooney, J. G. (2009). The Looming crisis of an inadequate pipeline for nursing faculty. In G. L. Dickson & L. Flynn (Eds.), *Nursing policy research: Turning evidence-based research into health policy* (pp. 209–218). New York, NY: Springer Publishing.

Cleary, B., Hofler, L., & Seamon, J. (2005). North Carolina Center for Nursing health policy fellowship: A strategy for developing nursing leaders for the future. *Policy, Politics & Nursing Practice, 6*(4), 327–330.

Cleary, B. (2001). The North Carolina Center for Nursing: A pioneering state nurse workforce policy initiative. *Policy, Politics & Nursing Practice, 2*(3), 210–215.

Cleary, B., & Rice, R. (2005). *Nursing workforce development strategic state initiatives.* New York, NY. Springer Publishing.

Cleary, B., Rice, R., Brunell, M. L., Dickson, G., Gloor, E., Jones, D., & Jones, W. (2005). Strategic state-level nursing workforce initiatives: Taking the long view. *Nursing Administration Quarterly, 29*(2), 162–170.

Courtney, K. L. (2005). Visualizing nursing workforce distribution: Policy evaluation using geographic information systems. *International Journal of Medical Informatics, 74*(11–12), 980–988.

Cox, K. S., Anderson, S. C., Teasley, S. L., Sexton, K. A., & Carroll, C. A. (2005). Nurses' work environment perceptions when employed in states with and without mandatory staffing ratios and/or mandatory staffing plans. *Policy, Politics & Nursing Practice, 6*(3), 191–197.

Cramer, M., Nienaber, J., Helget, P., & Agrawal, S. (2006). Comparative analysis of urban and rural nursing workforce shortages in Nebraska hospitals. *Policy, Politics & Nursing Practice, 7*(4), 248–260.

Dickson, G. L., & Flynn, L. (2009). *Nursing policy research: Turning evidence-based research into health policy.* New York, NY: Springer Publishing.

Diers, D., & Price, L. (2007). Research as a political and policy tool. In D. J. Mason, J. K. Leavitt, & M. W. Chaffee (Eds.), *Policy and politics in nursing and health care* (5th ed., pp. 195–206). St. Louis, MO: Saunders, Elsevier.

Donelan, K., Buerhaus, P. I., DesRoches, C., & Burke, S. P. (2010). Health policy thoughtleaders' views of the health workforce in an era of health reform. *Nursing Outlook, 58*(4), 175–180.

Florida Center for Nursing. (2010). *Workforce demand in nursing-intensive healthcare settings: 2009 vacancies and 2011 growth projections.* Retrieved September 17, 2010, from http://www.flcenterfornursing.org/files/2010_Demand_Report.pdf

Flynn, L. (2009). Workload, quality of care, and job satisfaction in home health nurses. In G. L. Dickson & L. Flynn (Eds.), *Nursing policy research: Turning evidence-based research into health policy* (pp. 143–154). New York, NY: Springer Publishing.

Foxall, M., Megel, M. E., Grigsby, K., & Billings, J. S. (2009). Faculty retirement: Stemming the tide. *The Journal of Nursing Education, 48*(3), 172–175.

Ganong, L. H. (1987). Integrative reviews of nursing research. *Research in Nursing & Health, 10*(1), 1–11.

Green, A., Fowler, C., Sportsman, S., Cottenoir, M., Light, K., & Schumann, R. (2006). Innovation in nursing education: A statewide grant initiative. *Policy, Politics & Nursing Practice, 7*(1), 45–53.

Green, A., Wieck, K. L., Willmann, J., Fowler, C., Douglas, W., & Jordan, C. (2004). Addressing the Texas nursing shortage: A legislative approach to bolstering the nursing education pipeline. *Policy, Politics & Nursing Practice, 5*(1), 41–48.

Hope, H. A. (2004). Working Conditions of the Nursing Workforce excerpts from a policy roundtable at AcademyHealth's 2003 Annual Research Meeting. *Health Services Research, 39*(3), 445–462.

Kaeding, T. H., & Rambur, B. (2004). Recruiting knowledge, not just nurses. *Journal of Professional Nursing: Official Journal of the American Association of Colleges of Nursing, 20*(2), 137–138.

Kalb, K. B., Cherry, N. M., Kauzloric, J., Brender, A., Green, K., Miyagawa, L., & Shinoda-Mettler, A. (2006). A competency-based approach to public health nursing performance appraisal. *Public Health Nursing (Boston, Mass.), 23*(2), 115–138.

Kemper, P., Brannon, D., Barry, T., Stott, A., & Heier, B. (2008). Implementation of the Better Jobs Better Care demonstration: Lessons for long-term care workforce initiatives. *The Gerontologist, 48 Spec No 1*, 26–35.

Kirschling, J. M., Harvey-McPherson, L., & Curley, D. (2008). Maine's nursing workforce legislation: Lessons from a rural state. *Nursing Outlook, 56*(2), 63–69.e2.

Kishi, A., & Green, A. (2008). A statewide strategy for nursing workforce development through partnerships in Texas. *Policy, Politics & Nursing Practice, 9*(3), 210–214.

Kotzer, A. M., & Arellana, K. (2008). Defining an evidence-based work environment for nursing in the USA. *Journal of Clinical Nursing, 17*(12), 1652–1659.

Lin, V. W., Juraschek, S. P., Xu, L., Jones, D., & Turek, J. (2008). California regional registered nurse workforce forecast. *Nursing Economics*, 26(2), 85–105, 121.

Longest, B. B. (2009). *Health policymaking in the United States* (5th ed.). Chicago, IL: Health Administration Press.

Loquist, R. S. (2002). State boards of nursing respond to the nurse shortage. *Nursing Administration Quarterly*, 26(4), 33–39.

Lundeen, S. P., Kaufmann, M., & Krause, C. (2007). *Educating the nursing workforce: The nurse faculty shortage in Wisconsin*. Retrieved September 19, 2010, from http://www.mstc.edu/nursing/pdf/EducatorReportSummary.pdf

Mason, D. J., Leavitt, J. K., & Chaffee, M. W. (2007). Policy & politics: A framework for action. In D. J. Mason, J. K. Leavitt, & M. W. Chaffee (Eds.), *Policy and politics in nursing and health care* (5th ed., pp. 1–16). St. Louis, MO: Saunders, Elsevier.

McHaney, D. F., & Varner, J. (2006). Accommodating the needs of the aging registered nurse workforce. *The Alabama Nurse*, 33(3), 24–25.

McKay, M. L., & Hewlett, P. O. (2009). Grassroots coalition building: Lessons from the field. *Journal of Professional Nursing: Official Journal of the American Association of Colleges of Nursing*, 25(6), 352–357.

North Carolina Institute of Medicine. (2004). *Task force on the North Carolina nursing workforce report*. Retrieved March 19, 2011, from http://www.nciom.org/publications/?task-force-on-the-north-carolina-nursing-workforce-report-7936

North Carolina Institute of Medicine. (2007). *Task force on the North Carolina nursing workforce report*. Retrieved September 17, 2010, from http://www.nciom.org/docs/nursing_workforce_update.pdf

Michigan Center for Nursing. (2009). *A profile of Michigan's nursing workforce 2009*. Retrieved September 18, 2010, from http://www.michigancenterfornursing.org/mimages/mi_nurse_profile09.pdf

Milstead, J. A. (2004). *Health policy and politics: A nurse's guide*. Sudbury, MA: Jones & Bartlett.

Palumbo, M. V., McIntosh, B., Rambur, B., & Naud, S. (2009). Retaining an aging nurse workforce: Perceptions of human resource practices. *Nursing Economics*, 27(4), 221–7, 232.

Palumbo, M. V. (2009). State funding for nurse faculty loan repayment: The Vermont experience. In G. L. Dickson & L. Flynn (Eds.), *Nursing policy research: Turning evidence-based research into health policy* (pp. 329–342). New York, NY: Springer Publishing.

Parkman, C. A. (1997). Health Care Workforce Regulation reform. *Nursing Management*, 28(9), 34–38.

Pennsylvania Department of Health Professions Study Group. (2004). *State health improvement plan: White paper the nurse workforce in Pennsylvania*. Retrieved September 17, 2010, from http://www.dsf.health.state.pa.us/health/lib/health/ship/nursewhitepaper.pdf

Quinn, B. C. (2008). The need for research and evaluation of state health reforms. *Health Services Research*, 43(1 Pt. 2), 341–343.

Roth, J. W. (2008). The North Carolina evidence-based transition-to-practice initiative. *Policy, Politics & Nursing Practice*, 9(3), 215–219.

Rudel, R., & Moulton, P. (2009). Nursing's long-term pipeline: A study of high school students using a unique data collection approach. In G. L. Dickson & Linda Flynn (Eds.), *Nursing policy research: Turning evidence-based research into health policy* (pp. 187–208). New York, NY: Springer Publishing.

Seago, J. A., Spetz, J., Coffman, J., Rosenoff, E., & O'Neil, E. (2003). Minimum staffing ratios: The California workforce initiative survey. *Nursing Economics*, 21(2), 65–70.

Shi, L., & Singh, D. A. (2008). *Delivering health care in America: A systems approach* (4th ed.). Sudbury, MA: Jones & Bartlett.

Simon, M., & Hoffman, L. (2004). *The next generation of workforce development project: A six-state policy academy to enhance connections between workforce and economic development policy.* Retrieved September 17, 2010, from http://www.nga.org/Files/pdf/0412DOLSIMON.PDF

Sparbel, K. J., & Anderson, M. A. (2000a). Integrated literature review of continuity of care: Part 1, conceptual issues. *Journal of Nursing Scholarship: An Official Publication of Sigma Theta Tau International Honor Society of Nursing / Sigma Theta Tau, 32*(1), 17–24.

Sparbel, K. J., & Anderson, M. A. (2000b). A continuity of care integrated literature review, part 2: Methodological issues. *Journal of Nursing Scholarship, 32*(2), 131–135.

Spetz, J. (2009). *Forecasts of the registered nurse workforce in California: Conducted for the California Board of Registered Nursing.* Retrieved September 18, 2010, from http://www.rn.ca.gov/pdfs/forms/forecasts2007.pdf

Sroczynski, M. (2003). *The nursing faculty shortage: A public health crisis.* Retrieved September 17, 2010, from http://www.nursema.org/downloads/faculty_crisis.pdf

State of Illinois Department of Finacial & Professional Regulation. (2007). *The 2007 Illinois nursing workforce survey report.* Retrieved September 18, 2010, from http://www.idfpr.com/nursing/PDF/2007NursingWorkforceSurveyFinal.pdf

Tanner, C. A., Gubrud-Howe, P., & Shores, L. (2008). The Oregon Consortium for Nursing Education: A response to the nursing shortage. *Policy, Politics & Nursing Practice, 9*(3), 203–209.

Tate, E. T., & Moody, K. (2005). The public good: Regulation of nursing students. *JONA'S Healthcare Law, Ethics and Regulation, 7*(2), 47–53; quiz 54.

Texas Center for Nursing Workforce Studies. (2006a). *The supply of and demand for registered nurses and nurse graduates in Texas.* Austin, Texas. Retrieved from http://www.dshs.state.tx.us/chs/cnws/SB132PP.ppt

Texas Center for Nursing Workforce Studies. (2006b). *Comprehensive strategic action plan to increase supply of registered nurses and nurse graduates to meet healthcare demands in Texas.* Austin, Texas. Retrieved September 17, 2010, from http://www.dshs.state.tx.us/chs/cnws/CSPlan06.pdf

Texas Center for Nursing Workforce Studies. (2008a). *2008 Long term care nurse staffing study.* Austin, Texas. Retrieved from http://www.dshs.state.tx.us/chs/cnws/Npublica.shtm

Texas Center for Nursing Workforce Studies. (2008b). *2008 Texas hospital nurse staffing survey.* Retrieved from http://www.dshs.state.tx.us/chs/cnws/Npublica.shtm

Texas Center for Nursing Workforce Studies. (2010). Comprehensive strategic plan for retention of nurses in the workforce. In Texas Statewide Health Coordinating Council (Ed.), *2011–2016 Texas state health plan: A roadmap to a healthy Texas* (pp. 189–192). Austin, Texas: Texas Department of State Health Services.

Texas Nurses Association. (2006). Policy recommendations for the nursing workforce head to legislature—A long-term investment is called for. *Texas Nursing, 80*(8), 6–7.

Texas Team Addressing Nursing Education Capacity. (2008, updated 2010). *A strategic plan for the state of Texas to meet nursing workforce needs* Austin, Texas: Retrieved from http://www.dshs.state.tx.us/chs/cnws/

University System of Georgia Board of Regents. (2009). *The Registered Nurse Workforce Shortage in Georgia.* Retrieved September 17, 2010, from http://www.usg.edu/health_workforce_center/documents/Shortage_of_RNs_2009_Policy_Brief.pdf

Wisconsin Nurse Faculty Task Force. (2007). *Wisconsin nurse faculty shortage task force report and recommendations.* Retrieved September 17, 2010, from http://www.mstc.edu/nursing/pdf/EducatorReportSummary.pdf

CHAPTER 5

An Integrative Review of Global Nursing Workforce Issues

Barbara L. Nichols, Catherine R. Davis, and Donna R. Richardson

ABSTRACT

Migration has been a way of life since the beginning of time, with migrants seeking other lands for personal and professional betterment. Today, in an era of globalization, trade agreements and technological advances, an increase in migration is inevitable. All professions have been affected, but the migration of health professionals, particularly nurses, has been the most dramatic. However, the migration of nurses across national and international borders comes with many challenges: systematic tracking of migration flows, harmonization of standards, recognition of professional credentials, fair and equitable distribution of the global health care workforce, and the effect of migration on the health care infrastructure of both source and destination countries. The international migration of nurses to address shortages in developed countries has, in some instances, left source countries with insufficient resources to address their own health care needs. The increasing complexity of health care delivery, aging of the population and the nursing workforce, and the escalating global demand for nurses create on-going challenges for policy makers. Strategically addressing global nursing workforce issues is paramount to sustaining the health of nations.

© 2011 Springer Publishing Company
DOI: 10.1891/0739-6686.28.113

Legend suggests that migration has been a social phenomenon since antiquity. Mythical men, such as Prometheus and Daedalus, were compelled to migrate because of disagreements with Zeus. It is also well known that Plato recruited talented individuals from ancient Athens and that the Ptolemies enticed scholars and scientists from Greece to Alexandria. In short, migration has been a fact of life from time immemorial (Mejia, Pizurki, & Royston, 1979).

In more recent times, people left their homes because of famine, rising taxes, and job shortages—often seeking personal freedom and relief from political and religious persecution as well. As we begin the second decade of the 21st century, migration is different in several ways. The chief difference is that migration is no longer cyclical, nor a mass movement of the poor, the wretched and the homeless, as the sonnet on the Statue of Liberty tablets suggests, but an on-going movement primarily of women and professionals migrating around the world to work (Kingma, 2006).

Modern patterns of migration also involve a considerable amount of temporary, return or circular migration, which includes elements of dual or multiple nationalities. Growing migration figures emphasize the fact that migration flows have become more complex and are comprised of heterogeneous groups of individuals (United Nations Development Programme, 2009).

This chapter presents an overview of the international nursing labor market. It highlights key trends in nurse migration, the workforce issues that arise as a result of migration, and the research and policy implications that flow from the interaction between migration and the nursing workforce. It suggests policy options that stress the need for international cooperation to address the issues. The chapter identifies major obstacles in discussing the international nursing labor market due to fragmented, inconsistent, and incomplete data; lack of standardized data elements and comparable databases; difficulty in comparing nursing roles in qualitatively-varying health care systems; and international differences in the use of the term nurse. For example, the International Council of Nurses (ICN) notes that there is no one, single definition of "nurse" or "nursing" throughout the world—different definitions are provided by different sources. Such disparity leads to varied interpretations of the scope of practice of nurses, which has an impact on effectiveness, efficiency, cost and quality of service.

The chapter draws from published data from the World Health Organization (WHO), ICN, the World Bank, the Organization for Economic Cooperation and Development (OECD), the International Labor Organization (ILO), the Institute on Migration, the Rockefeller Joint Learning Initiative, published literature in the field, CGFNS International research, and documents from CGFNS files. Research on nurse migration at the macro and micro levels has increased in the last decade, with researchers focusing on migration numbers and patterns, ethical recruitment, workforce composition, transition to practice, positive practice environments, and workplace challenges. Organizations such as WHO, OECD, ILO, ICN, and the World Bank have provided in-depth examination of the characteristics of nurse migration and its effect on the health care infrastructure in both supply and receiving countries. In-country researchers have focused on such topics as the effect of brain drain, the distribution of health care personnel, and the factors that promote migration and help to determine the destination country of choice.

However, the body of research that addresses the experience of the migrating nurse remains relatively small and somewhat fragmented. Anecdotal reports are common. Organizations such as ICN, CGFNS, AcademyHealth, and individual researchers have looked at not only domestic workforces and their augmentation with international nurses, but also the ethical recruitment of those nurses—as well as such transition to practice issues as communication, safety, and preparation for practice in a receiving country. Little research has been conducted on the experience of migration from the point of view of the international nurse or on the challenges faced by receiving staff that host international nurses.

MIGRATION AND THE GLOBAL HEALTH WORKFORCE
Global Context

International migration has always existed. However, the past decade has witnessed rapid increases in the migration of health personnel, fueled by shortages of skilled labor in developed countries and international trade agreements (OECD, 2008). Global estimates of international migrants place their numbers at approximately 214 million international migrants, 740 million internal migrants, and an unknown number of migrants in situations all over the world. These figures comprise a wide range of migrating populations, including such workers as refugees, students, documented and undocumented migrants, and health professionals (United Nations Development Program, 2009).

The WHO (2006a) states that, "The world is experiencing a serious human resource shortage in the health sector," which it calls, "a crisis in health." WHO (2006b) estimates that 4.3 million more health workers[1] are required to meet the Millennium Development Goals (MDGs),[2] which were adopted in 2000 and are due to be completed in 2015.

---

[1] WHO defines health workers to be all people engaged in action whose primary intent is to enhance health, such as doctors, nurses, midwives, and others.

[2] The MDGs include goals and targets on poverty, hunger, maternal and child mortality, disease, inadequate shelter, gender inequality, environmental degradation, and the Global Partnership for Development.

The human resource crisis described by WHO affects developed and developing countries, but globally affects developing countries disproportionately—not only because they have much smaller workforces but also because their needs are so much greater. These shortages are projected to increase over the next 20 years unless there is better international cooperation to improve recruitment, retention, integration, productivity and skill and staffing mix among systems, organizations and countries (OECD, 2008).

Major Obstacles to Creating International Labor Policy

The employment of people across national and international borders suggests that international labor policies should be enacted to ensure both sufficient workforce capacity and the effective and equitable distribution of the health workforce. However, the measurement of supply and demand has been challenging. For example, there are various methods used worldwide to calculate the number of nurses in the workforce. Some countries identify only employed nurses, while others report on all nurses who are eligible to practice. Some countries report head count, while others report full-time equivalence. Thus, reporting on nursing workforce data is not standardized across countries.

Many countries do not have detailed, sophisticated databases on their workforces, a limitation that impedes the measurement of nursing supply and demand across states, provinces, countries and nations—as well as specialty areas and provider types. Diversity among local jurisdictions, inconsistent use of terms, varying technologies, and lack of standardization often make it difficult to construct an accurate national database. Data collected in individual states in the United States, for example, have limited compatibility and comparability in the countries within the United Kingdom and the European Union (EU). Because data at the national level vary in detail and sophistication, information on the international labor market tends to be general and anecdotal rather than profession specific.

To address such variations, the ILO (2010a) has established 20 key indicators of the labor market, and encourages countries to use them as a basis for collecting and storing data in order to facilitate international comparisons. Currently, researchers are discussing definitions, and selecting indicators to guide collection of common data elements to be included in an international health service database.

The health workforce shortage limits governments' capability to provide adequate health care and promote better working conditions for all workers. Calculations based on the ILO Global Staff-Related Assess Deficit Indicator reveal that one-third of the global population has no access to health care due to gaps in the health workforce (ILO, 2010a).

Against this backdrop, international agencies, such as WHO, the World Bank and OECD, have focused on the growing challenge of ensuring that there is sufficient workforce capacity to enable health systems to function effectively. The growing concern about shortages of health personnel, in general, is magnified when one focuses on the registered nurse (RN) workforce in particular. For many countries, the on-going and most problematic challenge is the shortage of professional nurses (OECD, 2010). Nurses are the main professional component in most health systems, and their contributions are recognized as essential, not only to meeting the MDGs, but also to delivering safe and effective care.

Trends in Nurse Migration

In general, migration flow tends to be from rural to urban areas, from lower to higher income urban neighborhoods, and from developing to developed and industrialized countries. Migration is no longer a North American and Western European phenomenon, but now includes Asia, Africa, and the Caribbean (OECD, 2008). Generally, source countries (those that provide international nurses) include the Philippines, which prepares nurses for export, India, Korea, China, the Caribbean, and sub-Saharan Africa. Countries that are primarily destination or receiving countries include the United States, Canada, the United Kingdom, and Saudi Arabia. Migration within a given geographical area is often determined by economic factors. For example, the single, most pervasive cause of migration in sub-Saharan Africa and the English-speaking Caribbean is economic security—better salaries and wage differentials (Ojo, 1990; Vujicic, Ohiri, & Sparkes, 2009).

Causes and Consequences of Nurse Migration

There is widespread consensus that nurses migrate in search of incentives that usually fall within three categories: (1) improved learning and practice opportunities; (2) better quality of life, pay, and/or working conditions; and (3) personal safety (Davis & Richardson, 2009a; Kingma, 2006; OECD, 2008). For example, a recent Pan American Health Organization (PAHO) study of 200 nurses from Guyana found that between 1997 and 2010, nurses were motivated to leave the country not only for better pay but also for professional development, better quality of life and better working conditions. The top reasons given for migration included work environment, professional recognition, conditions of work that related to workloads and the degree of stress nurses work under, poor equipment and supplies, and the lack of orientation and in-service education (Alleyne, 2010).

CGFNS research supports these findings. In a 2007 CGFNS survey of its VisaScreen[3] applicants, nurses who had migrated to the United States indicated that poor wages (55.4%) and limited job prospects (23%) were the primary factors that prompted migration. Better wages (33.5%), a better way of life (26.8%), greater job opportunities (19.9%) and family in the United States (11.4%) were cited as the reasons for entering the country (Davis & Richardson, 2009a).

The 2010 OECD Policy Brief on recent migration trends discusses nurse migration and identifies main causes and consequences for destination and source countries. The Brief indicates that nurse migration to many countries has increased since 2000, although the United Kingdom and Ireland were exceptions, showing decreases of 4% and 2.7%, respectively (OECD, 2010). Permanent migration of foreign educated nurses to Australia increased six-fold since 2000 and tripled in Canada (OECD, 2010).

The 2008 National Sample Survey of Registered Nurses (Health Resources and Services Administration, 2010) estimated that foreign educated nurses comprised 5.6% of the U.S. registered nurse population in 2008, an increase from 3.4% in 2004. Just under half (48.7%) of those nurses were educated in the Philippines, 11.5% in Canada, and 0.3% in India.

Due to immigration retrogression[4] in the United States the number of foreign educated nurses has decreased significantly in the last 2 years, following large increases between 2001 and 2007 (Richardson & Davis, 2009). Retrogression has affected not only the supply of nurses in the United States but also in a number of source countries throughout the world. For example, the Philippines, which prepares nurses for export, has traditionally been the largest supplier of nurses to the United States. The inability to obtain a visa to practice in the United States because of retrogression, coupled with the recent proliferation of nursing schools, the large number of nursing graduates in the Philippines, and embargoes on migration to the United Kingdom and Ireland has led to estimates of over 400,000 Philippine nurses not being able to find employment in nursing in that country (Philippine Star, 2008).

In Ireland, Irish nursing graduates also are looking abroad for employment as the embargo on recruitment introduced by the Health Service Executive in September 2007 enters its third year. Annette Kennedy, Director of Professional

---

[3] VisaScreen is the CGFNS program that meets U.S. immigration law, which requires that foreign-educated nurses seeking U.S. employment must have their credentials evaluated in terms of comparability of education, English language proficiency, and licensure validity.

[4] Retrogression is the U.S. State Department term for the procedural delay in issuing an immigrant visa when there are more people applying for immigrant visas in a given year than the total number of visas available.

Development for the Irish Nurses Association, predicted that 90% of the 1,600 nurses who graduated in 2009 will emigrate due to better job prospects and conditions of employment available overseas. Concerns about the long term impact of the embargo, pension security, and continuation of employment contracts have resulted in retirements and the departure of overseas nurses recruited to Ireland between 2000 and 2006 (Fegan, 2009).

A recent report in the *Toronto Sun* warns that Canada is in danger of losing large numbers of nurses to other countries, particularly the United States, as provincial governments freeze or cut nursing jobs in response to budget pressures. Health experts caution that Canada could face a repeat of the 1990s when health care cuts by the provinces drove as many as 27,000 nurses to the United States to look for work (Spencer, 2010).

Japan, under the Economic Partnership Agreement (EPA), has accepted candidate nurses from Indonesia and the Philippines since 2008. However, the number of candidates from Indonesia in 2010 has decreased to one-third of the 2009 levels, with 58 nurse candidates and 83 care worker candidates accepted. This reduction is due to the deterioration of the domestic employment situation in Japan, which has increased the availability of Japanese employees, as well as to the large financial burden (e.g., cost of recruitment, orientation, language classes, and financial incentives) borne by health care institutions accepting foreign candidates (Japanese Nurses Association, 2009).

The ability to communicate effectively in health care settings across borders is critical to safe practice and highly valued by receiving countries and institutions (Davis & Richardson, 2009b). In a survey of U.S. nurse executives, Davis and Kritek (2005) found that English language proficiency was the single most important skill that foreign nurse graduates needed to practice safely in the United States. Many commercial and hospital recruiters now include English language classes in their preparation of nurses for U.S. employment.

Language has proven a significant barrier to foreign candidates seeking to pass the Japanese Nursing Licensure examination within the specified 3-year period. Language training is the responsibility of each health care institution in Japan, after employees enter the workforce; however, health care institutions and support groups have requested that the government improve support for candidates studying Japanese. As a result, the Japanese government is to provide more support for language training, including study fees charged by Japanese language schools. The Ministry of Health, Labor and Welfare regards accepting foreign nurses and care workers under the EPA as a special measure and does not believe it influences the domestic labor market (Japanese Nurses Association, 2009).

Circular Migration

Circular or return migration is a term used to describe the process through which nurses temporarily work abroad and then return to their country of origin, usually after a specified period of time. Such migration is often a matter of public policy to ensure a continuous feed of nurses to provide care in a host country. In some countries (e.g., India and China), it is used as an educational development model in that the nurse returns with international experience, which is then shared with colleagues at home to enhance the quality of both health care and nursing education (Nichols, Davis, & Richardson, 2010).

It has been argued that circular migration does not produce the same degree of loss to a country's skilled labor force as permanent migration. However, Hawkes, Kolenko, Shockness, and Diwaker (2009) indicate that the collective labor time spent outside of the country suggests that temporary migration may have a profound and underestimated impact on a nursing workforce. As an example, their study of 99 nurses at a private hospital in Kerala, India, found that 20% of the nursing workforce had temporarily worked outside of India, in such countries as Oman, Saudi Arabia, and Singapore, for a median of 6 years (range 2–15 years) before returning to India. This accounted for approximately 19% of their total work experience.

Effect on Patient Outcomes

In short, a worldwide demand for nurses that exceeds supply, chronic maldistribution of health care personnel, and movement of nurses across national and international boundaries, characterize the global nurse workforce. Various studies have documented the important link between nurse staffing levels, service delivery and health outcomes, suggesting that important issues exist with respect to how the nursing workforce is managed (Aiken & Cheung, 2008; Buchan, Baldwin, & Munro, 2008).

Increasingly, research has identified and quantified the essential role for nurses in maintaining health outcomes, particularly in acute care. The systematic review of international research, produced since 1990, involving acute care hospitals and adjusting for case mix, strongly suggests that the higher nurse staffing is associated with improved patient outcomes (Lankshear, Sheldon, & Maynard, 2005). Aiken et al. (2001) found that after adjusting for patient and hospital characteristics (size, teaching status, and technology), each reduction of nurse per patient ratio was associated with an increase in the likelihood of dying within 30 days of admission and in the odds of failure-to-rescue. In a multi-country study, European findings were very similar to the U.S. results (Stromberg et al., 2003). Other studies (Aiken, Clarke, Sloane, Sochalski, & Silber, 2002; Needleman, Buerhaus, Mattke, Stewart, & Zelevinsky, 2002) also have shown how failing to comply with the minimum staffing ratio for nurses in several hospitals was associated with significantly higher mortality and morbidity rates.

In conclusion, there is strong evidence that adequate staffing levels influence health outcomes. The migration of nurses augments staffing levels during periods of shortage, especially in developed countries such as the United States, Canada, and the United Kingdom. However, the recruitment and migration of nurses from developing countries, such as sub-Saharan Africa, can deplete a country's workforce and thus have major implications for the quality of care delivered (Munjanja, Kibuka, & Dovlo, 2005).

THE INTERNATIONAL NURSING LABOR MARKET

Long-Term Trends

Three long-term trends influence the international nursing labor market: demographic and epidemiological changes; complex technological changes; and globalization. Demographic changes, characterized by aging populations and increased prevalence of non-communicable diseases, shape the type and level of care and the number and type of nurses needed. Technological changes affect how and where nurses care for patients. Globalization influences nurses' mobility.

Demographic Changes

The current shortage of nurses is complicated by demographic characteristics. Population growth in many of the developed countries in North America and Northern Europe has slowed, ceased or even reversed (Buerhaus, Starger, & Auerbach, 2009; International Council of Nurses, 2008b). Populations in these countries are aging, have low birth rates, and are experiencing increased life expectancy. For example, in 2008 Europe was home to slightly more than 13% of the world population, decreased from 25% a century ago (United Nations, 2008). In the United States and Canada, persons 65 years and older represent 12.9% of the U.S. population—approximately 1 in 8 individuals—a figure that is expected to increase to 19% by 2030 (Administration on Aging, 2010). This same pattern holds true for Canada, where 14% of the population is 65 years of age and older and only 17% is 15 years of age or younger. Overall, the share of the population living in developed countries is projected to decrease from 18% in 2008 to less than 14% by 2050 (Population Reference Bureau, 2010).

In contrast, in much of the developing world, population growth and younger populations are the norm (ILO, 2010a; OECD, 2008). Africa's population, currently growing faster than any other region, is expected to make up 21% of the world population in 2050. Today, the share of the population 15 years of age and younger is 41% in the least developed countries compared to 17% in the more developed countries (Population Reference Bureau, 2010).

The nature of nursing services needed depends on the profile of the population to be served. Accordingly, the most rapid growth area for nursing care in developed countries will be in services for the elderly, for those with chronic physical and mental health conditions, and in primary care. Consequently, there is general consensus that more nursing services are required in community and long term care settings. For example, because of the shift of mental health care to the community, psychiatric mental health nurses in countries such as the United Kingdom have been required to expand their services beyond mental health institutions (Clinton, du Boulay, Hazelton, & Horner, 2001; OECD, 2008).

The age of the nursing workforce varies internationally. For example, Canada, like the United States, is experiencing an aging of its nursing workforce. It is estimated that in 2008, RNs between the ages of 50 and 54 made up 17% of the workforce in Canada, compared to 11% in 1994 (Canadian Institute for Health Information, 2010). That same pattern is seen in the United States, with 16.2% of RNs in the 50–54 age range (Health Resources and Services Administration, 2010).

In the United States, the average age of the RN population has been rising steadily over the past two decades. The average of all licensed nurses increased to 47.0 years in 2008, with the average age of the working nurse being 45.5 years (Health Resources and Services Administration, 2010). In Iceland one-quarter of the nurses are between 55 and the retirement age of 64 (Frindinnskottir & Johnsson, 2009). By contrast, the average age of the working nurse in India is 35 years (DiMarzio, 2010). The aging nursing workforces in developed countries such as the United States, Canada, and the United Kingdom, may be invigorated by integrating younger, migrant nurses. Their presence is fundamental to preparing the next cohort of clinical mentors, supervisors and managers (Kingma, 2006).

The lengths of nurses' professional careers also vary among countries. The average nursing career is 25–40 years in Asia, except in Japan and Korea, where the average career length is 14.8 and 10 years, respectively (International Council of Nurses, 2008b). In the United States, United Kingdom, and Australia, nurses' professional careers are shorter because of a higher proportion of mature nursing graduates, who spend less time in the workforce, and because of early retirement, particularly in the United States (Buerhaus et al., 2009; International Council of Nurses, 2008a). In Germany, the workforce is relatively young because few nurses remain in it for more than 3–4 years after graduation (Irwin, 2001).

Technological Changes

Growing use of technology in health care demonstrates that it can help nurses make better decisions at the point of care. It also can promote an organization's core business of care delivery and provide data about patient outcomes. Effective technology improves quality by improving patient care safety factors and by eliminating redundant work (American Nurse Today, 2010).

Technology does not replace nurses but can be used to enhance the nursing workforce by ensuring new ways of performing work to improve efficiency and reduce errors. For example, personal digital assistants (PDAs) are handheld instruments that provide a wealth of worldwide data that can be accessed by nurses at the point of care (Wilcox & La Tella, 2001). However, there is little research to demonstrate either their use by nurses or their effect on nursing care and patient outcomes. Garritty and El Emam (2006) conducted a systematic review of studies related to handheld devices in health care settings and found an increasing use of PDAs by health care professionals, primarily younger physicians, since 1999. Stroud, Erkel, and Smith (2005) surveyed 227 nurse practitioner students and faculty about their patterns of use and found that 67% used PDAs—primarily to support clinical decision making.

Globalization

Globalization, the international movement of technology, ideas, products, labor markets and professional education and standards, envisions a borderless world. International trade agreements facilitate the movement of goods and services—including nursing services—across national boundaries, and provide for the free movement of labor between and within countries. Globalization has led to a greater interdependency among nations and the increased mobility of labor among world regions.

The impact of trade agreements is far-reaching. The North American Free Trade Agreement (NAFTA) includes Canada, the United States, and Mexico; the EU is comprised of 27 member countries; and the Asia-Pacific Economic Cooperation (APEC) is comprised of 21 countries. These agreements create regional labor markets and have considerable influence on the movement of workers, including nurses. Many developed countries with similar nursing education and a common language recruit nurses from one another, including the United States, the United Kingdom, Canada, and Australia.

Although trade agreements encourage the movement of professional workers across borders, "barriers" often are formed by the various educational and regulatory requirements within individual countries. For example, NAFTA enables Canadian RNs to work in the United States. However, U.S. licensure standards, procedures and criteria, which vary from state to state, must be met before the

Canadian nurse can practice in a specific state. The same holds true for U.S. educated nurses seeking to practice under Trade NAFTA in any of the Canadian provinces (Richardson & Davis, 2009).

In Europe, all EU citizens have free mobility within participating countries, and all EU countries recognize regulated professionals from member states. However, individual countries may require additional assessments in an effort to bridge national differences in laws and language. For example, EU nurses may be required to demonstrate English language proficiency and to participate in adaptation programs prior to employment in the United Kingdom. Although there are various initiatives to upgrade nursing education, countries vary in their compliance with the European Commission directives (Zalalequi, Marquez, Nunin, & Mariscae, 2006).

The WHO also has identified challenges confronting nursing and midwifery services resulting from trade agreements under the World Trade Organization. WHO anticipates that the increased mobility of nurses and midwives will create shortages in less affluent geographical areas. Compounding this issue is the difficulty, if not impossibility, of tracking migration because of incomplete and incompatible data obtained from various in-country sources, which leads to an inaccurate representation of migration into or out of the country (Adams & Al-Gasseer, 2001). To address these issues, the 63rd World Health Assembly passed The Code of Practice on International Recruitment of Health Personnel. This Code contains a requirement for the collection of data regarding migrating health professionals. WHO and OECD have formed a Technical Workgroup of country representatives throughout the world to discuss the establishment of a minimum data set to allow for monitoring and reporting on health worker migration. The first meeting of the Technical Workgroup was held in June 2010. On-going meetings will occur to identify data collection approaches and minimum data sets.

It should be noted that the Bologna process,[5] which directly concerns Europe and its immediate neighbors and focuses on students, and EU Directive 36,[6] which focuses on professionals, both address standards of education and professional qualifications. To that end, both processes have generated global attention because of harmonization of nursing standards and the consolidation and recognition of

---

[5] The Bologna Process creates the European Higher Education Area by making academic degree and quality assurance standards more comparable and compatible throughout Europe. The Bologna Process currently has 46 participating countries committed to "Harmonizing the Architecture of the European Higher Education System." It is named after the place it was proposed, the University of Bologna, Bologna, Italy.

[6] EU Directive 36 regulates the recognition of professional qualifications for most regulated professions within the European Union.

professional qualifications across member countries. These two processes, when fully implemented, will enable cross-border harmonization and transferability of professional credentials, facilitate mobility across borders, and simplify the recognition process for nurses migrating within the EU (European Federation of Nurses Associations, 2010; Zalalequi et al., 2006).

Cyclical Changes

In addition to long-term trends, cyclical changes influence the international nursing labor market. These include reduction in demand, reduction in supply, and workplace instability. While the demand for nurses has been growing, the trend toward a large nursing workforce to meet that demand has not been continuous. Shortages, which result when a supply of nurses fails to keep pace with the demand, lead to increased recruitment and retention, usually followed by abatement in the shortage. Today, in developed countries such as the United States and Canada, aging of the population, including the nursing workforce, a faculty shortage, increase in career options open to women, and the anticipated retirement of the baby boomer generation (those born between 1946 and 1965) are expected to create significant shortages for years to come.

Chronic shortages and inequitable distribution of health workers has been a challenge worldwide for many years. Longer life expectancies, particularly in developed countries, suggest that the demand for health workers will continue to increase as shortages persist.

Reduction in Demand

After expanding in the 1970s and 1980s, the nursing workforce contracted in the 1990s when health care systems encountered an increase in demand for health services at the same time that cutbacks required them to contain costs (Buchan & Calman, 2004). Frequently restructuring and down-sizing the workforce meant increased emphasis on private enterprise, change in payment systems, shorter hospital stays, higher proportion of seriously ill, acute care patients, expansion of community-based services, including homecare, and greater emphasis on cost control (Cutshall, 2000).

Today, the demand for international nurses has decreased in several countries compared to the early 2000s. There is a reported surplus of nurses in many Asian countries due to either a decreased demand for, or a decreased reliance on, international nurses by a number of destination countries of choice, namely the United Kingdom, Canada, and the United States. For example, in Taiwan 44% of licensed nurses were not employed in nursing. It has been reported to CGFNS that over 400,000 RNs are unable to find jobs in the Philippines (Philippine Star, 2008). Without clinical experience, Philippine nurses are not eligible to leave the country to work abroad.

However, many agree that although there is currently not a shortage in the United States because of the downturn in the economy, the situation is only temporary. Shortage projections for the future are uniformly high. The Bureau of Labor Statistics (BLS, 2009) projects that more than 581,500 new RN positions will be created through 2018, which would increase the size of the RN workforce by 22%. Employment of RNs in the United States is expected to grow much faster than average, when compared to all other professions. Projections by Buerhaus et al. (2009) also indicate the beginning of a shortfall of nurses in 2018, which is expected to grow to a high of 260,000 nurses by 2025. A shortage of this magnitude would be twice as large as any nursing shortage experienced in the United States since the mid-sixties (American Association of Colleges of Nursing, 2010).

Reduction in Supply
Reduction in supply generally is related to such factors as historic fluctuations in nursing program enrollments, low recruitment into nursing programs, which exists worldwide, and embargos on international recruitment efforts introduced by governments. There are many factors that create decreased enrollment and recruitment to schools of nursing. For example, in many countries nursing school programs are publicly funded, and thus, compete for budgeted funds with other program areas. Thus, the decisions to reduce nursing student positions and/or the number of nursing schools relates to budget practices. In the United States, faculty shortages have led schools to decrease admissions to nursing programs.

Several destination countries of choice for migrating nurses, namely the United Kingdom and the United States, have made changes to immigration requirements and/or processes, thus affecting the migration of international nurses. As a consequence of budget constraints and increased nursing school graduation rates, the United Kingdom tightened immigration requirements for overseas nurses, thus limiting the number of nurses entering the country for employment. The United States instituted immigration retrogression for all countries in 2006 as a means of remedying backlogs in immigration processing, thus significantly decreasing the number of international nurses obtaining occupational visas.

Workplace Instability
Workload and work intensity impact the quality of the work environment and the deployment of human resources. Nursing's professional role and practice environments have deteriorated. Common issues have been reduced job security, changes in career structure, job location and job content, and a decrease in support services (ILO, 2010a).

In addition to dissatisfaction with the work environment, wages are an important issue. The International Council of Nursing (ICN, 2008a) cited wage discrimination against women as a cause of low salaries for nurses in both developing and developed countries. Given nurses' perception of their quality of work life and their wages, nursing workforce attrition is to be expected. Other reasons for leaving nursing include personal disability and care-giving responsibilities for aging family members. In many countries, nurses often leave the profession before or soon after they qualify. In the United Kingdom, for example, up to one-third of graduates from nursing programs never register as nurses at all (OECD, 2008). This creates job compression and increases market demands.

THE NATURE OF NURSING SHORTAGES

The impact of global nurse migration on developed and developing countries has fueled a worldwide nursing shortage in recent years.

> The issues surrounding nursing shortages and global nurse migration are inextricably linked. Global nurse migration has become a major phenomenon impacting health service delivery in both developed and developing countries. The phenomenon has created a global labor market for health professionals and has fueled international recruitment. International migration and recruitment have become dominant features of the international health policy debate. (Nichols, 2007)

The February 2010 OECD Policy Brief maintains that the recent economic crisis is unlikely to "drastically" affect the international migration of health personnel, as employment in the health sector is generally more resilient to cyclical economic downturns than most other sectors. The OECD also noted that the demand for nurses and other health care personnel has not decreased in many countries in the short term (OECD, 2010).

Unlike other sectors, aggregate health services employment levels have continued to increase when compared with the pre-global economic crisis. Compared to the same period in 2008, employment in health services registered an overall increase of 2.3%. Health services employment was strongest in Asia and the Pacific (China and India not included) at 6.2%, gains also continued in Europe and the Americas at 2.3% (ILO, 2010a; Khatiwada, 2009). The OECD does note, however, that in the medium-term, the number of health workers educated and recruited in the future could be affected due to the strain on public finances. However, there is little evidence of such an effect thus far (OECD, 2010).

The economic crisis has hit the health sector during a time of ongoing transformation. Globally, the economic crisis exacerbates chronic shortages and inequitable distribution of health workers and is another factor putting pressure on ministries of health to make tough health service allocations (ILO, 2010b). However, it is difficult to identify the precise nature of supply problems in the international arena. In estimating supply and demand, a simple headcount is insufficient. Factors that must be taken into account are the skill mix of nursing personnel and differences among specialties and health care sectors—including hospitals, home health care, nursing homes, and community care. Aggregate national data do not reveal local or regional differences in labor markets; thus, the problem of servicing isolated areas is particularly severe in countries such as Australia, China, and Africa.

Internationally, strategies to address the nursing shortage have been taken up by governments, employers and nursing associations. Traditionally, in most developed countries that recruit international nurses, more emphasis was placed on recruitment as an immediate answer than on retention. Faced with increasing difficulties in filling nursing vacancies, these countries implemented international recruitment strategies as a short term fix, rather than addressing long term investments in the supply of nurses.

That pattern is beginning to change. In the United States, Johnson and Johnson's Campaign for Nursing's Future addresses the nursing shortage by working with health care leaders and nursing organizations to bring more people into nursing, develop more nurse educators, and retain the talent already in the profession. The pharmaceutical company's partnership with the National League for Nursing supports faculty leadership and mentoring programs.

Canada also is addressing its reliance on international nurse recruitment. The Canadian Nurses Association (CNA) estimates that there will be a shortage of nearly 60,000 full-time equivalents by 2022 if no policy interventions are implemented (Nichols, Davis, & Richardson, 2010). CNA identified short term policy solutions to address the shortage that include increasing RN productivity and reducing absenteeism. Long term solutions focus on reducing RN exit rates, reducing attrition rates in entry level education programs, increasing enrollment in RN programs, and reducing international in-migration. The combined effects of the policy solutions are believed to be sufficient to eliminate the RN shortage in Canada within 15 years (Canadian Nurses Association, 2009).

RESEARCH AND POLICY IMPLICATIONS FOR THE INTERNATIONAL NURSING LABOR MARKET

The increasing complexity of health care delivery systems and the escalating demand for services create on-going challenges for policy makers. *The World Health Report, 2006: Working Together for Health* identified the centrality of human resources for health as fundamental and critical to the functioning of health systems. The challenge of training an adequate number of health workers, and deploying them, requires massive investment and a high level of political leadership and commitment (WHO, 2006a). Thus, scaling up the health workforce is viewed as a priority. The WHO report (2006a) presents several approaches for scaling up the health workforce, such as: significant investment in workforce production, infrastructure improvement, strengthening faculty, introducing new approaches and training methodologies, reducing attrition, and training other categories of health workers.

The global nursing workforce plays a critical role in addressing these challenges. However, over the next decade projections indicate that the shortage of RNs worldwide will deepen (Buerhaus et al., 2009; Health Resources and Services Administration, 2010; Vujicic, Ohiri, & Sparkes, 2009).

One response to the global nursing shortage is to educate large numbers of nurses in relatively short periods of time (WHO, 2006a). Scaling up the health workforce to achieve significant health gains is on the global agenda. However, the nursing shortage must be understood in terms of the broader themes of strengthening the health workforce, better knowledge of the composition and distribution of the workforce, and the regulatory and policy environment in which it exists. For sustainable solutions, policy interventions are required that (1) recognize that the delivery of health care in general, and nursing care in particular, is labor intensive and (2) utilize available nursing resources effectively.

In short, addressing global nursing workforce issues must include strategic examination of factors that create nursing shortages and the policies required to ensure that there are increased levels of retention; that competent health workers are available to poor and rural communities; and that common-element databases on the international workforce are available for supply and demand projections.

In presenting this snapshot of the global nursing workforce, issues and dynamic challenges were highlighted, such as the need for increasing training capacity and improving retention, addressing issues related to the international migration of nurses, and managing the health care delivery infrastructure—including local management of workload, staffing mix, and allocation of resources. Without effective and sustained interventions, global nursing shortages will persist—undermining global health care outcomes and the health of nations.

REFERENCES

Adams, O., & Al-Gasseer, N. (2001). *Strengthening nursing and midwifery: Process and future directions, 1996–2000, summary document.* Geneva, The Netherlands: World Health Organization. Retrieved September 12, 2010, from http://whqlibdoc.who.int/hq/2001/WHO_EIP_OSD_2001.5.pdf

Administration on Aging. (2010). *Aging statistics.* Retrieved October 22, 2010, from http://www.aoa. gov/aoaroot/aging_statistics/index.aspx

Aiken, L., & Cheung, R. (2008). *Nurse workforce challenges in the United States: Implications for policy.* OECD Health Working Paper No. 35. Retrieved September 10, 2010, from http://www.oecd. org/daraoecd/34/9/41431864.pdf

Aiken, L. H., Clarke, S. P., Sloane, D. M., Sochalski, J. A., Busse, R., Clarke, H.,...Shamian, J. (2001). Nurses' reports on hospital care in five countries. *Health Affairs (Project Hope),* 20(3), 43–53.

Aiken, L. H., Clarke, S. P., Sloane, D. M., Sochalski, J., & Silber, J. H. (2002). Hospital nurse staffing and patient mortality, nurse burnout, and job dissatisfaction. *The Journal of the American Medical Association,* 288(16), 1987–1993.

Alleyne, O. (2010). Workshop to devise 'action plan' to limit nurse loss. (March 2, 2010). *Stabroek News, Guyana.* Retrieved September 16, 2010, from http://www.stabroeknews.com/2010/ news/stories/02/03/workshop-to-devise-%E2%80%98action-plan%E2%80%99-to-limit-nurse-loss/

American Association of Colleges of Nursing. (2010). *Nursing shortage.* Retrieved October 26, 2010, from http://www.aacn.nche.edu/media/factsheets/nursingshortage.htm

American Nurse Today. (2010). Nurse leaders discuss the nurse's role in driving technology decisions. *American Nurse Today,* 5(1). January, 2010.

Buchan, J., Baldwin, S., & Munro, M. (2008). *Migration of health workers: The UK perspective.* OECD Health Working Paper No. 38. Retrieved September 15, 2010, from http://www.oecd.org/ dataoecd/48/2/41500789.pdf

Buchan, J., & Calman, L. (2004). *The global shortage of registered nurses: An overview of issues and actions.* Geneva, The Netherlands: International Council of Nurses.

Buerhaus, P., Starger, D., & Auerbach, D. (2009). *The future of the nursing workforce in the United States: Data trends and implications:* Boston, MA: Jones and Bartlett.

Bureau of Labor Statistics. (2009). Registered nurses. *Occupational Outlook Handbook 2010–2011 Edition.* Retrieved October 25, 2010, from http://www.bls.gov/oco/ocos083.htm

Canadian Institute for Health Information. (2008). *Regulated nurses: Trends 2003–2007, Table 13—Registered nurse workforce by highest education in nursing, by jurisdiction in Canada, 2003– 2007.* Retrieved September 2, 2010, from http://secure.cihi.ca/cihiweb/products/nursing_ report_2003_to_2007_e.pdf

Canadian Nurses Association. (2009). *Tested solutions for eliminating Canada's registered nurses shortage.* Ottawa, Canada: Author

Clinton, M., du Boulay, S., Hazelton, M., & Horner, B. (2001). *Mental health nursing education and health labour force: Literature review.* Retrieved September 8, 2010, from http://www.dest.gov. au/archive/highered/nursing/pubs/mental_health/1.htm

Cutshall, P. (2000). *Understanding cross border professional regulation: What nurses and other professionals need to know.* Geneva, The Netherlands: International Council of Nurses.

Davis, C. R., & Kritek, P. B. 2005. Foreign nurses in the U.S. workforce. *Healthy work environments: Foreign nurse recruitment best practices.* Washington, DC: American Organization of Nurse Executives, pp. 2–11. Retrieved October 22, 2010, from http://www.aone.org/aone/ pdf/ForeignNurseRecruitmentBestPracticesOctober2005.pdf

Davis, C. R., & Richardson, D. R. (2009a). Communicating in the U.S. healthcare system. In B. L. Nichols & C. R. Davis (Eds.), *The official guide for foreign-educated nurses: What you need to know about nursing and health care in the United States* (pp. 217–233). New York, NY: Springer.

Davis, C. R., & Richardson, D. R. (2009b). Preparing to leave your home country. In B. L. Nichols & C. R. Davis (Eds.), *The official guide for foreign-educated nurses: What you need to know about nursing and health care in the United States* (pp. 20–42). New York, NY: Springer.

DiMarzio, M. (2010). *Nursing and nursing education in India*. The Honor Society of Nursing, Sigma Theta Tau, Volunteer Connect. Retrieved September 1, 2010, from http://www.nursing society.org/VolunteerConnect/Pages/DiMarzioIndia.aspx

European Federation of Nurses Associations. (2010). *EFN Update, March 2010*. Retrieved September 20, 2010, from http://fineeurope.org/en/liens/EFN/EFN_march10.pdf

Fegan, C. (2009). Nurses forced to turn backs on Ireland for English jobs. December 16, 2009. *The Daily Mail*. Retrieved September 15, 2010, from http://www.pronurse.co.uk/news/articles/2114-nurses-forced-to-turn-backs-on-ireland-for-english-jobs

Frindinnskottir, E. B., & Johnsson, J. A. (2009). *The impact of the economic recession on nurses and nursing in Iceland*. Retrieved September 15, 2010, from http://www.hrhresourcecenter.org/node/2976

Garritty, C., & El Emam, K. (2006). Who's using PDAs? Estimates of PDA use by health care providers: A systematic review of surveys. *Journal of Medical Internet Research, 8*(2), April-June, 2006. Retrieved October 22, 2010, from http://www.ncbi.nlm.nih.gov/pmc/articles/PMC1550702/

Hawkes, M., Kolenko, M., Shockness, M., & Diwaker, K. 2009. Nursing brain drain from India. *Human Resources for Health*. Retrieved August 17, 2010, from http://www.human-resources-health.com/content/7/1/5

Health Resources and Services Administration. (2010). *The registered nurse population: Findings from the 2008 national sample survey of registered nurses*. Retrieved September 10, 2010, from http://bhpr.hrsa.gov/healthworkforce/rnsurvey/initialfindings2008.pdf

International Council of Nurses. (2008a). *An aging nursing workforce*. Geneva, The Netherlands: Author. Retrieved September 9, 2010, from http://www.ichrn.com/publications/factsheets/Ageing_Workforce-English.pdf

International Council of Nurses. (2008b). *Asia nursing workforce profile*. Geneva, The Netherlands: Author. Retrieved September 15, 2010, from http://www.icn.ch/images/stories/documents/pillars/sew/sew_asia_workforce_profile_2008.pdf

International Labor Organization (ILO). (2010a). *Key indicators of the labour market*. Retrieved September 20, 2010, from http://www.ilo.org/empelm/what/langen/WCMS_114240

International Labor Organization (ILO). (2010b). *The global economic crisis: Trends in employment and working conditions by economic activity*. Retrieved September 15, 2010, from http://www.ilo.org/wcmsp5/groups/public/dgreports/dcomm/documents/publication/wcms_124478.pdf

Irwin, J. (2001). Cross border health care: Migration patterns of nursing in the EU. *EuroHealth, 7*(4), 13–15. Retrieved September 15, 2010, from http://test.cp.euro.who.int/Document/Obs/Eurohealth7_4.pdf

Japanese Nurses Association. (2009). *JNA News Release*, Volume 1. Retrieved September 15, 2010, from http://www.nurse.or.jp/jna/english/news/pdf/2009nr_1.pdf

Khatiwada, S. (2009). *Stimulus packages to counter global economic crisis: A review*. Discussion Paper Series No. 196, International Labor Organization. Retrieved September 17, 2010, from http://www.ilo.org/public/libdoc/ilo/2009/109B09_49_engl.pdf

Kingma, M. (2006). *Nurses on the move: Migration and the global health care economy*. Ithaca, NY: Cornell University Press.

Lankshear, A. J., Sheldon, T. A., & Maynard, A. (2005). Nurse staffing and healthcare outcomes: A systematic review of the international research evidence. *Advances in Nursing Science, 28*(2), 163–174.

Mejia, A., Pizurki, H., & Royston, E. (1979). *Physician and nurse migration: Analysis and policy implications*. Geneva, The Netherlands: World Health Organization.

Munjanja, O., Kibuka, S., & Dovlo, D. (2005). *The nursing workforce in sub-Saharan Africa*. Geneva, The Netherlands: International Council of Nurses. Retrieved October 2, 2010, from http://www.ghdonline.org/uploads/The_nursing_workforce_in_sub-Saharan_Africa.pdf

Needleman, J., Buerhaus, P., Mattke, S., Stewart, M., & Zelevinsky, K. (2002). Nurse-staffing levels and the quality of care in hospitals. *The New England Journal of Medicine, 346*(22), 1715–1722.

Nichols, B. 2007. *The impact of global nurse migration on health services delivery* (a white paper). Philadelphia, PA: CGFNS International, Inc.

Nichols, B., Davis, C. R., & Richardson, D. R. (2010). *International models of nursing.* Commissioned paper for the Robert Wood Johnson Foundation Initiative on the Future of Nursing at the Institute of Medicine.

Ojo, O. (1990). International migration of health manpower in sub-Saharan Africa. *Social Science Medicine, 31*(6), 1–7.

Organization for Economic Cooperation and Development (OECD). (2008). *The looming crisis in the health workforce: How can OECD countries respond?* Retrieved September 10, 2010, from http://www.oecd.org/document/47/0,3343,en_2649_37407_36506543_1_1_1_37407,00.html

Organization for Economic Cooperation and Development (OECD). (2010) *International migration of health workers.* OECD Observer. Paris: Author.

Philippine Star. (2008). *Nowhere to train.* September 8, 2008. Retrieved September 2, 2010, from http://www.bizlinksphilippines.net/090808.htm

Population Reference Bureau. (2010). *2008 world population data sheet.* Retrieved October 22, 2010, from http://www.prb.org/pdf08/08WPDS_Eng.pdf

Richardson, D. R., & Davis, C. R. (2009). Entry into the United States. In B. L. Nichols & C. R. Davis (Eds.), *The official guide for foreign-educated nurses: What you need to know about nursing and health care in the United States* (pp. 1–19). New York, NY: Springer.

Spencer, C. (2010). Experts warn of nursing shortage (March 20, 2010). *The Toronto Sun.* Retrieved September 12, 2010, from http://www.torontosun.com/news/canada/2010/03/20/13303221.html

Stromberg, A., Martensson, J., Fridlund, B., Levin, L. A., Karlsson, J. E., & Dahlstrom, U. (2003). Nurse-led heart failure clinics improve survival and self-care behaviors in patients with heart failure: Results from a prospective randomized trial. *EUR Heart Journal, 24*(11), 1014–1023. Retrieved October 22, 2010, from http://eurheartj.oxfordjournals.org/content/24/11/1014.short

Stroud, S., Erkel, E., & Smith, C. (2005). The use of personal digital assistants by nurse practitioner students and faculty. *Journal of the American Academy of Nurse Practitioners, 17*(2), 67–75. Retrieved October 22, 2010, from http://onlinelibrary.wiley.com/doi/10.1111/j.1041-2972.2005.00013.x/full

United Nations. (2008). *World population prospects: The 2008 revision population database.* Retrieved October 22, 2010, from http://esa.un.org/unpp/

United Nations Development Programme. (2009). Overcoming barriers: Human mobility and development. *Human Development Report 2009.* Retrieved October 21, 2010, from http://hdr.undp.org/en/media/HDR_2009_EN_Complete.pdf

Vujicic, M., Ohiri, K., & Sparkes, S. (2009). *Working in health; Financing and managing the public sector health workforce.* Washington, DC: World Bank.

Wilcox, R. A., & La Tella, R. R. (2001). The personal digital assistant, a new medical instrument for the exchange of clinical information at the point of care. *The Medical Journal of Australia, 175*(11–12), 659–662.

World Health Organization (WHO). (2006a). *The world health report 2006: Working together for health.* Geneva, The Netherlands: Author.

World Health Organization (WHO). (2006b). *Migration of health workers.* Fact sheet No. 301, April, 2006. Geneva, The Netherlands: Author.

Zalalequi, A., Marquez, M., Nunin, R., & Mariscae, I. (2006). Changes in nursing education in the European Union. *Journal of Nursing Scholarship, 38*(2), 114–118.

CHAPTER 6

Bullying, Harassment, and Horizontal Violence in the Nursing Workforce

The State of the Science

Judith A. Vessey, Rosanna DeMarco, and Rachel DiFazio

ABSTRACT

In the complex health care workplace of nurses, intra/interprofessional ideals intersect with the expectations of patients, families, students, and coworkers in a context of managed care environments, academia, and other health care enterprises. Integral to quality assessment, management, and assurance is collegial and respectful communication. Decades of reported descriptive and anecdotal data on intra/inter professional and on client communication, describe the antithesis of these ideals. Specifically, increasing frequency and rates of persistent bullying, harassment, or horizontal violence (BHHV) have shown to yield detrimental effects on workplace satisfaction, workforce retention, and the psychological and physical health of nurses as well as implied effects on quality of patient care and risk of poor health outcomes. Persistent BHHV among nurses is a serious concern. In advancing the science of description and explanation to a level of prevention intervention, explanatory models from biology, developmental psychology, intra/interpersonal interactionism are described along with theoretical explanations for the prevalence of BHHV in nurse workplaces. Making

© 2011 Springer Publishing Company
DOI: 10.1891/0739-6686.28.133

the connection between explanatory models and creative solutions to address BHHV through multiple levels of behavioral influence such as individual, environmental, interpersonal, and cultural contexts is key to advancing the science of the relationship between professional behavior and client/family/community health care outcomes.

Quality patient-centered care requires cooperation among nurses, other health-care personnel, patients, and their families. A prerequisite for such partnerships includes respectful, collaborative, working relationships among members of the nursing workforce. Without these collaborative relationships, the open exchange of health care information is jeopardized, putting patients at risk for negative health outcomes. While there will always be challenges in nurses' interactions, today's increasingly complex and stress-laden hospitals can cause poor interactions to deteriorate further into persistent bullying, harassment, or horizontal violence (BHHV) among nurses (Clark, Leddy, Drain, & Kaldenberg, 2006). When BHHV occurs, all meaningful communication is essentially stopped.

BHHV is a problem; within and across all health care professional groups the preponderance of evidence supports that BHHV is the greatest problem intra-professionally within nursing, both in its prevalence and level of distress it causes (Farrell, 1997, 1999; Randle, 2003; Woelfle & McCaffrey, 2007). Intraprofessional BHHV also permits, and even encourages, interprofessional BHHV to flourish (Duddle & Boughton, 2007).This review will focus on intraprofessional (nurse to nurse) BHHV, particularly as it is manifested in acute care settings. Its description, explanatory models, epidemiology, and impact will be explicated. Finally, the identification of interventions and solutions including primary and secondary prevention strategies designed to rapidly identify and manage BHHV will be described.

METHOD
Inclusion Criteria
In order to allow for the greatest representation of BHHV and to later analyze, synthesize, and generalize key constructs (Cooper, Hedges, & Valentine 2009), all articles that were written by nurses or included nurses in their target population in which bullying, harassment, horizontal (lateral) violence, and/or social aggression were key concepts were reviewed. Inclusion criteria were not limited to data-based articles in refereed journals; the nursing literature is replete with clinically focused articles about BHHV in the nursing workforce but actual research evidence is scant. To impose this limitation would severely truncate this

review. Instead, using the rubric of evidence-based practice (Melnyk & Fineout-Overholt, 2005), review and clinically focused refereed articles and professional organizational white papers and briefs were considered to be the evidence of professional expertise. The full array of unpublished studies was not included due to difficulties with identification and retrieval. Research and reviews published in refereed electronic journals were included if it was retrievable. Because BHHV occurs across the international nursing workforce, all articles written in English were included, regardless of origin.

Search Strategies and Critique Methods

The accessible literature base was identified using the following search strategies: keyword and author search of journals indexed in the following databases: CINAHL (1982–2010), Medline (1966–2010), and PsycAbstracts/PsycINFO (1987–2010). Manual searches of the reference lists of identified research and review articles were also conducted. Although attempts were made to be as inclusive as possible, the conclusions were drawn only from the retrieved literature and thus may not be totally representative of all aspects of BHHV within the nursing workforce, especially for nurses working outside of the acute care arena where there is significantly less information available.

All articles were reviewed chronologically and conceptually to ascertain how each contributed to our understanding of BHHV. Articles were coded as to whether they were research, and if so, by the conceptual framework that was used, the study methodology, and the analytic techniques employed. Nonresearch literature was evaluated on the evidence provided that supported the authors' assertions and the quality of the journal in which the article appeared. Finally, in order to better explicate its theoretical underpinnings, supportive literature that addressed explanatory models of BHHV behaviors across biological and psychosocial sciences was reviewed to yield frameworks that described specific physiological, developmental, intrapersonal and interpersonal aspects of BHHV.

FINDINGS: THE STATE OF THE SCIENCE

Definition

The World Health Organization (2002) has defined violence as "the intentional use of physical force or power, threatened or actual, against oneself, another person, or against a group or community that either results in or has a high likelihood of resulting in injury, death, psychological harm, mal-development or deprivation." BHHV are one subset that meets this definition. Although there is a considerable literature on workplace violence and BHHV, there is lack of standardized definitions among these three terms and numerous other related terms (e.g., social, relational, and passive aggression; workplace trauma) that are used in the literature (Broome, 2008; National Advisory Council on Nurse Education and Practice [NACNEP], 2007; Wiskow, 2002). Commonalities across these terms include offensive, abusive, intimidating, or insulting behaviors that cause psychological and/or physical distress to the recipient. Careful concept analyses to distinguish among the terms were conducted and a standardized nomenclature was created by the authors to normalize terms across the literature. For example, horizontal and lateral violence were determined to share all of the same root characteristics; the same can be said for the term bullying, also known as mobbing in the international community.

Bullying differs from horizontal violence in that a real or perceived power differential between the instigator and recipient must be present in bullying, while horizontal violence occurs among peers. With bullying, anyone can be a potential target while harassment generally is associated with the notion of difference—whether due to gender, race, ethnicity, age or disability (Gillen, 2002; Normandale & Davies, 2002). In the literature, these terms are frequently used interchangeably or bullying is used as an umbrella term to describe all interpersonal violence in the workplace (Gilmour & Hamlin, 2003). Due to the conceptual overlap and the fact that these terms are often used interchangeably in the literature, for this review, the terms BHHV will be examined together as a single construct. BHHV is then defined as repeated, offensive, abusive, intimidating, or insulting behavior, abuse of power, or unfair sanctions that makes recipients upset and feel humiliated, vulnerable, or threatened, creating stress and undermining their self-confidence.

Explanatory Models for the Occurrence of BHHV

Explanatory models abound in the literature about social contexts that contribute to BHHV; an inclusive view of why BHHV may occur needs to include an understanding of a variety of models that move beyond just defining BHHV. Evidence-based explanatory models elucidate the influence of human interactions in biological, developmental, intrapersonal, and environmental spheres of nurses in the workplace. Models from these three paradigms are critiqued in terms of their explanatory power in explaining the occurrence of BHHV.

Biological Models

Biologic or biobehavioral models help identify plausible reasons for direct or covert aggressive behaviors in the workplace. These models also can help explain why some individuals could be easy targets. Biologic models that are used to explain the biobehavioral responses of perpetrators or victims of BHHV all have limitations. This is primarily due to the fact that cognitive or mental processes occur as antecedents to biobehavioral responses and effect behavior over time (Lupien, McEwen, Gunnar, & Heim, 2009). Genetics (temperament) and early experiences in growth and development effect neurological development and future cognitive performance (Cirulli et al., 2010); response antecedents may vary as a selective filter for different individuals based on their experiences with stress and coping (Olff, Langeland, & Gersons, 2005).

Despite these limitations, early studies demonstrated through animal and human experiments that the removal or lowering of the levels of testosterone decrease aggression and/or dominance and biobehavioral responses to stress. In women, this takes the form of befriending the perpetrator rather than a fight or flight response that is often connected with the activation of testosterone (Albert, Walsh, Gorzalka, Siemens, & Louie, 1986). Women tend to use attachment behaviors to quell aggression and these are triggered by oxytocin, not testosterone (Campbell, 2008; Jack, 1993, 1999). Terburg, Morgan, and van Honk (2009) supported the claim that female aggression exists, but that it is less mediated by testosterone and thus aggression is not overt but social or relational in nature. For example, adult victims of "mobbing" have altered circadian cycles of cortisol levels which may negatively influence the social climate by affecting, sensory acuity, learning, and memory in the workplace (Kudielka & Kern, 2004). Finally, dehydroepiandrosterone (DHEA) is an endogenous hormone secreted by the adrenal gland that can protect the individual from exposure to cortisol and thus mitigate its effect on behavior. Testosterone, cortisol, and DHEA in combination with environmental influences have an interactive role in the development of behavior (Kudielka, 2004).

Developmental Models

The larger domain of social aggression has as a key characteristic the intent on the part of a perpetrator to do social harm while one subtype, relational aggression, focuses on harm directed to the individual or in the case of BHHV the peer specifically (Archer & Coyne, 2005). Galen and Underwood (1997) describe relational aggression as a direct or indirect form of social aggression used to damage a peer's self esteem, social status or both. Archer et al. (2005) in analyzing the differences in goals and strategies across indirect, social, and relational aggression state that forms of aggression change across age. In all cases, indirect forms of aggression historically have been used primarily by girls. With the advent of the cyberbullying, a type of indirect aggression, early work suggests that equal gender participation is the norm (Kiriakidis & Kavoura, 2010).

From a developmental perspective, indirect aggression as a learned experience by girls may be reinforced developmentally for women over time. Jack (1999) explored the origins, meanings, and experiences of women's aggression through interviews with women from varying socio-economic backgrounds. She argues that aggression arises from failures in relationships with other people and can take the form of veiled/indirect approaches, control in getting back at others, or indirect resisting victimization. Jack's main argument is that women are not aggressive because of human nature, but that indirect aggression develops in a cultural and interpersonal context. She states: "the basic pattern behind the differing forms [of aggression in women] remains the same: attempts to hurt, to oppose, or to express anger go underground to reach others through hidden channels, while surface behaviors mask the intent" (Jack, 1999, p. 188).

Intrapersonal Models
Unique situational issues that can affect individuals, help explain why BHHV may be a response to situations occurring in the workplace environments. Hershcovis and colleagues (2007) identified use of drugs and alcohol, interpersonal/family and economic stressors outside of the workplace, and circadian effects related to time of day one works (shifts in the case of hospital settings) as key components of aggression in the workplace. Balducci, Alfano, and Fraccaroli (2009) investigated the relationships between the individuals' experience of mobbing (bullying) at work ($N = 107$) and personality traits and symptom patterns as assessed by the Minnesota Multiphasic Personality Inventory (MMPI-2). Individuals who were the recipients of the mobbing scored highly on the neurotic and paranoid components of the MMPI-2. A pattern of positive and significant correlations was found between the frequency of exposure to mobbing behaviors and the MMPI-2 clinical, supplementary, and content scales, including the Post-traumatic Stress Diagnostic Scale (McCarthy, 2008). Half of the participants in this study, and who were recipients of mobbing, showed a level of posttraumatic stress symptoms consistent with posttraumatic stress disorder. In addition, the frequency of exposure to mobbing predicted suicidal ideation and behavior, with depression only partially mediating this relationship.

Jack's (1993) seminal research on silencing the self behaviors and Jack and Ali's (2010) more recent work, explain that women silence or suppress certain thoughts, feelings, and actions that may contradict another's view. The "other" to which Jack (1993) originally referred to was often an intimate partner, but others have identified the concept and behaviors in the workplace of nurses (DeMarco, 1997, 2002; DeMarco & Roberts, 2003; Roberts, DeMarco, & Griffin, 2009). "Silencing the self" is an intrapersonal behavior based on a relational situation, i.e., women trying to avoid conflict to maintain relationships and/or ensure their psychological or physical safety (Jack, 2010). One schema that describes the result of silencing the self is the inner stress and strain women expressed in Jack's original work (1993) about how divided women often felt about outwardly trying to keep peace and not disrupt relationships ("not rocking the boat") while inwardly feeling more and more anger. The anger often comes from a violation of justice in that one is held back from doing the right thing (telling others directly what they need and feel). Over time anger and self-blame become a struggle behind the mask of compliance for women (Jack, 1999).

Interpersonal Models

Behaviors like aggression or withdrawal can create roles (bully versus victim) and can influence how others behave in the context of these roles. Emotional and cognitive reactions to BHHV begin to be part of a work culture in which self-esteem, feelings of injustice, resentment, and frustration results in what Bowling and Beehr (2006) call "reciprocation" (p. 1001) within the work environment. Reciprocation takes the form of retaliatory behaviors that are intended to "get even" with others or the organization. Whether the perpetrator stands alone or is assisted with others in the group or institution directly or indirectly can vary across work environments, cultures, and normative beliefs about behavior.

Each disciplinary perspective appears to recognize that, like in other types of workplaces, BHHV takes on the form of relational aggression in the workplace. Galen and Underwood (1997) define relational aggression as a subtype of social aggression where a perpetrator targets a victim. The key characteristic of social aggression is the intent on the part of a perpetrator of BHHV to do social harm while relational aggression in BHHV focuses on the peer. Social aggression is described as a direct or indirect form of relational aggression used to damage a peer's self esteem, social status or both.

The process of social aggression is both overt and covert (passive) in nature, as are the responses of the victims. The overriding effects of the interpersonal aggression can be identified at the individual, workgroup, and organizational level in the health care setting. Beyond developmental perspectives of how individuals develop over time and learn to tacitly accept cultural imperatives about appropriate and nonappropriate behavior discussed in the ontogenetic section of the ecological model, Archer and Coyne (2005) found that girls may be just as aggressive as boys when using manipulative forms of aggression, such as gossiping and spreading rumors in all types of environmental settings (home, school, and later at work). These forms of aggression are known by the term social aggression including subtypes of relational aggression previously mentioned as indirect or passive aggression. A functional explanation for indirect aggression in the work environment includes behavior that is an alternative strategy to direct aggression, generally used when the costs of direct aggression are high and when the aim of the behavior is to socially exclude, or harm the social status of, a victim while simultaneously inflating one's own social status (Jack, 1999). In this way, BHHV have the characteristic of being additive in that they accumulate burden on the individual similar to that of a toxin in an unhealthy environment. Although extremely subtle, BHHV may have not only an additive but synergistic effect in relationship to consequent behaviors.

Crick and colleagues (2006) use the term relational aggression to characterize girls' and later women's indirect practice of "harming others through purposeful manipulation and damage of their peer relationships" by exclusion in the context of the work environment, individuals can withdraw friendship, or control behavior, spreading rumors so peers will reject others. Boys/men use physical, verbal aggression or intimidation as forms of aggression whereas women try to affect the relational space between individuals. Examples of relational aggression in nurse workplaces can include nurses creating "in-groups" that share information, activities, friendship, confidences and workloads, but clearly do not do the same with others in the workplace who are at the same peer level. Those who are excluded from the "in-group" are put in a position of feeling like outsiders, "less-than," not welcome and generally feel stigmatized in some way (Underwood, 2003).

In trying to understand why direct or indirect aggression among nurses occurs in the work environment, an explanatory model that intersects gender studies, social science, psychology, and individual/environment interactions is that of *Oppressed Group Behaviors* (Roberts, 1983). Roberts (1983) was the first nurse who described BHHV as outcomes of structural or social contexts of work environments of nurses based on the original work, *Pedagogy of the Oppressed*, by Paulo Freire (2000) and conceptualizing her own observations of nurses in the workplace "oppressed group behaviors." Freire's (2000) primary contribution to Roberts' understanding and interpretation of BHHV was in the area of critical pedagogy. As an educator who was highly influenced by Marxist principles in Brazil, Friere explored how oppression is often justified in a normative manner by a mutual process between the "oppressor" and the "oppressed." Freire theorized that the powerless in societies where oppression proliferates can be frightened of freedom, i.e., freedom to address negative behavior of an oppressor as opposed to supporting a culture of BHHV. Friere beckoned those that were oppressed to pursue constantly and responsibly BHHV as defined in this paper. According to Freire, freedom is the result of action not inaction. Roberts (1983, 1996, 1997) identified in her work that inaction on the part of nurses when BHHV were present in the workplace was related to a history of gender oppression as well as marginalization from the discipline of medicine. Using the work of Freire, she described the ability of dominant groups who identify norms as the "right" ones.

Individual, workgroup, and larger work cultures or systems are related and perpetuate acceptance of BHHV as normative while supporting inaction—decreased acts of freedom—when BHHV are not named and ignored for reasons of maintaining power and control. When nurse managers and administrators do not address BHHV it may lead to "silencing the self" as a force of "inaction" that maintains power and control for nurse managers and administrators. It also perpetuates the sub-oppression that Freire (2000) identified when one who was oppressed has power (DeMarco, 2003). Hutchinson, Vickers, Jackson, and Wilkes (2006) developed an organizational model and matching outcome measures to evaluate specific domains of the workplace that accounted for antecedents of bullying behavior. These researchers identified organizational tolerance, informal organizational alliances and misuse of legitimate authority processes and procedures as antecedents to bullying acts. These bullying acts were at the personal reputation and competence level as well as attacks through work process. The individual/environmental consequences identified in this model of bullying acts included (1) normalization of bullying, (2) distress and avoidance of bullying in the workplace, (3) negative health effects, and (4) interruption to work and career trajectory.

Prevalence of BHHV

There are incomplete global epidemiologic data of BHHV due to the difficulty tracking events secondary to definitional inconsistencies and measurement problems, including the "the lack of systematic and coordinated data collection procedures and scant research" (NACNEP, 2007, p. 18). Although the exact prevalence is not known, BHHV is accepted as a common and pernicious problem and a persistent, occupational hazard within the global nursing workforce (Clark, 2006; Farrell, Bobrowski, & Bobrowski, 2006; Gunnarsdottir, Sveinsdottir, Bernburg, Fridriksdottis, & Tomasson, 2006; Hegney, Eley, Plank, Buikstra, & Parker, 2006; Kwok, Law, Li, Ng, Cheung, Fung, et al., 2006; Quine, 2001; Rutherford & Rissel, 2004; Stevens, 2002; Yildirim, 2009).

Five studies conducted in the international arena reveal that between 17% and 76% of professional nurses report experiencing BHHV (Clark, 2006; Farrell, 2006; Gunnarsdottir, 2006; Hegney, 2006; Kwok, 2006; Quine, 2001; Rutherford, 2004; Stevens, 2002); marked differences in study methodologies likely account for this large range. Data for the U.S. nursing workforce is sparse. Simons' (2008) study of measured negative acts consistent with bullying in Massachusetts registered nurses (RNs; $N = 511$); 31% reported being bullied (with bullying subjectively defined as >1 negative act) and bullying was a significant ($p < .0005$) factor in intent to leave the workplace. Stanley, Martin, Nemeth, Michel, and Welton (2007) studied lateral violence of staff RNs ($N = 601$) at one hospital; 46% indicated that lateral violence was a very or somewhat serious problem, although an explicit definition of lateral violence was not provided. In a cross-sectional study, Australian nurses (N = 2,487) reported that in across their last five shifts, 1.1% had experienced nurse-on-nurse physical violence, 2% had threats of violence, and another 14.7% experienced emotional abuse (Roche, Diers, Duffield, & Catling-Paull, 2010). An American Association of Critical-care Nurses (AACN) study (2006) indicates that 88% of nurses (N = 4,000) work with a colleague that engages in low intensity behaviors (e.g., verbal abuse, gossip, self-promotion at another's expense) consistent with BHHV. Lastly, new, and as yet unpublished data from a federally funded lateral violence project, reports that 88% of nurses have been recipients of similar low-intensity forms of lateral violence while in a staff nurse position ("Upstate Lateral Violence," n.d.). More concerning is that 76% report witnessing such behaviors directed at one or more colleagues on a weekly basis; this is supported by Stanley et al.'s (2007) work, where 6% reported frequently observing lateral violence behaviors among coworkers.

These studies, however, lack methodological rigor (AACN, 2006; Stanley et al., 2007; "Upstate Lateral Violence," n.d.), lack clear definitions (AACN, 2006; "Upstate Lateral Violence," n.d.), did not include the full scope of BHHV behaviors (AACN, 2006; Simons, 2008; Stanley et al., 2007; "Upstate Lateral Violence," n.d.), used nonspecific sampling criteria (AACN, 2006), used instrumentation with insufficient psychometric evaluation (AACN, 2006; Simons, 2008; Stanley et al., 2007; "Upstate Lateral Violence," n.d.), or had a poor response rates—54.4% (Simons, 2008) and 36% (Stanley et al., 2007) indicating that sampling bias may be an issue. The reason for the absence of robust prevalence studies in not understood although the influence of culture, government-controlled or fragmented and competitive health systems, fears of litigation, or acceptance of longstanding attitudes (e.g., "nurses eat their young") and roles of professional nurses in the larger society cannot be discounted.

As with other forms of victimization, significant underreporting is likely (Ferns & Chojnacka, 2005; NACNEP, 2007). Frequent low-grade BHHV goes unnoticed by others and the recipient may not report such incidents for fear of appearing petty. In part, this may be because these behaviors are learned in the schoolyard where most bullying among girls is relational, covert and socially toxic—ostracism, insults, divisive gossip, and so on—the same behaviors that are demonstrated in the workplace (Farrington, 1993; Rayner & Hoel, 1998; Vessey, DeMarco, Gaffney, & Budin, 2009). BHHV, surrounded by a "culture of silence," fears of retaliation, and the perception that "nothing will be changed," can also effectively shut down the exchange of information (DeMarco, 1998; 2002; Ferns, 2005; Stearley, 1997). Data support these assertions. Out of two British studies and one U.S. study on bullied nurses who reported that they had tried to take action, only 22–43%

was satisfied with the result (Quine, 1999; Royal College of Nursing, 2002; Vessey, 2009).

Perpetrators and Recipients of BHHV

For some nurses, BHHV is viewed as a normal part of the job and therefore tolerated (Dunn, 2003; Lewis, 2006). This view is reinforced by the hierarchical organizational culture within hospitals which limits reporting of BHHV-related behaviors (Alexy & Hutchins, 2006; Lewis, 2006). What constitutes BHHV varies, in part, according to people's ideas and perceptions about workplace culture. BHHV is commonly a 'learned behavior' among practicing nurses (Lewis, 2006). Issues are rarely handled during the early stages of conflict and when they do emerge, nurse managers try to keep them contained (Lewis, 2006; MacIntosh, 2005). Workplace BHHV thrives on organizationally dysfunctional units. BHHV tends to be more common in settings where technical expertise is valued over interpersonal competence (Cole, 1996; Corr, 2000). Some individuals and unit cultures may support or condone BHHV; staff who thrive in such environments are seen by their colleagues as strong and resilient (Hughes, 2003).

BHHV increases in high-intensity, stressful environments and has become more prevalent among the nursing workforce over the last decade along with escalating patient acuity, attempts to 'right-size' the nursing workforce, and subsequent increases in staff turnover (Gilmour, 2003; Jackson, Clare, & Mannix, 2002; Long, 1996; Mayhew & Chappell, 2002a, 2002b). Research has demonstrated that nurses who have just entered the workforce are at greater risk of being targeted for BHHV as they are often younger, less experienced, somewhat insecure in their new role, and less aware of the a unit's cultural norms than their more seasoned colleagues (Griffin, 2004; McKenna, Smith, Poole, & Coverdale, 2003; Simons & Mawn, 2010). When BHHV is unnoticed or unchecked by nurse managers or supervisors, the instigator considers such behaviors appropriate (Hughes, 2003). In descriptive studies of nurses working in acute care settings, 50%–76% of nurses report regularly witnessing BHHV (Quine, 2001; Stanley et al., 2007; "Upstate Lateral Violence," n.d.), but frequently have little idea as to how they might best intervene. In qualitative interviews, nurses ($n = 29$) revealed that witnessing BHHV between colleagues was actually more distressing than physical assault from patients (Farrell, 1997). Over time, bystanders who observe BHHV but choose not to intervene, even if they abhor BHHV behaviors, it is postulated that they become complicit and begin to create reasons to justify the BHHV they have witnessed (Deans, 2004; Stevens, 2002).

Nursing management is implicated as being the most frequent initiator of BHHV (Deans, 2004; Long, 1996; Quine, 1999; Vessey, 2009). For example, in the Vessey et al. (2009) survey, 37% of U.S. nurses ($N = 314$) reported nursing management engaged in bulling behaviors. Similar findings were reported in the (British) Royal College of Nursing (2002) nationwide survey ($N = 778$), with findings indicating that 41% of the nursing workforce was bullied by management in the six months prior to their study. Lastly, McMillan (1995) reported that 61% of British nurses identified line managers as a source of constant bullying (1995), noting that because managers are in positions of power, they are as likely to target strong as well as weak subordinates just in the process of exercising power and advancing themselves, which may come at the expense of others. The Royal College of Nursing (2002) noted that nurses who found their supervisors intimidating became less sensitive and more morally disengaged over time; these nurses' disenchantment was also contagious to other staff members. A synthesis of available data supports that a crisis of leadership occurs in many hospitals when nurse managers are promoted to their posts based on clinical competence rather than the appropriate educational background and necessary organizational and leadership skills required for the position (Hauge, Skogstad, & Einarsen, 2007; Long, 1996; Pearson et al., 2004).

Psychological and Physical Impact of BHHV

BHHV has been shown to be deleterious to the recipient's psychological and physical health (Cortina & Magley, 2003; Gilmour, 2003; Gunnarsdottir, 2006; MacIntosh, 2005). Recipients of BHHV experience stress directly from the attacks. They constantly edit their behaviors to avoid what they perceive as further aggravation of the instigators; avoidance and withdrawal behaviors have been repeatedly documented (Gilmour, 2003; Graveson, 1998; Hansen et al., 2006; McVicar, 2003) as has the increased use of tobacco, alcohol and other substances (Kivimaki, Elovainio, & Vahtera, 2000; Normandale, 2002). Psychological distress symptoms that have been reported across studies including anxiety, irritability, panic attacks, tearfulness, depression, loss of confidence and self-esteem, mood swings, and irritability (Cortina, 2003; Gilmour, 2003; Graveson, 1998; Gunnarsdottir, 2006; Yildirim, 2009). Physical symptoms include sleep disturbances, headaches, increased blood pressure, anorexia, gastrointestinal upset, and loss of libido. Lastly, sleep disorders, posttraumatic stress disorder, suicide ideation and suicide have been documented in the research literature (Gilmour, 2003; Graveson, 1998; Normandale, 2002; Hansen, 2006; Royal College of Nursing, 2002; Vessey, 2009).

International studies that have explored the biological effects of BHHV underlying psychological and physical symptomatology experienced by on recipients indicate compelling effects on the body. Di Rosa and colleagues (2009) postulated that victims of workplace mobbing were at increased risk for psychological diagnosable disorders. Comparing healthy individuals with those experiencing mobbing by measuring oxidative stress, these researchers found victims of mobbing had higher serum levels of protein carbonyl groups and of nitrosylated proteins which are biological markers of oxidative stress conditions. Monteleone and colleagues (2009) found hypoactivity of the hypothalamo-pituitary-adrenal axis in victims of BHHV and conjectured through further analysis that there is a relationship between brain function and victim's temperament and chronicity of the work-related psychological distress as a result of BHHV.

Cortina and Magley (2003) demonstrated in their large scale survey (n = 1167) of nonnurse public employees, that the impact of BHHV on recipients is exacerbated further if, when seeking redress, recipients experience retaliation from their supervisors. This has significant implications for nursing as it is known that collectively, symptomatology related to BHHV lowers nurses' confidence and competence (Deans, 2004; Leivers, 2004) and thus can influence the quality of nursing care rendered and subsequently, patient care outcomes.

Impact of BHHV on Quality of Care

BHHV interrupts critical components of teamwork; communication, the exchange of crucial health information, and collaborative decision-making, all of which are associated with increased medical errors and poorer patient outcomes (Hughes, 2003; ISMP, 2009; Joint Commission, 2008; Longo, 2007; Quine, 2001). However, strong correlational or causal impacts of BHHV on patient safety/quality of care are just beginning to be specifically explicated in the empirical literature. Nurses' reactions to BHHV have resulted from situations in which their contributions are ridiculed, their sense of professional mastery threatened, and ultimately, deeply eroding their self-esteem. Nurse recipients report avoiding staff interactions that target them for insult and abuse (Macintosh, 2005; McVicar, 2003; Quine, 1999, 2001; Stevens, 2002). Because BHHV is not limited solely to a dysfunctional dyadic relationship, staff who are bystanders are affected and teamwork is undermined (Hughes, 2003). Hutchinson, Wilkes, Jackson & Vickers, (2010) have recently used structural equation modeling and confirmatory factor analysis to test a multidimensional model of bullying using data from 370 surveys completed by Australian nurses. Organizational characteristics, including misuse of authority/policies/procedures, organizational tolerance, and informal alliances were confirmed as critical antecedents to bullying, its frequency, and intra- and interpersonal consequences.

Results of BHHV—poorer job satisfaction, professional disengagement, and increased turnover—are related to poorer quality of care (American Organization of Nurse Executives [AONE], 2000; Armstrong & Laschinger, 2006; Moyad, Daraiseh, Shell, & Salem, 2006; Rowe & Sherlock, 2005). Numerous studies have consistently identified the linkages between BHHV and poor job satisfaction (Graveson,

1998; Hegney, 2006; Leer, 2006; Mayhew, 2002a, 2002b; Yildririm, 2009). Across studies, recipients of verbal abuse report declines in morale (67–81%), decreased productivity (41–71%), and decreased nursing care delivery (36–54%), although the survey methodologies employed were not particularly rigorous. Other studies have successfully identified the relationship between poor job satisfaction and negative patient outcomes (American Nurses Association [ANA], 2001; Blegen, 1993; Hegyvary & Haussman, 1976; Weisman & Nathanson, 1985). A study conducted by the Institute for Safe Medication Practices (2009), examined the role intimidating behaviors had on medication errors. Within the RN subsample ($n = 1,565$), 7% stated that intimidation lead to a medication error within the past year (translating to 110 avoidable medication errors); however, the instigator of intimidation (i.e., RN, MD, PharmD) was not specified.

In other studies, nurses self-reported a range of in increase in patient safety errors from 51% to 87%, but the type of error and specific antecedents were not explicated (Braun, Christle, Walker, & Tiwanak, 1991; Cox, 1987; Sofield & Salmond, 2003). Roche and colleagues (2010) also demonstrated positive correlations between workplace violence and patient falls, delayed medication administrations, and medication errors, however, the definition of violence employed encompassed more than just nurse to nurse BHHV, including violence between nurses and physicians or patients and their families. All of these organizational, staffing, and patient care outcomes consequences result in substantial direct and indirect financial costs, although these are difficult to calculate.

Available Evidence-based Interventions and Instrumentation

Despite the presence of BHHV and its impact on workforce indicators and as a root cause of preventable medical errors, evidence-based strategies for its detection and prevention have not been specifically addressed in organizational white papers/reports/materials that posit solutions for contextual nursing workplace issues associated with BHHV(AACN 2006; American Association of Colleges of Nursing, 2004; American Hospital Association Commission on Workforce for Hospitals and Health Systems, 2002; AONE, 2000; National Institute for Occupational Safety and Health, 2002; U.S. Health Resources Services Administration, 2002). The two exceptions are the Center for American Nurses (2008) policy statement on lateral violence and bullying and the Joint Commission's 2008 Sentinel Event Alert *Behaviors that Undermine a Culture of Safety* (2008). The American Nurses' policy statement outlines broad actions that need to be taken at the interpersonal and organizational levels, with specific calls for more research on all aspects of BHHV in the workplace. The Joint Commission's Sentinel Event Alert outlines the need for institutions to develop the following primary and secondary prevention activities: (1) skills-based training and coaching, (2) ongoing, nonconfrontational surveillance, (3) a system for assessing staff perceptions of the seriousness and extent of unprofessional behaviors, and (4) policies that support early reporting without fear of intimidation.

There is little evidence that organizational leadership has the tools to routinely employ interventions to thwart the development of BHHV or engage in system-wide screening when BHHV is most amenable to intervention. While a plethora of articles (>130) describe the problem of BHHV; a review of the literature revealed five instruments to measure constructs related to BHHV, all of which have limitations (see Table 6.1). None of these instruments embrace the full range of behaviors seen in BHHV. Additionally, such 'stand-alone', single construct instruments, while appropriate for research, may not be amenable for clinical use due to their negative tone and possible ramifications that could negatively influence the workplace climate. In the era of multiple staff surveys to continuous quality assessment, hospital administrators may be reluctant to employ them for ongoing surveillance due to their costs respondent fatigue resulting in poor response rates.

A variety of interventions strategies have been proposed including no tolerance policies (Bigony et al., 2009) and application of restorative/shared responsibility approaches (Hutchinson, 2009). Documentation of the number of health care facilities that have policies specific to BHHV is limited. In some countries, there are specific laws that address BHHV and the organization's responsibility for monitoring and addressing such incidents (Rocker, 2008). In the United States, federal legislation prohibits harassment based on the notion of difference—race, ethnicity, gender—but not for bullying per se. In a small study conducted on nursing administrators (N = 108) in New York, 55% of the facilities that they represented had policies that addressed horizontal violence but they were only enforced approximately 43% of the time (Sellers, Millenbach, Kovach, & Yingling, 2009–2010).

In addition, only three small studies were identified that focused on intervention. Griffin (2004) investigated the use of cognitive rehearsal with newly licensed RNs (N = 26). After a two hour didactic teaching session, cueing cards for handling lateral violence were provided to the participants. At one year postintervention, qualitative data indicated that cognitive rehearsal helped them deal with lateral violence; no quantitative data were collected. DeMarco, Roberts, and Chandler (2005) pilot-tested a group writing intervention designed to decrease negative workplace behaviors with a sample of graduate nursing students (N = 5). The goal was to evaluate the efficacy of the intervention; no data regarding the effectiveness of the intervention was documented.

The third study by Barrett, Piatek, Korber, and Padula (2009) used a quasi-experimental, pretest/posttest design. The researchers implemented two team

TABLE 6.1

Instruments to Measure Constructs Related to BHHV

Instrument	Construct	Description and Psychometric Properties
Bullying Acts Inventory for the Nursing Workplace (Hutchinson, Wilkes, Vickers, & Jackson, 2008)	Bullying	• 17 items, 7-point Likert scale, 3 subscales: attack upon competence/reputation (6 items), personal attack (6 items), attack through work tasks (5 items) • Normed on nurses ($N = 102$) of varying ages, race/ethnicity n/a; diverse practice areas; 20% response rate • Overall Cronbach's α = .83; 93, .89, & .88 for respective subscales • Content Validity by expert panel • Used to test a multidimensional model of bullying in the workplace. Results indicated that the characteristics of the organization are antecedents of bullying and influence the occurrence of bullying and the resultant consequences (Hutchinson et al., 2010).
Lateral Violence in Nursing Survey (Stanley et al., 2007)	Lateral violence	• 23 dichotomous items organized by perceived seriousness, oppressors, mediators, and open-ended questions • Normed on RNs ($n = 601$) from 1 U.S. SE hospital; licensed from <1 to >30 years, race/ethnicity: 82% White; 36% response rate • No reliability or validity reported • No reports of the use of this tool in other studies identified
Negative Acts Questionnaire–Revised (Simons, 2008)	Horizontal violence	• Adapted from *Norwegian Negative Acts Questionnaire* • 22 items descriptive of bullying behaviors if repetitive over time, 3-point Likert scale • Trialed with MA RNs ($n = 511$), 78% licensed w/in past 3 years; race/ethnicity: 84% White; 6.7% male • Cronbach's α = .88; no validity indicated • Note: Original scale also revised for use in Japan (Abe & Henly, 2010)

(Continued)

TABLE 6.1

Instruments to Measure Constructs Related to BHHV   (Continued)

Instrument	Construct	Description and Psychometric Properties
Sabotage Savvy Questionnaire (Briles, 1999)	Sabotage	• 40 items, 3-point scoring; victim & saboteur subscales • Perioperative RNs ($n = 145$). Race/ethnicity: 86.2% White • No initial reliability and validity reported • Used in one other study, Dunn, 2003; reported Cronbach's α .86 & .72 for victim & saboteur subscales
Violence Climate Survey (Kessler, Spector, Chang, & Parr, 2008)	Safety/ violence	• 18-item measure assessing workplace climate; 3 subscales: policies, practices, pressures • Full-time employees ($n = 216$), diverse work settings not specific to nursing; 82% female, race/ethnicity data not provided • Cronbach's α's for policies, practices, & pressures subscales: .95, .90, & .90 respectively; Face validity indicated • No reports of the use of this tool in other studies identified

building sessions, each lasting two hours with RNs ($N = 145$) from four diverse patient care areas. Each unit served as their own control. Significant ($p = .037$) differences were noted between pre- and posttest scores on the Group Cohesion Scale using the Mann-Whitney U test. No statistical findings were reported for the differences in the pre- and posttest scores for the RN-RN interaction subscale of the NDNQI Adapted Index of Work Satisfaction, although the authors state that some improvements on the units were seen. Unfortunately, the response rates on pre- and posttest measures were only 41% and 31% in the pre- and posttest measures respectively, indicating potential sampling bias. Moreover, the dose of intervention was not likely to result in long-term change as BHHV is an engrained problem, rarely responsive to brief interventions. The reasons for the lack of intervention research are complex and include but are not limited to methodological difficulties, lack of standardized and measurable definitions, the lack of reliable and valid instrumentation, difficulty achieving institutional access, and limited available funding.

STRATEGIES FOR ADDRESSING BHHV

A model (see Figure 6.1) that can advance incremental and significant traction to address the challenge of BHHV is the stages of prevention model (Wallace, 2008). When applied to BHHV, primary prevention refers to reducing the number of BHHV incidents by intervening before BHHV occurs. Primary prevention requires identifying the risk and protective factors for BHHV, eliminating or against the development of BHHV and its adverse consequences; an approach advocated by nursing leaders (Embree & White, 2010). Organization wide awareness reducing associated risks and strengthening those individual, interpersonal, and organizational factors, campaigns, policy development, and the use of risk markers to target high-risk groups and/or individuals for educational interventions and follow up are exemplars of such activities.

Secondary prevention focuses on early problem detection of BHHV when these behaviors are still 'under the radar'. It helps stop BHHV from worsening and prevents or ameliorates long-term sequelae from developing. Lead time is the time for potential discovery of BHHV by screening compared to the time when BHHV becomes obvious. Screening allows for early detection of BHHV when it is most amenable to intervention. The longer the lead-time, the greater the opportunity for screening. No empirical data are available regarding lead time of BHHV, but anecdotal reports indicate that due to its subtle nature, it is often years before it is addressed, if ever (Cortina, 2003; ISMP, 2009; MacIntosh, 2005; Stevens, 2002). Screening tools would help nursing leadership teams and occupational health nurses who may speculate about which nursing units are experiencing BHHV, but have limited options for objectively identifying them and for tracking improvements after interventions have been initiated.

Tertiary prevention is required when there is failure to address issues of BHHV until after full-blown problems have erupted. Such interventions,

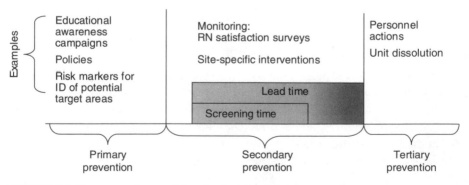

FIGURE 6.1 The prevention model as the study's guiding framework.
© Judith A. Vessey.

including disciplinary action, terminations, and in the worst case scenario, unit reorganization or dissolution, are palliative in nature, result in suboptimal outcomes. Tertiary prevention activities can usually be avoided with appropriate primary and secondary prevention.

SUMMARY

Intraprofessional BHHV is a global issue. It is detrimental to nurses' well-being and organizational culture. It results in nursing dissatisfaction, increasing disengagement and absenteeism, intent to leave, and interrupts intraprofessional communication, and is a crucial component in medical errors and patient outcomes. The overall quality of available evidence on BHHV is limited; there particularly are few data-based intervention studies that provide foundational information useful for adoption by clinical settings. Although the reasons for this are open to conjecture, in part it may be due to the historic lack of public acknowledgement and/or unwillingness by hospital administrators to recognize or address BHHV. Future well-conducted studies are needed.

REFERENCES

Abe, K., & Henly, S. J. (2010). Bullying (ijime) among Japanese hospital nurses: Modeling responses to the revised Negative Acts Questionnaire. *Nursing Research, 59*(2), 110–118.

Albert, D. J., Walsh, M. L., Gorzalka, B. B., Siemens, Y., & Louie, H. (1986). Testosterone removal in rats results in a decrease in social aggression and a loss of social dominance. *Physiology & Behavior, 36*(3), 401–407.

Alexy, E. M., & Hutchins, J. A. (2006). Workplace violence: A primer for critical care nurses. *Critical Care Nursing Clinics of North America, 18*(3), 305–312.

American Association of Colleges of Nursing. (2004). *Hallmarks of quality and patient safety.* Retrieved from http://www.aacn.nche.edu/publications/pdf/Qual&PatientSafety.pdf

American Association of Critical-care Nurses. (2006). *Silence kills. The seven crucial conversations for healthcare.* Retrieved February 9, 2009, from www.aacn.org/WD/Practice/Docs/PublicPolicy/SilenceKills.pdf

American Hospital Association Commission on Workforce for Hospitals and Health Systems. (2002). *In our hands: How hospital leaders can build a thriving workforce.* Retrieved from http://www.eric.ed.gov/ERICDocs/data/ericdocs2sql/content_storage_01/0000019b/80/1b/03/62.pdf

American Nurses Association. (2001). *Analysis of the American Nurses Association staffing survey.* Warwick, RI: Cornerstone Communications Group.

American Organization of Nurse Executives. (2000). *Perspectives on the nursing shortage: A blueprint for action.* Washington, DC: Author.

Archer, J., & Coyne, S. M. (2005). An integrated review of indirect, relational, and social aggression. *Personality and Social Psychology Review, 9*(3), 212–230.

Armstrong, K. J., & Laschinger, H. (2006). Structural empowerment, Magnet hospital characteristics, and patient safety culture: Making the link. *Journal of Nursing Care Quality, 21*(2), 124–32, quiz 133.

Balducci, C., Alfano, V., & Fraccaroli, F. (2009). Relationships between mobbing at work and MMPI-2 personality profile, posttraumatic stress symptoms, and suicidal ideation and behavior. *Violence and Victims, 24*(1), 52–67.

Barrett, A., Piatek, C., Korber, S., & Padula, C. (2009). Lessons learned from a lateral violence and team-building intervention. *Nursing Administration Quarterly, 33*(4), 342–351.

Bigony, L., Lipke, T. G., Lundberg, A., McGraw, C. A., Pagac, G. L., & Rogers, A. (2009). Lateral violence in the perioperative setting. *AORN Journal, 89*(4), 688–96; quiz 697.

Blegen, M. A. (1993). Nurses' job satisfaction: A meta-analysis of related variables. *Nursing Research, 42*(1), 36–41.

Bowling, N. A., & Beehr, T. A. (2006). Workplace harassment from the victim's perspective: A theoretical model and meta-analysis. *The Journal of Applied Psychology, 91*(5), 998–1012.

Braun, K., Christle, D., Walker, D., & Tiwanak, G. (1991). Verbal abuse of nurses and non-nurses. *Nursing Management, 22*(3), 72–76.

Briles, J. (1999). *Women to women 2000: Becoming sabotage savvy in the new millennium.* Far Hills, NJ: New Horizon Press.

Broome, B. A. (2008). Dealing with sharks and bullies in the workplace. *The ABNF (Association of Black Nursing Faculty) Journal, 19*(1), 28–30.

Campbell, A. (2008). Attachment, aggression and affiliation: The role of oxytocin in female social behavior. *Biological Psychology, 77*(1), 1–10.

Center for American Nurses. (2008). *Bullying and lateral violence in the workplace.* Retrieved from http://centerforamericannurses.org/associations/9102/files/Position%20StatementLateral%20Violence%20and%20Bullying.pdf

Cirulli, E. T., Kasperaviciute, D., Attix, D. K., Need, A. C., Ge, D., Gibson, G., & Goldstein, D. B. (2010). Common genetic variation and performance on standardized cognitive tests. *European Journal of Human Genetics, 18*(7), 815–820.

Clark, P. A., Leddy, K., Drain, M., & Kaldenberg, D. (2007). State nursing shortages and patient satisfaction: More RNs–better patient experiences. *Journal of Nursing Care Quality, 22*(2), 119–27; quiz 128.

Cole, A. (1996). Fighting the bully. *The Health Service Journal, 106*(5485), 22–24.

Cooper, H. M., Hedges, L. V., & Valentine, J. C. (2009). *The handbook of research synthesis and meta-analysis* (2nd ed.). New York, NY: Russell Sage Foundation.

Corr, M. (2000). Reducing occupational stress in intensive care. *Nursing in Critical Care, 5*(2), 76–81.

Cortina, L. M., & Magley, V. J. (2003). Raising voice, risking retaliation: Events following interpersonal mistreatment in the workplace. *Journal of Occupational Health Psychology, 8*(4), 247–265.

Cox, H. C. (1987). Verbal abuse in nursing: Report of a study. *Nursing Management, 18*(11), 47–50.

Crick, N. R., Ostrov, J. M., & Werner, N. E. (2006). A longitudinal study of relational aggression, physical aggression, and children's social-psychological adjustment. *Journal of Abnormal Child Psychology, 34*(2), 131–142.

Deans, C. (2004). Nurses and occupational violence: The role of organizational support in moderating professional competence. *Australian Journal of Advanced Nursing, 22*(2), 15–18.

DeMarco, R. (1997). The relationship between family life and workplace behaviors: Exploring the gendered perceptions of staff nurses through the framework of systemic organization. (Doctoral Dissertation, Wayne State University, 1997). *Dissertation Abstracts International, 58* (3B), 9725823.

DeMarco, R. F. (1998). Caring to confront in the workplace: An ethical perspective for nurses. *Nursing Outlook, 46*(3), 130–135.

DeMarco, R. F. (2002). Two theories/a sharper lens: The staff nurse voice in the workplace. *Journal of Advanced Nursing, 38*(6), 1–8.

DeMarco, R. F., & Roberts, S. J. (2003). Negative behaviors in nursing. *The American Journal of Nursing, 103*(3), 113–116

DeMarco, R. F., Roberts, S. J., & Chandler, G. E. (2005). The use of a writing group to enhance voice and connection among staff nurses. *Journal for Nurses in Staff Development, 21*(3), 85–90; quiz 91.

Di Rosa, A. E., Gangemi, S., Cristani, M., Fenga, C., Saitta, S., Abenavoli, E.,…Cimino, F. (2009). Serum levels of carbonylated and nitrosylated proteins in mobbing victims with workplace adjustment disorders. *Biological Psychology, 82*(3), 308–311.

Duddle, M., & Boughton, M. (2007). Intraprofessional relations in nursing. *Journal of Advanced Nursing, 59*(1), 29–37.

Dunn, H. (2003). Horizontal violence among nurses in the operating room. *AORN Journal, 78*(6), 977–988.

Embree, J. L., & White, A. H. (2010). Concept analysis: Nurse-to-nurse lateral violence. *Nursing Forum, 45*(3), 166–173.

Farrell, G. A. (1997). Aggression in clinical settings: Nurses' views. *Journal of Advanced Nursing, 25*(3), 501–508.

Farrell, G. A. (1999). Aggression in clinical settings: Nurses' views—A follow-up study. *Journal of Advanced Nursing, 29*(3), 532–541.

Farrell, G. A., Bobrowski, C., & Bobrowski, P. (2006). Scoping workplace aggression in nursing: Findings from an Australian study. *Journal of Advanced Nursing, 55*(6), 778–787.

Farrington, D. (1993). Understanding and preventing bullying. *Crime and Justice, 17,* 381–458.

Ferns, T., & Chojnacka, I. (2005). Reporting incidents of violence and aggression towards NHS staff. *Nursing Standard (Royal College of Nursing [Great Britain]: 1987), 19*(38), 51–56.

Freire, P. (2000). *Pedagogy of the oppressed.* New York, NY: Continuum.

Galen, B. R., & Underwood, M. K. (1997). A developmental investigation of social aggression among children. *Developmental Psychology, 33*(4), 589–600.

Gillen, P. (2002). A concept analysis of bullying in midwifery. *Midwifery, 2*(2), 46–51.

Gilmour, D., & Hamlin, L. (2003). Bullying and harassment in perioperative settings. *British Journal of Perioperative Nursing: the Journal of the National Association of Theatre Nurses, 13*(2), 79–85.

Graveson, G. (1998). Workplace bullying–the abuse of power. *The British Journal of Theatre Nursing, 7*(11), 21–23.

Griffin, M. (2004). Teaching cognitive rehearsal as a shield for lateral violence: An intervention for newly licensed nurses. *Journal of Continuing Education in Nursing, 35*(6), 257–263.

Gunnarsdottir, H. K., Sveinsdottir, H., Bernburg, J. G., Fridriksdottir, H., & Tomasson, K. (2006). Lifestyle, harassment at work and self-assessed health of female flight attendants, nurses and teachers. *Work (Reading, Mass.), 27*(2), 165–172.

Hansen, A. M., Hogh, A., Persson, R., Karlson, B., Garde, A. H., & Ørbaek, P. (2006). Bullying at work, health outcomes, and physiological stress response. *Journal of Psychosomatic Research, 60*(1), 63–72.

Hauge, L. J., Skogstad, A., & Einarsen, S. (2007) Relationships between stressful work environments and bullying: Results of a large representative study. *Work & Stress, 21,* 220–242.

Hegney, D., Eley, R., Plank, A., Buikstra, E., & Parker, V. (2006). Workplace violence in Queensland, Australia: The results of a comparative study. *International Journal of Nursing Practice, 12*(4), 220–231.

Hegyvary, S. T., & Haussman, R. K. (1976). Correlates of the quality of nursing care. *The Journal of Nursing Administration, 6*(9), 22–27.

Hershcovis, M. S., Turner, N., Barling, J., Arnold, K. A., Dupré, K. E., Inness, M., . . . Sivanathan, N. (2007). Predicting workplace aggression: A meta-analysis. *The Journal of Applied Psychology*, 92(1), 228–238.

Hughes, A. (2003). Being bullied what an insight. *British Journal of Perioperative Nursing*, 13(4), 166–8, 171.

Hutchinson, M. (2009). Restorative approaches to workplace bullying: Educating nurses towards shared responsibility. *Contemporary Nurse: A Journal for the Australian Nursing Profession*, 32(1–2), 147–155.

Hutchinson, M., Vickers, M., Jackson, D., & Wilkes, L. (2006). Workplace bullying in nursing: Towards a more critical organisational perspective. *Nursing Inquiry*, 13(2), 118–126.

Hutchinson, M., Wilkes, L., Vickers, M., & Jackson, D. (2008). The development and validation of a bullying inventory for the nursing workplace. *Nurse Researcher*, 15(2), 19–29.

Hutchinson, M., Wilkes, L., Jackson, D., & Vickers, M. H. (2010). Integrating individual, work group and organizational factors: Testing a multidimensional model of bullying in the nursing workplace. *Journal of Nursing Management*, 18(2), 173–181.

Institute for Safe Medication Practices. (2009). *Results from ISMP Survey on Workplace Intimidation*. Retrieved January 9, 2009, from https://www.ismp.org/Survey/surveyResults/Survey0311. asp

Jack, D. C. (1993). *Silencing the self: Women and depression*. New York, NY: Harper Perennial.

Jack, D. C. (1999). *Behind the mask: Destruction and creativity in women's aggression*. Cambridge, MA: Harvard University.

Jack, D. C., & Ali, A. (2010). *Silencing the self across cultures: Depression and gender in the social world*. New York, NY: Oxford.

Jackson, D., Clare, J., & Mannix, J. (2002). Who would want to be a nurse? Violence in the workplace–a factor in recruitment and retention. *Journal of Nursing Management*, 10(1), 13–20.

Joint Commission. (2008, July 9). Sentinel Event alert. *Behaviors that undermine a culture of safety*. Retrieved August 10, 2008, from http://www.jointcommission.org/SentinelEvents/SentinelEventAlert/sea_40.htm

Kessler, S. R., Spector, P. E., Chang, C., & Parr, A. D. (2008). Organizational violence and aggression: Development of the three-factor violence climate survey. *Work and Stress*, 108–224.

Kiriakidis, S. P., & Kavoura, A. (2010). Cyberbullying: A review of the literature on harassment through the internet and other electronic means. *Family & Community Health*, 33(2), 82–93.

Kivimäki, M., Elovainio, M., & Vahtera, J. (2000). Workplace bullying and sickness absence in hospital staff. *Occupational and Environmental Medicine*, 57(10), 656–660.

Kudielka, B. M., & Kern S. (2004). Cortisol day profiles in victims of mobbing (bullying at the work place): Preliminary results of a first psychobiological field study. *Journal of Psychosomatic Research*, 56(1), 149–50.

Kwok, R. P., Law, Y. K., Li, K. E., Ng, Y. C., Cheung, M. H., Fung, V. K., . . . Leung, W. C. (2006). Prevalence of workplace violence against nurses in Hong Kong. *Hong Kong Medical Journal*, 12(1), 6–9.

Leer, R. E. (2006). *Effective nursing management: A solution for nurses' job dissatisfaction and low retention rate?* Doctoral dissertation, Capella University, Minneapolis.

Leivers, G. (2004). Harassment by staff in the workplace: The experiences of midwives. *MIDRS Midwifery Digest*, 14, 19–24.

Lewis, M. A. (2006). Nurse bullying: Organizational considerations in the maintenance and perpetration of health care bullying cultures. *Journal of Nursing Management*, 14(1), 52–58.

Long, J. (1996). Battle of the bullies. *Nursing Management*, 3(6), 10–11.

Longo, J. (2007). *Bullying in the workplace: Reversing a culture*. Silver Spring, MD: Center for American Nurses.

Lupien, S. J., McEwen, B. S., Gunnar, M. R., & Heim, C. (2009). Effects of stress throughout the lifespan on the brain, behaviour and cognition. *Nature Reviews Neuroscience, 10,* 434–445.

MacIntosh, J. (2005). Experiences of workplace bullying in a rural area. *Issues in Mental Health Nursing, 26*(9), 893–910.

Mayhew, C., & Chappell, D. (2002a). Bullying and the healthcare workforce. *Lamp, 59*(7), 29–30.

Mayhew, C., & Chappell, D. (2002b). *Occupational violence in the NSW health workforce: Establishment of baseline data, report to the Taskforce on the Prevention and Management of Violence in the Health Workforce.* NSW Department of Health, Sydney.

McCarthy, S. (2008). Post-traumatic Stress Diagnostic Scale (PDS). *Occupational Medicine (Oxford, England), 58*(5), 379.

McKenna, B. G., Smith, N. A., Poole, S. J., & Coverdale, J. H. (2003). Horizontal violence: Experiences of Registered Nurses in their first year of practice. *Journal of Advanced Nursing, 42*(1), 90–96.

McMillan, J. (1995). Losing control. *Nursing Times, 91,* 40–43.

McVicar, A. (2003). Workplace stress in nursing: A literature review. *Journal of Advanced Nursing, 44*(6), 633–642.

Melnyk, B. M., & Fineout-Overholt, E. (2005). *Evidence-based practice in nursing & healthcare: A guide to best practice.* Philadelphia, PA: Lippincott Williams & Wilkins.

Monteleone, P., Nolfe, G., Serritella, C., Milano, V., Di Cerbo, A., Blasi, F., . . . Maj, M. (2009). Hypoactivity of the hypothalamo-pituitary-adrenal axis in victims of mobbing: Role of the subjects' temperament and chronicity of the work-related psychological distress. *Psychotherapy and Psychosomatics, 78*(6), 381–383.

Moyad, F. A., Daraiseh, N., Shell, R. & Salem, S. (2006). Workplace bullying: A systematic review of risk factors and outcomes. *Theoretical Issues in Ergonomics Science, 7,* 311–327.

National Advisory Council on Nurse Education and Practice. (2007). *Violence against nurses. An assessment of the causes and impacts of violence in nursing education and practice* (5th ed.). Retrieved February 1, 2009, from http://bhpr.hrsa.gov/nursing/NACNEP/reports/fifth/status.htm

National Institute for Occupational Safety and Health. (2002). *Violence. Occupational hazards in hospitals* (DHHS [NIOSH] Publication # 2002–101). Retrieved from http://www.cdc.gov/niosh/2002-101.html

Normandale, S., & Davies, J. (2002). Bullying at work. *Community Practitioner, 75,* 474–477.

Olff, M., Langeland, W., & Gersons, B. P. (2005). Effects of appraisal and coping on the neuroendocrine response to extreme stress. *Neuroscience and Biobehavioral Reviews, 29*(3), 457–467.

Pearson, A., Laschinger, J., Porritt, K., Jordan, Z., Tucker, D., & Long, L. (2004). A comprehensive systematic review of evidence on developing and sustaining nursing leadership that fosters a healthy work environment in health care. *Health Care Reports, 2*(7), 129–192.

Quine, L. (1999). Workplace bullying in NHS community trust: Staff questionnaire survey. *BMJ (Clinical Research Ed.), 318*(7178), 228–232.

Quine, L. (2001). Workplace bullying in nurses. *Journal of Health Psychology, 6,* 73–84.

Randle, J. (2003). Bullying in the nursing profession. *Journal of Advanced Nursing, 43*(4), 395–401.

Rayner, C., & Hoel, H. (1998). A summary review of literature relating to workplace bullying. *Journal of Community and Applied Social Psychology, 7,* 181–191.

Roberts, S. J. (1983). Oppressed group behavior: Implications for nursing. *ANS. Advances in Nursing Science, 5*(4), 21–30.

Roberts, S. J. (1996). Breaking the cycle of oppression: Lessons for nurse practitioners? *Journal of the American Academy of Nurse Practitioners, 8*(5), 209–214.

Roberts, S. J. (1997). Nurse executives in the 1990s: Empowered or oppressed? *Nursing Administration Quarterly, 22*(1), 64–71.

Roberts, S., DeMarco, R. F., & Griffin, M. (2009). The effect of oppressed group behavior on the culture of the nursing workplace: A review of evidence and interventions for change. *Journal of Nursing Management, 17*(3), 288–293.

Roche, M., Diers, D., Duffield, C., & Catling-Paull, C. (2010). Violence toward nurses, the work environment, and patient outcomes. *Journal of Nursing Scholarship, 42*(1), 13–22.

Rocker, C. F. (2008). Addressing nurse-to-nurse bullying to promote nurse retention. *Online Journal of Issues in Nursing, 13*(3). Retrieved from http://www.nursingworld. org/MainMenuCategories/ANAMarketplace/ANAPeriodicals/OJIN/TableofContents/ vol132008/No3Sept08/ArticlePreviousTopic/NursetoNurseBullying.aspx

Rowe, M. M., & Sherlock, H. (2005). Stress and verbal abuse in nursing: Do burned out nurses eat their young? *Journal of Nursing Management, 13*(3), 242–248.

Royal College of Nursing. (2002). *Working well: A call to employers. A summary of the RCN's Working well survey into the wellbeing and working lives of nurses.* London: RCN.

Rutherford, A., & Rissel, C. (2004). A survey of workplace bullying in a health sector organisation. *Australian Health Review, 28*(1), 65–72.

Sellers, K., Millenbach, L., Kovach, N., & Yingling, J. K. (2009). The prevalence of horizontal violence in New York State registered nurses. *The Journal of the New York State Nurses' Association, 40*(2), 20–25.

Simons, S. (2008). Workplace bullying experienced by Massachusetts registered nurses and the relationship to intention to leave the organization. *ANS. Advances in Nursing Science, 31*(2), E48–E59.

Simons, S. R., & Mawn, B. (2010). Bullying in the workplace—A qualitative study of newly licensed registered nurses. *American Association of Occupational Health Nurses, 58*(7), 305–311.

Sofield, L., & Salmond, S. W. (2003). Workplace violence. A focus on verbal abuse and intent to leave the organization. *Orthopaedic Nursing/National Association of Orthopaedic Nurses, 22*(4), 274–283.

Stanley, K. M., Martin, M. M., Nemeth, L. S., Michel, Y., & Welton, J. M. (2007). Examining lateral violence in the nursing workforce. *Issues in Mental Health Nursing, 28*(11), 1247–1265.

Stearley, H. (1997). Desensitization to nurse abuse. *Revolution (Staten Island, NY), 7*(4), 23–27.

Stevens, S. (2002). Nursing workforce retention: Challenging a bullying culture. *Health Affairs (Project Hope), 21*(5), 189–193.

Terburg, D., Morgan, B., & van Honk, J. (2009). The testosterone-cortisol ratio: A hormonal marker for proneness to social aggression. *International Journal of Law and Psychiatry, 32*(4), 216–223.

Underwood, M. K. (2003). *Social aggression among girls.* New York: The Guilford Press.

Upstate Lateral Violence in Nursing Project (C. Luciano, PD). Department of Health and Human Services, Health Services Resource Administration, Bureau of Health Professions, Nurses Education, Practice, and Research (NEPR) grant (award # is 5 D11HP08361).

U.S. Health Resources Services Administration. (2002). *Projected supply, demand, and shortages of registered nurses: 2000–2020.* Retrieved from http://bhpr.hrsa.gov/healthworkforce/rnproject

Vessey, J. A., Demarco, R. F., Gaffney, D. A., & Budin, W. C. (2009). Bullying of staff registered nurses in the workplace: A preliminary study for developing personal and organizational strategies for the transformation of hostile to healthy workplace environments. *Journal of Professional Nursing, 25*(5), 299–306.

Wallace, R. B. (Ed.). (2008). *Wallace/Maxcy-Rosenau-Last public health & preventive medicine* (15th ed.). Philadelphia, PA: McGraw-Hill.

Weisman, C. S., & Nathanson, C. A. (1985). Professional satisfaction and client outcomes. A comparative organizational analysis. *Medical Care, 23*(10), 1179–1192.

Wiskow, C. (2002). *Framework guidelines for addressing workplace violence in the health sector.* Geneva, Switzerland: The International Labour Office, the World Health Organization, The International Council of Nurses, and Public Services International. Retrieved January 22, 2009, from http://www.ilo.org/public/english/dialogue/sector/papers/health/guidelines.pdf

Woelfle, C. Y., & McCaffrey, R. (2007). Nurse on nurse. *Nursing Forum, 42*(3), 123–131.

World Health Organization. (2002). *World report on violence and health.* Geneva, Switzerland: Author.

Yildirim, D. (2009). Bullying among nurses and its effects. *International Nursing Review, 56*(4), 504–511.

CHAPTER 7

Interdisciplinary Teamwork and Collaboration

An Essential Element of a Positive Practice Environment

Patricia Reid Ponte, Anne H. Gross,
Yolanda J. Milliman-Richard, and Kara Lacey

ABSTRACT

Interdisciplinary collaboration is critical to excellence in patient care delivery. There is a growing consensus that the basic education for all clinical professionals should include the knowledge, skills, and attitudes required to effectively participate in interdisciplinary teams, and that health care organizations should continue this education in the practice setting. The authors examine the large and growing evidence base regarding interdisciplinary collaboration and teamwork and explore the relationship between interdisciplinary collaboration and patient, workforce, and organizational outcomes. Antecedents and attributes of the construct are presented, as well as structures, models, and programs that are being implemented by health care organizations and academic settings to facilitate and advance interdisciplinary collaboration in clinical practice.

Over the past decade, nursing and other clinical professions have embraced the principles of interdisciplinary collaboration. Within health care organizations,

© 2011 Springer Publishing Company
DOI: 10.1891/0739-6686.28.159

interdisciplinary collaboration is critical to patient care as well as strategic planning and quality and safety initiatives. Within both service and academe, there is a growing consensus that the basic education for all clinical professionals should include the knowledge, skills, and attitudes required to effectively participate in interdisciplinary teams, and that health care organizations should continue this education in the practice setting. And within the research community, there is a growing focus on advancing interdisciplinary research with the understanding that this approach yields stronger idea generation, methods, and study outcomes (Woods & Magyary, 2010).

Interdisciplinary collaboration is also a central feature of many programs and initiatives advanced by professional associations. The American Nurses Credentialing Center's (ANCC) Magnet Recognition Program; the Malcolm Baldrige National Quality Award; the American Association of Critical-Care Nurses Beacon Award; the American Organization of Nurse Executives Principles of a Healthful Practice Environment; the Agency for Healthcare Research and Quality (AHRQ) TeamSTEPPS Program; and the Institute for Healthcare Improvement/ Robert Wood Johnson Transforming Care at the Bedside initiative are just some of the programs promoting standards and frameworks that advance practice and organizational cultures steeped in inclusion, shared decision making, equity, and teamwork.

Underlying this push for greater interdisciplinary collaboration is the premise that safety, quality, and efficiency in patient care delivery is bolstered by structures and processes that equalize the status of clinicians on the care team, and that promote interdisciplinary collaboration and teamwork while reducing or eliminating traditional hierarchical systems and cultures. This premise is supported by research on positive practice environments conducted by Aiken and colleagues (2002, 2009), Drenkard (2010), Havens (2001), McClure, Poulin, Sovie, and Wandelt (2002), and Kalisch (2010). Additionally, the application of crew resource management (CRM) concepts in the aviation industry resulted in important understanding about human behavior, risk mitigation, safety and human factors that contribute to error. This knowledge was transferred into the health care industry following the tragic deaths of patients from a chemotherapy overdose in 1995 (Clarke & Aiken, 2003; Connor et al., 2007; Conway et al., 2007). The premise is further endorsed by a series of reports from the Institute of Medicine (IOM, 1999, 2001, 2004) that identify interdisciplinary collaboration as a key element of a culture of safety and quality improvement efforts.

In this article, the authors examine the large and growing evidence base regarding interdisciplinary collaboration and teamwork. In addition to exploring the relationship between interdisciplinary collaboration and patient, workforce, and organizational outcomes, it examines antecedents and attributes of the construct, as well as structures, models, and programs that are being implemented by health care organizations and academic settings to facilitate and advance interdisciplinary collaboration in clinical practice.

LITERATURE REVIEW METHODS

Several terms are used in the current literature to address similar concepts related to collaboration across disciplines. These include: interdisciplinary, multidisciplinary, transdisciplinary, and interprofessional. Each term was closely examined in preparation for this literature review.

Tress, Gunther, and Fry (2006) and Cronin (2008) provide definitions for these concepts within the context of the research process. They define *disciplinary* studies as those that take place within the bounds of a single currently recognized academic discipline, while *multidisciplinary* studies involve several different academic disciplines researching one theme or problem but with multiple disciplinary goals. In multidisciplinary studies, participants exchange knowledge, but do not aim to cross subject boundaries to create new knowledge and theory. The research process progresses as parallel disciplinary efforts without integration but usually with the aim to compare results. *Interdisciplinary* studies involve connections being made across disciplinary boundaries; several unrelated academic disciplines are involved in a way that forces them to cross subject boundaries to create new knowledge and theory and solve a common research goal. *Transdisciplinary* studies integrate academic researchers from unrelated disciplines, and nonacademic participants such as land managers and the public, to research a common goal and create new knowledge and theory. Transdisciplinary research involves a range of approaches that may result in the breaking down of disciplinary boundaries and the introduction of nondisciplinary knowledge from external stakeholders. Klein (2007) notes that because of these diverse perspectives transdisciplinary research has the potential to create new knowledge frameworks and an overarching synthesis, which may in turn lead to a "transcendent" process of knowledge production.

The concept of *interprofessional* collaboration is explored by Clarke (2006) in the context of the educational process. Interprofessional collaboration occurs when students from various professions learn from and about each other to improve collaboration and the quality of care. The students' interactions are characterized by integration and modification reflecting participants' understanding of the core principles and concepts of each contributing discipline and familiarity with the basic language and mindsets of the various disciplines.

Within the clinical context, *interdisciplinary* collaboration has been defined as "a group of discipline-specific clinicians who relate on a routine basis to each other for the purpose of patient- and family-centered care delivery within a particular practice, unit, or program. These clinicians are typically: nurses, physicians, social workers, pharmacists, psychologists, chaplains, nutritionists, physical therapists, and occupational therapists. Given its link to clinical practice, the authors chose the construct "interdisciplinary" as the operational definition for this review; however, because interdisciplinary, multidisciplinary, transdisciplinary, and interprofessional are sometimes used interchangeably in the literature, all of these terms were used to identify eligible articles for review.

INCLUSION CRITERIA

The literature review focused on articles published in the past decade (2000–2010). Consistent with the authors' practice setting and experience and the overall aim of this paper, the articles selected for inclusion focused on one of the following three areas: (1) training and development necessary to assure that clinicians have the required knowledge, skills, and attitudes to provide interdisciplinary care and work as a team to deliver care; (2) health care organizational initiatives to advance interdisciplinary care and teamwork in the delivery of care; (3) research studies that demonstrated or attempted to demonstrate the relationship between effective interdisciplinary care and teamwork and patient, workforce, or organizational outcomes.

SEARCH STRATEGIES AND CRITIQUE METHODS

Searches of the CINAHL and PubMed databases using EBSCO were conducted using the following keywords: interdisciplinary, multidisciplinary, trans-disciplinary, inter-professional, collaboration, teamwork, teaming, team training, outcomes, practice, and care. Each article was reviewed, summarized, and categorized according to: year of publication, the country of origin, the title of the paper and first author, the purpose of the paper and in the case of research studies and improvement projects, the purpose, population, design, methods/ instruments utilized and major themes/findings. A more limited search of the Medline database was also conducted to identify additional papers describing organizational structures and initiatives to advance interdisciplinary care and teamwork in the care delivery setting.

The authors assessed the quality of 68 papers using a rating system adapted from Cesario, Morin, and Santa-Donato (2002). Most of the papers were descriptive, describing programs of education or professional development, a quality improvement project, or a qualitative study that used interventions such as team training to improve team effectiveness. Outcome and process measures believed to be related to effective interdisciplinary teamwork and collaboration were usually used to assess the intervention's success. The authors ranked the papers using the following criteria: from 0 = *minimal new information or evidence*; 2 = *supports or adds to current evidence or practice*; 3 = *innovative or new approaches to assuring competency by clinicians in effective teamwork or collaboration*, or b) interventions resulted in positive patient outcomes (i.e., decreased length of stay, decreased hospital readmission rates, improved medication adherence, quality of life, symptom management); positive workforce outcomes (reduced turnover of staff, improved staff satisfaction, or perceptions of improved teamwork); or positive organizational outcomes (such as reduced medication errors, improved safety culture, decrease in missed nursing care, and decreased cost).

TRAINING AND DEVELOPMENT IN THE ACADEMIC AND SERVICE SETTINGS

Physicians, nurses, pharmacists, and other clinicians have historically worked in teams to care for patients and families, yet academic programs and healthcare organizations have only recently begun providing education and training to assure effective and efficient teamwork. The current literature offers numerous examples of approaches to teaching interdisciplinary teamwork for the purposes of increasing overall team satisfaction, efficiency, and quality of care. The recent increase in educational programming is likely related to recommendations made by the IOM in its 2003 report (IOM, 2003), *Health Professions Education: A Bridge to Quality*. In the report, the IOM identified the ability to work in effective interdisciplinary teams when caring for patients and families as a core competency for clinicians. The report's recommendations are based on the IOM's assessment of competencies needed by clinicians practicing in the current health care system environment to assure patient safety and clinical quality in the care they deliver.

One of the studies addressing teaching strategies in the academic setting was conducted by Hobgood, Sherwood, Frush, Hollar, and Maynard (2010) and involved a randomized controlled trial ($N = 438$). In the study, the researchers assessed changes in knowledge, skill, and attitude associated with four different pedagogical methods for delivering teamwork training adapted from the AHRQ TeamSTEPPS Patient Safety Program: didactic (control), audience response didactic, role play, and human patient simulation. Participants included 203 senior nursing students and 235 fourth year medical students. Each student was randomly assigned into one of the teaching methods and all students completed pre- and posttest surveys. All four cohorts demonstrated an increase in attitude and knowledge of teamwork; however, no single technique emerged as superior and none of the groups achieved a change in skill level. The study had several limitations in the area of design and measurement. Participants' content knowledge at pretesting was higher than anticipated and a tool for measuring specific team behaviors within the context of the TeamSTEPPS tool was not available. Additionally, the intervention's longitudinal effect on content retention by participants was not measured.

Simulation technology, which is now commonly used as a teaching and learning strategy in the nursing and medical professions, has also been used to develop collaboration skills among nursing and medical students. In a study conducted by Reese, Jeffries, and Engum (2010), 15 third-year medical students and 13 senior nursing students at a mid-western university in the United States were paired together in a simulation lab. The students were assigned to jointly assess and care for a patient who was deteriorating as a result of postoperative complications for a 20-minute period. Each student completed postsimulation surveys that used the Simulation Design Scale (Jeffries, 2007). High scores (mean 4.4 out of 5) were obtained for student perceptions that working well with another health care professional helped them provide higher quality care to the patient. Limitations of the study included sample size and design. Because there was no follow-up measurement of physician and nurse collaboration in real patient situations, the researchers were unable to evaluate whether the simulation intervention improved teamwork at the bedside. Hallin, Kiessling, Waldner, and Henriksson (2009) studied the effect of clinical teamwork training on perceived interprofessional competence. The study involved 616 undergraduate students enrolled in nursing, medicine, physiotherapy, and occupational therapy programs in Sweden between 2002 and 2005. Each of the students participated in an interprofessional training course on a patient care unit and completed pre and post training course surveys, measuring perceived interprofessional competence (response rate = 96%). The environment where the learning occurred was also assessed. Results indicated that all groups perceived an increase in their level of knowledge about each others' work ($p = .000$), and believed the training had contributed to their understanding of the importance of teamwork and communication in patient care ($p = .000$). The study's authors also concluded that the clinical unit where care was provided was an effective learning environment and conducive to increasing collaboration and professional competence in teamwork. However, measurement of interdisciplinary collaboration post intervention was not part of the study.

Dumont, Briere, Morin, Houle, and Iloko-Fundi (2010) studied faculty perceptions of inter-professional collaboration training, conducting an intervention among faculty in the school of Health Sciences at Laval University in

Quebec. The aim of the study was to increase faculty knowledge of interprofessional collaboration training and enhance their point of view regarding its benefits. Pre- and posttest results indicated an increase in faculty point of view following the intervention.

In the clinical setting, examples of adapting teamwork training methods from other industries to the health care environment are also beginning to emerge, with a focus on reducing medical error through improved communication, collaboration, and role clarification. Mann, Marcus, and Sachs (2006) successfully adapted concepts of CRM team training in the inpatient obstetrics environment. Neily and colleagues (2010) also successfully adapted CRM concepts in a team training initiative across 74 facilities in the Department of Veterans Affairs and reported an overall 18% decrease in surgical mortality rates after the intervention. Dodds et al. (2010) incorporated principles of interdisciplinary practice into their leadership curriculum for maternal and child health practitioners at the University of North Carolina, Chapel Hill, promoting increased competence and commitment to interdisciplinary practice among fellows who complete the program. Goldsmith, Wittenberg-Lyles, Rodriguez, and Sanchez-Reilly (2010) reported findings from a qualitative study of six interdisciplinary clinician team members in the geriatric and palliative care setting. One conclusion of this study was that using reflective narratives as a pedagogical tool can be a rich and beneficial means for helping team members understand one another's experiences and perceptions of teamwork. Of note were the divergent views within various disciplines about the effectiveness of teamwork and effectiveness within their group. These divergent views were also noted by Hansson, Arvemo, Marklund, Gedda, and Mattsson (2009) in their study of district nurses and general medical doctors providing primary care in Sweden. Mills, Neily, and Dunn (2008) also uncovered divergent views of level of collaboration and teamwork across disciplines when they administered the Medical Team Training (MTT) questionnaire to the members of a surgical team. The researchers noted that using the MTT questionnaire can help focus team training sessions on areas of need.

These and other studies highlight the benefits of interprofessional education and the importance of interprofessional learning for improved collaboration, communication, and teamwork. At the same time, it is worth noting an observation offered by Henderson, O'Keefe, and Alexander (2010), who cite the benefits of interprofessional education while cautioning that over-emphasizing it or over-attributing its successes should be done with reservation until clearer outcomes are available.

To provide the reader with ease of access to examples of current curricula and training methods found in the literature, Table 7.1 follows.

TABLE 7.1
Curricula

Author	Program	Organization	Content Development	Content and Structure	Evaluation
Dodd et al. (2009)	Maternal Child Health (MCH) Leadership Training Consortium	University of North Carolina, Chapel Hill (UNC-CH)	Faculty from various disciplines in the MCH Consortium	Instructional over academic year include orientation, leadership workshop, conflict resolution/facilitation, cultural competence, family-professional collaboration, leadership reflection.	Qualitative feedback from participants and faculty.
Dumont et al. (2010)	Patient-Centered Care: Better Training for Better Collaboration Program	University of Laval, Quebec City Canada	Faculty in Schools of Nursing, Medicine and Social Work	45 hours of classroom time; designed for students to acquire knowledge, skills and attitudes specific to five prioritized skill sets: (1) participation and partnership with patients and families; (2) interaction skills; (3) professional roles and responsibilities; (4) collaboration; (5) reflection.	Student self-administered Likert questionnaire using a 5-point scale.
Hallin et al. (2009)	Interprofessional Clinical Education Ward (CEW) Teamwork Training	Karolinska Institute, Danderyd Hospital, Stockholm, Sweden	Faculty in schools of medicine, nursing, occupational therapy and physiotherapy	2-week training course on clinical unit; training occurred on specified CEWs with real patients receiving care; students were divided into teams with faculty from each discipline serving as mentors.	Student evaluations questionnaires at the end of each training.

AHRQ.gov, November 12, 2010	TeamSTEPPS	Agency for Healthcare Research and Quality (AHRQ)	Department of Defense Patient Safety Program in conjunction the AHRQ	3-Phase approach which can be "dosed" according to organization's need: (1) Organizational Assessment, (2) Planning, Training, Intervention, (3) Sustainment. The Training program consists of a 2.5 day "Train the Trainer" workshop followed by a 4–6 hour "Fundamentals" workshop for clinical staff and a 1–2 hour "Essentials" workshop for nonclinical staff.	Pre- and post-training measurement of staff satisfaction and knowledge; ongoing measurement of impact on processes and outcomes.
	Veterans Health Administration (VHA) Medical Team Training	VHA	Adaptation of crew resource management theory from the aviation industry and in coordination with the VHA Surgical Quality Improvement Program	Learning session (lecture, interaction, video instruction); 4 quarterly follow-up structured telephone interviews for 1 year to provide coaching, support, and assessment of the medical team training implementation.	Measurement of pre- and post-training surgical mortality rates.

ORGANIZATIONAL MODELS AND STRUCTURES THAT ADVANCE INTERDISCIPLINARY COLLABORATION AND TEAMWORK

There is increasing reference in the literature to the role of interdisciplinary leadership in shaping an environment of transparency, collaboration, and equal partnering and accountability in the oversight of clinical services. Reid Ponte, Gross, Winer, Connaughton, and Hassinger (2007) describe the role of a triad model of leadership (physician, nurse, and administrator) in supporting effective team collaboration, decision making, priority setting, patient safety, and patient- and family-centered care. Richardson and Storr (2010) focused on the role of leadership, interdisciplinary working, advocacy, empowerment, and collaboration in assuring patient safety, and identified gaps in the level of influence, leadership, and empowerment held by nurses and the potential for improving this inequity.

Other researchers have focused on identifying models that promote collaboration and partnership at the level of the care team. In a descriptive study using exemplars from staff on several inpatient units at the Hospital of the University of Pennsylvania, Dietrich and colleagues (2010) identify shared governance and peer review as models that are helpful in promoting partnership and learning and improving quality of care. O'Leary et al. (2010) conducted a controlled trial to evaluate the impact of structured interdisciplinary rounds. In the study, usual communication methods were maintained on one unit (the control unit), while interdisciplinary rounds were implemented on another (the intervention unit).In post intervention surveys, staff on the intervention unit reported improvements in the quality of interdisciplinary communication and collaboration. Vogwill and Reeves (2008) observed multidisciplinary rounds on an inpatient unit in a large medical center in Canada and concluded that communication among interdisciplinary colleagues could be streamlined and enhanced with the use of structured processes to facilitate the exchange of information. Lown and Manning (2010) examined the effects of Schwartz Center Rounds, an interdisciplinary forum where attendees discuss psychosocial and emotional aspects of patient care. Through retrospective surveys, they found that clinicians participating in Schwartz Center Rounds reported better teamwork and a heightened appreciation of the roles and contributions of colleagues. The researchers also found that the more rounds individuals attended, the greater was the impact on teamwork.

While these articles offer some information about organizational structures and models that promote interdisciplinary collaboration, the literature review makes it clear that such models are in a nascent form industry-wide. Additional research is needed to identify other structures that advance interdisciplinary collaboration, as well as tools capable of measuring important attributes, antecedents, and consequences.

INTERDISCIPLINARY TEAMWORK AND COLLABORATION AND PATIENT, WORKFORCE, AND ORGANIZATIONAL OUTCOMES

Understanding the costs, effectiveness, and impact of interdisciplinary collaboration and teamwork in the health care arena has been a topic of interest and research for at least three decades across multiple disciplines. In 2001, Schmitt reviewed past research efforts on the effectiveness of team care, summarizing methodological and conceptual challenges encountered by researchers, gaps in the available evidence, and directions for future research. The summary included 10 studies on the effectiveness of team care, conducted between 1950 and 1985, and described the study settings and outcomes relative to costs and patient morbidity and mortality. Eleven studies of geriatric team care interventions were also included, with descriptions of the settings, participant characteristics, and cost and mortality outcomes. With each study, Schmitt critiqued the methods, design, subject selection, measurement of collaboration, and outcome evaluation. Schmitt also provided a brief summary of selected studies reported in the literature between 1985 and 2000. The Schmitt review revealed slow progress between the 1950s and 1990s in advancing theoretical models of interdisciplinary teams, conducting rigorous research on the efficacy of these models, and effectively measuring their outcomes. The limitations that were identified related to the conceptualization and measurement of team collaboration. There was variable reporting of outcomes, possibly due to the difficulty of consistently measuring the amount, type, and duration of team interventions. Although a body of knowledge on team effectiveness began to emerge by 2000, it focused largely on the inpatient, hospital-based setting, with much of the work being conducted in intensive care units. Randomized clinical trials were scarce, issues with measuring collaboration remained a problem, and outcome measurement was still an area for improvement. These methodological issues continue today.

More recently, Manser (2009) conducted a review of current teamwork research in areas of high risk medical care such as operating rooms, intensive care units, emergency departments, and trauma resuscitation teams. This review supported the relationship between effective teamwork and patient safety and recommended further study in the following areas: (1) investigations of interdisciplinary collaboration and teamwork factors that contribute to adverse events; (2) staff perceptions of teamwork within their teams; and (3) observational studies of teamwork behaviors related to high clinical performance and outcomes.

Petri (2010) offers an overview of the meaning of interdisciplinary collaboration in health care settings using Rodger's Evolutionary View of Concept Analysis to identify attributes, antecedents, and consequences of interdisciplinary collaboration, and also calls for future research on the development of robust measures to evaluate it. Fennell, Prabhu Das, Clauser, Petrelli, and Salner (2010) described the impact of various types of multidisciplinary care team structures on quality of treatment and care and proposed a conceptual model for effective multidisciplinary oncology care teams using Donabedian's (2000) approach of structure, process, and outcome as a foundation for measuring the impact of multidisciplinary teams on patient outcomes.

Individual studies examining the effects of interdisciplinary collaboration on patient outcomes include one by O'Mahony, Mazur, Charney, Wang, and Fine (2007), which assessed the impact of interdisciplinary rounds and determined that adjusted average length of stay decreased after rounds were introduced. Chung and Nguyen (2005) found that introducing an interdisciplinary team focused on pain management yielded improvements in patient satisfaction after only three months. Pratt and colleagues (2007) adapted the CRM concepts to team training in the obstetrics environment and reported a 23% reduction the incidence of adverse outcomes over four years as well as an improvement in the satisfaction of all team members.

Table 7.2 outlines literature that explores organizational models and training approaches to interdisciplinary teamwork.

INSTRUMENTATION

Instruments designed to measure perception of teamwork by team members, measures of effective interdisciplinary collaboration by individuals (some proxy measures) and team member's knowledge and skill in teamwork behavior are beginning to emerge in the health care literature. Many of the available instruments and the programs that have been designed to use them are adapted from the TeamSTEPPs program developed by the Department of Defense and the AHRQ and/or based on CRM principles developed and promulgated from the aviation industry. Table 7.3 outlines instruments that measure outcomes of effective interdisciplinary collaboration and teamwork.

DISCUSSION

Research conducted in the last decade has broadened our understanding of interdisciplinary collaboration, including how it can be promoted and advanced by educational and organizational structures and how it affects patient outcomes. However even with this progress, much additional work is needed.

In the area of education, formalized models and programs of training in the principles and practices of interdisciplinary team collaboration, including the Team STEPPS approach, unit-based interprofessional training programs, and simulation lab team training, are increasingly being incorporated into the curricula of academic programs and offered by continuing education departments

TABLE 7.2

Organizational Models and Training Approach

Author	Purpose	Population	Research Design	Instruments or Methods	Findings
Dodds et al. (2010)	To describe the University of North Carolina/Chapel Hill, Maternal Child Health (UNC-CH MCH) Leadership Consortium—collaboration among five MCH-funded training programs—and to delineate the evolution of the leadership curriculum developed by the Consortium created to cultivate interdisciplinary MCH leaders.	The UNC-CH MCH Leadership Consortium	Descriptive Report of an Educational training and Improvement Initiative ($N = 150$ trainees).	Quantitative and qualitative process evaluations	The interdisciplinary leadership curriculum developed by the Consortium has allowed fellows to emerge as competent practitioners and leaders who are committed to interdisciplinary practice and through continuous quality improvement methods of evaluation, the program has adapted to meet the changing needs of trainees who participate in the program.
Dumont et al. (2010)	Describe the purpose, implementation, results, and evaluation of a series of courses for faculty in interprofessional collaboration.	215 faculty from the School of Health Sciences at Laval University, Quebec	Intervention study using pre/posttest measurement to describe the effect of an educational intervention on knowledge and skills regarding the benefits of interprofessional collaboration.	Investigator derived curricula based on inventory of existing courses and methodologies of teaching teamwork	Postintervention surveys showed an increase in point of view regarding knowledge and benefit of interprofessional collaboration training.

(Continued)

TABLE 7.2

Organizational Models and Training Approach *(Continued)*

Author	Purpose	Population	Research Design	Instruments or Methods	Findings
Goldsmith et al. (2010)	To examine the nature and process of interdisciplinary teamwork in geriatric and palliative care settings.	Six interdisciplinary care team members participating in a one year fellowship in Interdisciplinary teamwork (IDT).	Qualitative study; semistructured, taped interviews with each team member utilizing open-ended questioning to promote reflective narrative.		The functional reflective narrative analysis revealed specific themes that demonstrated divergent experience/perception amongst team members in their conceptualization of teamwork and effectiveness and described the collaborative nature of teams. Reflective narratives are a useful tool in team training.
Hallin et al. (2010)	To evaluate whether students perceived that they had achieved interprofessional competence after participating in clinical teamwork training.	616 students from four undergraduate educational programs (medicine, nursing, physiotherapy, and occupational therapy) at a university hospital in Stockholm, Sweden.	Quantitative study	Study outcomes were measured by responses from student evaluation questionnaires following the completion of unit-based interprofessional trainings. The study commenced in the autumn term 2002 and was completed in the spring term	Active patient-based learning by working together in a real unit-based context seemed to be an effective means to increase collaboration and professional competence.

			Commentary	
Henderson et al. (2010)	To explore the value of interprofessional education (IPE) in Australia, which has been described as a response to widespread calls for improved communication and collaboration between health care professionals.			Although there is much that is commendable in IPE, the authors caution that the benefits may be overstated if too much is attributed to, or expected of, IPE activities. Engagement with clinicians in the clinical practice setting who are instrumental in assisting students make sense of their knowledge through practice, is imperative for sustainable outcomes.
Hobgood et al. (2010)	To test student acquisition of knowledge, skill, and attitudes in each of four pedagogical methods for delivering teamwork training.	203 senior nursing students and 235 fourth year medical students.	Randomized controlled trial utilizing one of four education methods: didactic (control), audience response didactic, role-play, human patient simulation, to teach teamwork training to nursing and medical students. The methods were evaluated	All four cohorts demonstrated improvement in attitude and knowledge. However, no educational technique appeared to be superior nor resulted in a change in teamwork skill.

(Continued)

TABLE 7.2

Organizational Models and Training Approach (*Continued*)

Author	Purpose	Population	Research Design	Instruments or Methods	Findings
			using a series of 4 surveys (pre/post training) measuring attitudes, knowledge, skills and performance.		
Interdisciplinary Teams: Models/Components					
Dietrich et al. (2010)	To describe the components necessary to form successful partnerships using the Hospital of the University of Pennsylvania Nursing Excellence Professional Practice (HUP-NEPP) model, at HUP.	Multiple units at University of Pennsylvania Hospital (HUP).	Hospital-based reporting of components of effective partnerships through nursing exemplars	Exemplars of several units describing different approaches and models from weak partnerships in a hierarchical model to those that is stronger and more complex in a hierarchical model.	Partnerships are necessary for communication through the disciplines, exchanging of ideas, and peer review process to maintain quality outcomes. Authoritarianism is not an easy concept to relate, especially in institutions that have followed a paternalistic doctrine for years, but it is possible to have effective partnerships and alter the old way of doing things, given the effort, commitment, collaboration, communication, trust and respect of the relationship of authentic leaders with their employees.

Oliver, Tatum, Kapp, & Wallace (2010)	To explore the experiences of hospice medical directors within the context of collaboration.	17 hospice medical directors who were previously involved in a larger survey study on the same topic.	Qualitative, descriptive study	Semistructured interviews with thematic analysis.	Medical directors in the hospice setting reported positive collaborative experiences. Assisting medical directors to find time and financial opportunities for professional development and support in their role was found to be an opportunity to further improve collaboration.
Petri (2010)	To explore the meaning of interdisciplinary collaboration within the context of health care.	Literature review to clarify the current use of interdisciplinary collaboration in health care.		Rodgers' Evolutionary View of Concept Analysis to identify attributes, antecedents, and consequences of interdisciplinary collaboration.	A comprehensive definition of interdisciplinary collaboration within the context of health care is presented as an outcome of this analysis. Further inquiry should focus on the development of valid measures to accurately evaluate this subject.

(Continued)

TABLE 7.2

Organizational Models and Training Approach (Continued)

Author	Purpose	Population	Research Design	Instruments or Methods	Findings
Interdisciplinary Teams: Impact/Outcomes					
Cashman, Reidy, Cody, & Lemay (2004)	To report the results of a longitudinal study of an intervention to enhance interdisciplinary team functioning in a primary care setting.	Health care team members: physician, nurse practitioner, physician's assistant, registered nurse, health assistant (*N* = 5) at a federally funded community health center in New England, USA.	Intervention study	The System for the Multiple Level Observation of Groups (SYMLOG) was used to evaluate team members' assessments of progress towards expressing values consistent with an effective team.	Intentional team training and development, coupled with dedicated time for team meetings, can result in team members' expressing values consistent with high functioning teams. Team members' objective assessments, as well as their lived experiences, provide detailed reaffirmation that to sustain effective team functioning, organizational structures and reward systems must support the team's vision and goals. Methods for reducing team turnover are needed to ensure growth and sustainability.

Fennell et al. (2010)	Review of various types of multidisciplinary care (MDC) teams and their impact on the quality of treatment care for cancer patients. The authors also outline a conceptual model of the connection between team context, structure, process, and performance and their subsequent effects on cancer treatment care processes and patient outcomes	MDC teams caring for oncology patients.	Target of the health care, organizational behavior and management literature.	Despite advances in research on MDC in oncology many gaps for future research remain; in what situations do which structures work best: what characteristics of physicians and other team members assure optimal team performance; what external/regulatory influences prohibit or enhance the sustainability of MDC teams; which type of MDC lead to best patient quality of life, outcomes, and experience.
Woods & Magyary (2010)	Describes the imperative of interdisciplinary collaboration in translational research with special emphasis on contributions of nurses in these collaborations.		Opinion piece based on review of literature	
Hansson et al. (2009)	To measure attitudes toward collaboration among General Practitioners (GP) and RNs and to investigate whether	A cohort of 600 GPs and RNs in Vastra Gotaland region of Sweden	Quantitative study	The Jefferson Scale of Attitudes toward Physician Nurse Collaboration and the Professional	RNs were slightly more positive about collaboration than GPs. A positive attitude toward collaboration did not seem to be a part of the GP's

(Continued)

177

TABLE 7.2

Organizational Models and Training Approach (*Continued*)

Author	Purpose	Research Design	Population	Instruments or Methods	Findings
	there is a correlation between a positive attitude toward collaboration and high self-esteem in the professional role.			Self-Description Form (PSDF) were used.	professional role to the same extend as it is for RNs. Professional norms seem to have more influence on attitudes than do gender roles. RNs seem more confident in their profession than GPs.
Kydona, Malamis, Giasnetsova, Tsiora, & Gritsi-Gerogianni (2010)	To investigate the level of collaboration, as part of organizational culture in the environment of an ICU in Hippokratio Hospital, Thessaloniki, Greece.	Descriptive study	ICU personnel, and other cooperating clinical departments and labs in the Hospital (N = 196).	Questionnaire was administered to measure teamwork and patient safety attitudes in high-risk areas; participants were also asked to describe personal perception of the quality of collaboration and communication.	Teaching teamwork skills and team concepts should become a significant part of medical and nursing education and training if we want to achieve a substantial improvement in quality of health care services, especially in high risk areas such as ICU's.
Mann et al. (2006)	To describe how the application of crew resource management, a	Descriptive study	220 staff (MDs, RNs, residents, and support staff) in the	Occurrence of adverse events on the L&D unit	Teaching clinicians to behave as teammates will improve staff attitudes and enhance

	concept used by military and commercial flight teams, on L&D units can improve patient safety and reduce patient lawsuits.	Labor and Delivery Unit at an academic medical center in Boston, MA.	whose etiology related to failures in communication and/or teamwork	performance in an L&D unit, which can improve maternal and neonatal outcomes and reduce malpractice claims.
Manser (2009)	To examine current research on teamwork in highly dynamic domains of health care such as ORs, ICUs, EDs, or trauma and resuscitation teams with a focus on aspects relevant to the quality and safety of patient care.	Broad review of various health-related databases yielded 277 articles fulfilling the inclusion criteria which were further categorized and refined, resulting in 101 publications chosen for in-depth review.		Evidence from three main areas of research supports the relationship between teamwork and patient safety: (1) Studies investigating critical incidents and adverse events have shown that teamwork plays an important role in the causation and prevention of adverse events. (2) Research focusing on health care providers' perceptions of teamwork demonstrated that (a) staff perception of teamwork and attitudes toward safety-relevant team behavior were related to the quality and safety of patient care and (b) perceptions of teamwork and leadership style are associated with staff well being, which may impact clinician ability to provide safe patient care.

(Continued)

TABLE 7.2

Organizational Models and Training Approach *(Continued)*

Author	Purpose	Population	Research Design	Instruments or Methods	Findings
					(3) Observational studies on teamwork behaviors related to high clinical performance have identified patterns of communication, coordination, and leadership that support effective teamwork.
Merali et al. (2008)	To evaluate the effectiveness of a medication safety project to (1) identify areas of exposure to risk and make recommendations to enhance medication safety within the hospital and (2) to inform the development of a medication safety checklist specific to the OR setting.	Anesthesiologists, nurses, and pharmacists from the OR at a large teaching hospital in Ontario, Canada.	Descriptive study	An interdisciplinary team of consultants from the Institute of Safe Medication Practice (ISMP) Canada and a representative from the US performed a targeted systematic review of medication use in the OR and related patient care areas. Direct observation was used in each area. System weaknesses	Enhancing working relationships among anesthesiologists, pharmacists, and nurses is pivotal for safe medication practices in the OR setting. Strategies developed and implemented during the project were aimed at reducing the risk of injury induced by medication errors.

					were identified, and 75 specific recommendations were made to enhance medication safety.
Mills et al. (2008)	To assess the effectiveness of cooperation and communication among surgical teams and ICU teams.	Clinicians and administrators from the operating rooms and ICUs in 6 Veterans Administration medical centers (VAMCs) in the US.		The Medical Team Training (MTT) questionnaire	The MTT was helpful in identifying hidden problems with communication before formal team training, learning sessions. It revealed a pattern of discrepancies among physicians and nurses in which surgeons perceive a stronger organizational culture of safety, better communication, and better teamwork than either nurses of anesthesiologists do.
Neily et al. (2010)	To determine if an association existed between Veterans Health Administration (VHA) Medical Team Training and surgical outcomes.	Surgical staff at 74 VHA facilities across the US received the training and 108 facilities were analyzed.	Retrospective health services cohort study using a contemporaneous control group.	VHA data on risk adjusted mortality rates, aggregated by facility as Team Training intervention was instituted by facility (i.e., unit of analysis = facility)	The 74 facilities where team training occurred reported an 18% reduction in annual mortality (rate ratio, 0.82; 95% confidence interval, 0.76–0.91; $p = .01$).

(Continued)

TABLE 7.2

Organizational Models and Training Approach *(Continued)*

Author	Purpose	Population	Research Design	Instruments or Methods	Findings
O'Leary et al. (2010)	To assess ratings of teamwork and barriers to collaboration by providers on inpatient medical units and barriers to collaboration.	RNs, PCPs, and medical subspecialty consultant physicians on 4 general medical units at a 753-bed academic hospital in Chicago, IL	Cross-sectional study with a qualitative review of comments.	Likert scale-based survey to assess teamwork ratings, barrier ratings. Qualitative review of comments.	In the general medical inpatient setting, discrepancies among RNs and MDs existed in the ratings of collaboration and barriers to teamwork. Whereas MDs rated the quality of teamwork with RNs favorably, RNs perceived teamwork as suboptimal.
O'Leary et al. (2010)	To assess the impact of an intervention, Structured Inter-Disciplinary Rounds (SIDR) on nurses' ratings of collaboration and teamwork.	Two hospitalist staffed units at an 897 tertiary care teaching hospital in Chicago, IL	Controlled trial of an intervention.	A 5-point ordinal scale survey was used to rate the nurses' assessment of collaboration and communication.	SIDR had a positive effect on nurses' ratings of teamwork and collaboration on a hospitalist unit; however there was no effect on length of stay or cost.
Reid Ponte et al. (2007)	To describe the implementation of a new interdisciplinary governance and management structure at an ambulatory, academic, comprehensive cancer center.		Qualitative, descriptive study.	Leadership interviews	Four years into the project, the structure of interdisciplinary governance is firmly in place. Change in accomplished more readily than prior to the implementation. A culture that promotes accountability,

	Aim	Sample	Design	Measures	Findings
					communication, respect and collaboration has been established. Collaborative simulations may improve interdisciplinary communication and ultimately improve patient care.
Reese et al. (2010)	To investigate the use of a framework for the collaborative medical and nursing management of a surgical patient with complications.	Senior level baccalaureate nursing students and third-year medical students for a large Midwestern university.	Descriptive study	The Simulation Design Scale and the Satisfaction and Self-Confidence Scale. Collaboration was measured using a collaboration scale developed by the researchers.	
Richardson & Storr (2010)	To identify to what extent and in what way nursing leadership, collaboration and empowerment can have a demonstrable impact on patient safety.	Literature review of abstracts and papers focused on leadership, advocacy, interdisciplinary working, empowerment, and collaboration.	Review of literature		Significant gaps exist in relation to knowledge of the extent and nature of the role of RNs in patient safety improvement. Huge potential exists for improvement through nursing empowerment, leadership and the development of tools to strengthen and support RNs influential role in the quality and safety movement.

(Continued)

183

TABLE 7.2

Organizational Models and Training Approach *(Continued)*

Author	Purpose	Population	Research Design	Instruments or Methods	Findings
Schmitt et al. (2001)	Describe the state of the science and summarize the literature on interdisciplinary collaboration with emphasis on geriatric teams from 1950–1995.	Review article			Progress has been made in moving from rhetoric to solid science, with the development of theoretical frameworks, rigorous design and methods and focused measurement.
Vogwill & Reeves (2008)	To explore the interprofessional communication practices and needs cf nurses and physicians in multidisciplinary m meetings (bullet rounds).	Medicine, nursing, OT, PT, social work, and pharmacy staff at a general internal medicine unit in a large teaching hospital in Canada.	Qualitative	Content analysis approach. Field notes coded using an adapted version of the Team Observation Protocol (TOP) taxonomy.	Insight was provided into the complex process of managing and exchanging information in bullet rounds. Researches suggested introducing structure to the process of information exchange for study.

TABLE 7.3

Instruments

Author	Instrument	Content Development	Content and Structure	Evaluation
Bales & Cohen (1979); Robert Freed Bales, social psychologist	System for the Multiple Level observations of Groups (SMYLOG)	Based on theory developed from observations of three main bipolar dimensions: dominant vs. submissive; friendly vs. unfriendly; acceptance vs. nonacceptance.	26-item questionnaire assessing factors known to contribute to team effectiveness Evaluation: Teams participate in targeted discussion regarding results of questionnaire to evaluate perceptions of team functioning and changes needed for increased effectiveness; Neily et al (2010).	Teams participate in targeted discussion regarding results of questionnaire to evaluate perceptions of team functioning and changes needed for increased effectiveness.
Mills et al. (2008); Mills, Peter; Neily, Julia; Dunn, Edward; Veterans Health Administration	Medical Team Training Questionnaire	Adapted from the VHA Team Training questionnaire to elicit specific information from members of clinical teams.	26 item questionnaire measuring perception of: organizational culture, communication, teamwork, and human factors awareness using a Likert scale.	Subscale Cronbach alpha scores all >0.70; overall Cronbach alpha = 0.881.
O'Leary et al. (2010)	Teamwork and barriers to collaboration assessment	Survey development based on previous tools to assess teamwork attitudes and perceived barriers using a Likert scale, with comment section at the end for open-ended feedback on teamwork and communication. Administered electronically through a web-based mechanism.	Two parts: (1) Assessment of provider teamwork attitudes and quality of communication and collaboration within their own discipline and across disciplines. (2) Rating of barriers to communication and teamwork.	No evaluation of the survey tool reported.

in health care institutions. The success of these programs has been largely measured using pre and post testing methods to demonstrate effectiveness, as well as satisfaction surveys and other qualitative measures of perceived improvements in working relationships and collaboration. Studies evaluating the longer term impact of training programs on interdisciplinary collaboration in the work setting are needed. Narrowing and standardizing the "dose" of teamwork training applied across study groups is also a challenge and must be accomplished to build a body of knowledge regarding the effectiveness of educational interventions.

Although the role of health care leaders in promoting interdisciplinary collaboration is widely discussed, very little research has been conducted to assess the impact of different leadership and organizational structures on assuring and advancing teamwork and collaboration. Research in this area is especially important if organizations are to create the kind of work environments promoted by the IOM and the ANCC's Magnet Recognition Program, environments that are characterized by inclusiveness, transparency, teamwork, and collaboration.

Outcome data demonstrating actual improvements in the quality of patient care as a result of interdisciplinary teamwork are beginning to emerge, but remain scarce in the literature and should be a focus of future research. Because of the myriad interactions that occur in the health care environment among clinicians and between clinicians and patients, it is challenging to isolate and measure the impact of specific interactions on patient outcomes. Like all other areas related to collaboration, studies in this area would benefit from greater methodological rigor and improved instrumentation.

Developing programs and models to assure and advance interdisciplinary collaboration among practicing clinicians is especially important in light of ongoing efforts to reform the U.S. health care system and enhance health care quality, safety, and cost effectiveness. Interdisciplinary collaboration is integral to many of the programs supported by the reform legislation, including the development and implementation of accountable care organizations, "health home" initiatives, and other programs aimed at improving the care of patients with complex conditions. Answering the following research questions will heighten nurses' understanding of interdisciplinary collaboration and support them in developing structures that make a difference in the patient and family experience and patient, workforce, and financial outcomes.

1. When interdisciplinary team members collaborate effectively, what effect does it have on clinical outcomes over time?
2. How does effective interdisciplinary collaboration among clinicians caring for patients with chronic conditions affect the experience and perceptions of family members?

3. Is an interdisciplinary care team delivery model more or less costly in terms of human resources, use of ancillary services, medication management?
4. Do interdisciplinary care teams that function effectively provide safer care?
5. What organizational structures are most effective in assuring that interdisciplinary collaboration and teamwork actually happen consistently and effectively?

Answering these and other questions will help organizations advance interdisciplinary collaboration and teamwork and maximize its impact on patient safety, organizational effectiveness, the practice environment, and patient, workforce, and organizational outcomes.

REFERENCES

Aiken, L. H., Clarke, S. P., Sloane, D. M., Sochalski, J., & Silber, J. H. (2002). Hospital nurse staffing and patient mortality, nurse burnout, and job dissatisfaction. *JAMA: the Journal of the American Medical Association, 288*(16), 1987–1993.

Aiken, L. H., Havens, D. S., & Sloane, D. M. (2009). The Magnet Nursing Services Recognition Program: a comparison of two groups of magnet hospitals. *The Journal of Nursing Administration, 39*(7–8 Suppl.), S5–14.

Bales, R. F., & Cohen, S. P. (1979). *SMYLOG: A systematic multiple level observation of groups.* New York, NY: Free Press.

Cashman, S., Reidy, P., Cody, K., & Lemay, C. (2004). Developing and measuring progress toward collaborative, integrated, interdisciplinary health care teams. *Journal of Interprofessional Care, 18*(2), 183–196.

Cesario, S., Morin, K., & Santa-Donato, A. (2002). Evaluating the level of evidence of qualitative research. *Journal of Obstetric, Gynecologic, and Neonatal Nursing: JOGNN/NAACOG, 31*(6), 708–714.

Chung, H., & Nguyen, P. H. (2005). Changing unit culture: An interdisciplinary commitment to improve pain outcomes. *Journal for Healthcare Quality, 27*(2), 12–19.

Clarke, P. G. (2006). What would a theory of interprofessional education look like? Some suggestions for developing a theoretical framework for teamwork training. *Journal of Interprofessional Care, 20*(6), 577–589. doi:10.1080/13561820600916717

Clarke, S. P., & Aiken, L. H. (2003). Failure to rescue: Needless deaths are prime examples of the need for more nurses at the bedside. *American Journal of Nursing, 103*(1), 42–47.

Connor, M., Duncombe, D., Barclay, E., Bartel, S., Borden, C., Gross, E., . . . Ponte, P. R. (2007). Creating a fair and just culture: One institution's path toward organizational change. *Joint Commission Journal on Quality and Patient Safety/Joint Commission Resources, 33*(10), 617–624.

Conway, J., Nathan, D., Benz, E., Shulman, L., Sallan, S., Reid Ponte, P., . . . Weingart, S. (2006). *Key learning from the Dana-Farber Cancer Institute's ten-year patient safety journey.* American Society of Clinical Oncology. 42nd Annual Meeting, Atlanta, GA, 615–619.

Cronin, K. (2008). *Transdisciplinary research (TDR) and sustainability.* Report prepared for the Ministry of Research, Science and Technology (MoRST).

Dietrich, S. L., Kornet, T. M., Lawson, D. R., Major, K., May, L., Rich, V. L., & Riley-Wasserman, E. (2010). Collaboration to partnerships. *Nursing Administration Quarterly, 34*(1), 49–55.

Dodds, J., Vann, W., Lee, J., Rosenberg, A., Rounds, K., Roth, M.,... Margolis, L. H. (2010). The UNC-CH MCH Leadership Training Consortium: building the capacity to develop interdisciplinary MCH leaders. *Maternal and Child Health Journal, 14*(4), 642–648.

Donabedian, A. (2000). Evaluating physician competence. *Bulletin of the World Health Organization, 78*(6), 857–860.

Drenkard, K. (2010). The business case for Magnet. *The Journal of Nursing Administration, 40*(6), 263–271.

Dumont, S., Briere, N., Morin, D., Houle, N., & Iloko-Fundi, M. (2010). Implementing an inter-faculty series of courses on interprofessional collaboration in prelicensure health science. *Education for Health, 23*(1), 395.

Fennell, M., Prabhu Das, I., Clauser, S., Petrelli, N., & Salner, A. (2010). The organization of multidisciplinary care teams: Modeling internal and external influences on cancer care quality. *Journal of the National Cancer Institute Monographs, 40*, 72–80.

Goldsmith, J., Wittenberg-Lyles, E., Rodriguez, D., & Sanchez-Reilly, S. (2010). Interdisciplinary geriatric and palliative care team narratives: collaboration practices and barriers. *Qualitative Health Research, 20*(1), 93–104.

Hallin, K., Kiessling, A., Waldner, A., & Henriksson, P. (2009). Active interprofessional education in a patient based setting increases perceived collaborative and professional competence. *Medical Teacher, 31*(2), 151–157.

Hansson, A., Arvemo, T., Marklund, B., Gedda, B., & Mattsson, B. (2010). Working together–primary care doctors' and nurses' attitudes to collaboration. *Scandinavian Journal of Public Health, 38*(1), 78–85.

Havens, D. S. (2001). Comparison of nursing department infrastructure and outcomes: ANCC magnet and nonmagnet CNEs report. *Nursing Economics, 19*(6), 258–266.

Henderson, A. J., O'Keefe, M. F., & Alexander, H. G. (2010). Interprofessional education in clinical practice: not a single vaccine. *Australian Health Review, 34*(2), 224–226.

Hobgood, C., Sherwood, G., Frush, K., Hollar, D., & Maynard, L. (2010). Teamwork training with nursing and medical students: Does the method matter? Results of an interinstitutional, interdisciplinary collaboration. *Quality and Safety in Health Care. 19*(6), e25.

Institute of Medicine. (1999). *To err is human: Building a safer health system.* Washington, DC: National Academies Press.

Institute of Medicine. (2001). *Crossing the quality chasm.* Washington, DC: National Academies Press.

Institute of Medicine. (2003). *Health professions education: A bridge to quality.* Washington, DC: National Academy Press.

Institute of Medicine. (2004). *Keeping patients safe: Transforming the work environment of nurses.* Washington, DC: National Academies Press.

Jeffries, P. R., (Ed). (2007). *Simulation in nursing education: From conceptualization to evaluation.* New York: National League for Nursing.

Kalisch, B. (2010, October/November). The impact of the level of nursing teamwork on the amount of missed nursing care. *Nursing Outlook.*

Klein, J. T. (2007). Interdisciplinary approaches in social science research. In W. Outwaite & S. P. Turner (Eds.), *The Sage handbook of social science methodology* (pp. 32–49). Los Angeles, CA: Sage Publications.

Kydona, C. H. K., Malamis, G., Giasnetsova, T., Tsiora, V., & Gritsi-Gerogianni, N. (2010). The level of teamwork as an index of quality in ICU performance. *Hippokratia, 14*(2), 94–97.

Lown, B. A., & Manning, C. F. (2010). The Schwartz Center Rounds: Evaluation of an interdisciplinary approach to enhancing patient-centered communication, teamwork, and provider support. *Academic Medicine: Journal of the Association of American Medical Colleges, 85*(6), 1073–1081.

Mann, S., Marcus, R., & Sachs, B. (2006). Lessons learned from the cockpit: How team training can reduce errors in L&D. *Contemporary OBGYN*, 1–7.

Manser, T. (2009). Teamwork and patient safety in dynamic domains of healthcare: a review of the literature. *Acta Anaesthesiologica Scandinavica*, 53(2), 143–151.

McClure, M., Poulin, M., Sovie, M., Wandelt, M. (2002). *Magnet Hospitals: Attraction and retention of professional nurses.* American Nurses Association. Silver Spring, MD: Nursesbooks.

Mills, P., Neily, J., & Dunn, E. (2008). Teamwork and communication in surgical teams: implications for patient safety. *Journal of the American College of Surgeons*, 206(1), 107–112.

Merali, R., Orser, B. A., Leeksma, A., Lingard, S., Belo, S., & Hyland, S. (2008). Medication safety in the operating room: teaming up to improve patient safety. *Healthcare Quarterly (Toronto, Ont.)*, 11(3 Spec No.), 54–57.

Neily, J., Mills, P. D., Young-Xu, Y., Carney, B. T., West, P., Berger, D. H., . . . Bagian, J. P. (2010). Association between implementation of a medical team training program and surgical mortality. *JAMA: The Journal of the American Medical Association*, 304(15), 1693–1700.

O'Leary, K. J., Haviley, C., Slade, M., Shah, H., Lee, J., & Williams, M. (2010). Improving teamwork: Impact of structured interdisciplinary rounds on a hospitalist unit. *Journal of Hospital Medicine*, 1–4.

O'Leary, K. J., Ritter, C. D., Wheeler, H., Szekendi, M. K., Brinton, T. S., & Williams, M. V. (2010). Teamwork on inpatient medical units: assessing attitudes and barriers. *Quality & Safety in Health Care*, 19(2), 117–121.

Oliver, D. P., Tatum, P., Kapp, J. M., Wallace, A. (2010). Interdisciplinary collaboration: The voices of hospice medical directors. *American Journal of Hospice and Palliative Care Medicine*, 1–8. OnlineFirst, published May 3, 2010, as doi:10.1177/ 1049909110366852.

O'Mahony, S., Mazur, E., Charney, P., Wang, Y., & Fine, J. (2007). Use of multidisciplinary rounds to simultaneously improve quality outcomes, enhance resident education, and shorten length of stay. *Journal of General Internal Medicine*, 22(8), 1073–1079.

Petri, L. (2010). Concept analysis of interdisciplinary collaboration. *Nursing Forum*, 45(2), 73–82.

Pratt, S. D., Mann, S., Salisbury, M., Greenberg, P., Marcus, R., Stabile, B., . . . Sachs, B. P. (2007). John M. Eisenberg Patient Safety and Quality Awards. Impact of CRM-based training on obstetric outcomes and clinicians' patient safety attitudes. *Joint Commission Journal on Quality and Patient Safety/Joint Commission Resources*, 33(12), 720–725.

Reese, C. E., Jeffries, P. R., & Engum, S. A. (2010). Learning together: Using simulations to develop nursing and medical student collaboration. *Nursing Education Perspectives*, 31(1), 33–37.

Reid Ponte, P., Gross, A. H., Winer, E., Connaughton, M. J., & Hassinger, J. (2007). Implementing an interdisciplinary governance model in a comprehensive cancer center. *Oncology Nursing Forum*, 34(3), 611–616.

Richardson, A., & Storr, J. (2010). Patient safety: A literature [corrected] review on the impact of nursing empowerment, leadership and collaboration. *International Nursing Review*, 57(1), 12–21.

Schmitt, M. H. (2001). Collaboration improves the quality of care: methodological challenges and evidence from US health care research. *Journal of Interprofessional Care*, 15(1), 47–66.

Tress, B., Gunther, R., & Fry, G. (2006). Defining concepts and the process of knowledge production in integrative research. Chapter 2 in Tress, B. et al. *From Landscape Research to Landscape Planning—Aspects of integration, education and application.* Wageningen UR Frontis Series 12 ISBN 1402039786 pp 13–26. Retrieved July 25, 2008, from http://library.wur.nl/frontis /landscape_research/02_tress.pdf

Vogwill, V., & Reeves, S. (2008). Challenges of information exchange between nurses and physicians in multidisciplinary team meetings. *Journal of Interprofessional Care*, 22(6), 664–667.

Woods, N. F., & Magyary, D. L. (2010). Translational research: Why nursing's interdisciplinary collaboration is essential. *Research and Theory for Nursing Practice*, 24(1), 9–24.

CHAPTER 8

The Health Care Work Environment and Adverse Health and Safety Consequences for Nurses

Jeanne Geiger-Brown and Jane Lipscomb

ABSTRACT

Nurses' working conditions are inextricably linked to the quality of care that is provided to patients and patients' safety. These same working conditions are associated with health and safety outcomes for nurses and other health care providers. This chapter describes aspects of the nursing work environment that have been linked to hazards and adverse exposures for nurses, as well as the most common health and safety outcomes of nursing work. We include studies from 2000 to the present by nurse researchers, studies of nurses as subjects, and studies of workers under similar working conditions that could translate to nurses' work environment. We explore a number of work organization factors including shift work and extended work hours, safety climate and culture, teamwork, and communication. We also describe environmental hazards, including chemical hazards (e.g., waste anesthetics, hazardous drugs, cleaning compounds) and airborne and bloodborne pathogen exposure. Nurses' health and safety outcomes include physical (e.g., musculoskeletal disorders, gastrointestinal, slips, trips and falls, physical assault) and psychosocial outcomes (e.g., burnout, work-family conflict). Finally, we present recommendations for future research to further

© 2011 Springer Publishing Company
DOI: 10.1891/0739-6686.28.191

protect nurses and all health care workers from a range of hazardous working conditions.

Nurses' working conditions are inextricably linked to the quality of care that is provided to patients and patients' safety. These same working conditions are associated with health and safety outcomes for nurses and other health care providers, and as such, research focused on the health and safety of nurses is critically important. Health care workers comprise more than 10% of those employed in the United States (14 million) and their numbers are projected to increase in the future, accounting for 20% of all new jobs. Among this population, 80% are female, and there are a greater percentage of African Americans and Asians in health care work compared to other industry sectors. While notable for its size and demographics, the health care workforce is also distinguished by the large number of hazards these workers face and their high injury and illness rates. The 2008 Bureau of Labor Statistics (BLS) data show that the occupational injury and illness rate of hospital employees was 7.6 per 100 full-time workers compared with a rate of 3.9 per 100 workers in the private sector (BLS, 2009). While the rate of occupational injuries and illnesses across other sectors has declined over past years, only a modest decrease has been seen in the health care sector. Incidence rates for three of the four most prevalent nonfatal illness and injury types (overexertion injuries, falls, and workplace violence) are 65–260% higher in health care than in private industry (Figure 8.1).

Most research addressing the nurse and health care work environment, including those cited in this chapter, focus on the hospital environment, yet only 62% of employed registered nurses (RNs) work in a hospital setting (Health Resources and Services Administration [HRSA], 2010). In general, the hospital environment includes hazards and exposure levels greater than with other health care settings because of the high acuity of the patient population, heavy use of technology, and the high physical and emotional demands of professional care giving. Yet hospitals also have resources that can control the dose of workers' exposure to these hazards. For example, nurses who provide care in a client's home face many of the same hazards as their counterparts in the hospital environment; but do so in an environment where they have less control of the physical work environment; lack policies, equipment and training specific to this environment; and a different social role of caregiver in the client's home. These factors may intensify the occupational risk for illness or injury in the home care setting and in other nontraditional settings such as in military nursing.

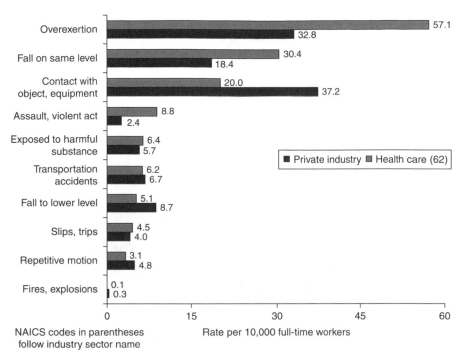

FIGURE 8.1 Incidence rates of nonfatal occupational injuries and illnesses involving days away from work by selected events of exposures leading to injury or illness, health care and social assistance sector and private industry, 2005. *Source*: BLS, 2005.

Two major theoretical frameworks serve as underpinnings for this chapter. First, Karasek's job strain model has been widely used to assess a range of jobs that vary by the intensity of work demands (physical and psychosocial) and the degree of control a worker has over their work environment (skill discretion and decision authority; Karasek, 1979). Jobs characterized by high demands and low control (job strain) have been associated with many adverse health outcomes, in particular increased cardiovascular disease (CVD; Dobson & Schnall, 2009), musculoskeletal disorders (Schoenfisch & Lipscomb, 2009) and poorer psychological outcomes (van Der Doef & Maes, 1999). Spence Laschinger (2001) found that nurses working in high job strain settings were less satisfied with their jobs and had less commitment to the organization. She suggested that structural empowerment (access to information, resources, and support to be autonomous) may contribute to reducing job strain.

When the construct of social support is added to job demands and controls, models have further explanatory power for a number of these outcomes

(Johnson & Hall, 1988). The second conceptualization of work stress and health outcomes is based on the theory of effort-reward imbalance (ERI), which proposes that we should receive comparable rewards for the effort expended (Siegrist, 1996). Workers who experience failed reciprocity at work (high ERI) are at twice the risk of CVD, depression and alcohol dependence compared to those not exposed (Siegrist, 2005). The ERI theory appears to be the better framework for assessing work stress in occupations related to the service and professional work, such as health care workers (Calnan, 2000; Marmot, Siegrist, Theorell, & Feeney, 1999).

In the sections that follow, we describe aspects of the nursing work environment that have been linked to hazards and adverse exposures for nurses, as well as the most common health and safety outcomes of nursing work. We include studies by nurse researchers, studies of nurses as subjects, and studies of workers under similar working conditions that could translate to nurses' work environment. Because each study describes an exposure and an outcome, the placement of studies into sections of this report is somewhat arbitrary. To avoid duplication we include a study only once in a section of the report where it seems to fit best. We included literature from 2000 till present, with addition of seminal studies where they were relevant. We explore a number of work organization factors including shift work and extended work hours, safety climate and culture, teamwork, and communication. We also describe environmental hazards, including chemical hazards (e.g., waste anesthetics, hazardous drugs, cleaning compounds) and airborne and bloodborne pathogen exposure. Nurses' health and safety outcomes include physical (e.g., musculoskeletal disorders, gastrointestinal, slips, trips and falls, physical assault) and psychosocial outcomes (e.g., burnout, work–family conflict [WFC]). Finally, we present recommendations for future research to further protect nurses and all health care workers from a range of hazardous working conditions.

WORK ORGANIZATION

Health care employers have control over how work is organized for their employees (Figure 8.2). Decisions made at the organizational level have influence over workers' health and safety.

Employers control the relative proportion of RNs to support staff and technicians; the scheduling paradigm; the quality and intensity of supervision, the availability and quality of protective equipment, and the human resource policies that define salaries and benefits. At the unit level an individual nurse's quality of work life depends on unit teamwork and communication, how physical and psychosocial job demands are managed to accomplish the work at hand, the nurse's

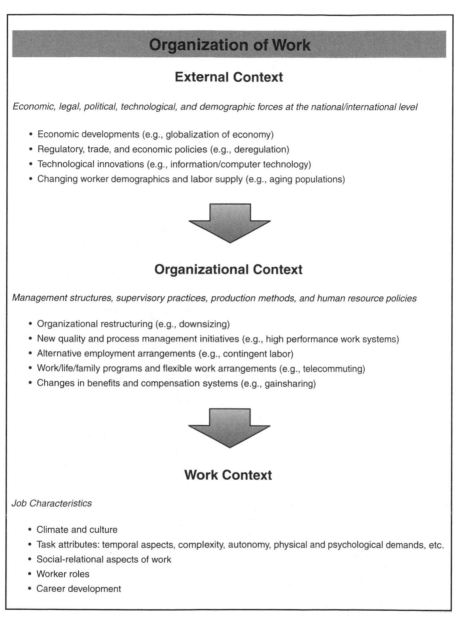

FIGURE 8.2 Organization of work.
Source: Sauter et al., 2002.

autonomy in the role, the degree of social and supervisory support available, and the actual negotiated work schedule. In this section, we will describe features of nurses' work schedules, safety culture and climate and teamwork and communication, as they influence nurses' health and safety.

Work Schedule

Nurses' work schedules are a source of job control (decision latitude) when self-scheduling is available, but this often breaks down when nurses are called to come in during time away from work. Although the use of mandatory overtime has largely been replaced by "on call," being called in to work decreases time for recovery (Trinkoff, Geiger-Brown, Brady, Lipscomb, & Muntaner, 2006). Several features of nurses' work schedules create health hazards including extended work hours (12-hour, or longer, shifts), early start times, and shift work/shift rotation (Boivin, Tremblay, & James, 2007).

Extended Work Hours

Many nurses who provide direct patient care choose or are required to work extended work hours (shifts of 12 hours or more; Josten, Ng, & Therry, 2003). These are often accompanied by compressed schedules (e.g., 3–4 successive 12-hour days before rest days). In Trinkoff, Geiger-Brown, et al.'s (2006) recent study of RNs she found that more than one-third of staff nurses routinely work 12 or more hours per day, with critical care nurses nearly always working sustained workdays. Even a nominal 12-hour duty rotation is sometimes close to 13 hours because additional demands (intershift report, medication counting, unfinished patient care and paperwork) can increase the duration of work (Heller, 1998). Hughes and Rogers (2004) found that nurses left work at the end of their scheduled workday less than 20% of the time, with overruns of 55 minutes on average. Some of these sustained shifts are worked during off-hours, which can increase the stressful effect of sustained work.

Lengthening of the shift duration from 8 to 12 hours significantly restricts the opportunity for sleep and produces sleep deficiency (Dawson & McCulloch, 2005). In a study of male chemical workers, where 8- and 12-hour shifts were compared, 12-hour shifts were associated with a mean sleep duration of only 6–6.6 hours and more disturbed sleep (Tucker, Barton, & Folkard, 1996). In comparison to these physically active workers, nurses also experience a high level of psychosocial demands and often have additional responsibilities for housework, childcare or eldercare during nonwork hours; thus they may have less time to sleep. This was shown in a recent study of objectively measured sleep (actigraphy) in 12-hour shift nurses where nurses achieved a mean of 5.5 hours (SD 1 hour) between shifts, with night shift nurses having considerable fragmentation of sleep (Geiger-Brown, Rogers, Trinkoff, Kane, & Scharf, 2010). Using subjective sleep measures, British RNs reported that 62% of nurses complained of getting insufficient sleep, with mean sleep durations of 6.3–7.1 hours (Edell-Gustafsson, Kritz, & Bogren, 2002). In a sample of U.S. critical care nurses, 87% of whom worked 12-hour workdays, 68% met the criteria for poor sleep quality (a metric that combines duration and other subjective perceptions of sleep disturbance; Ruggiero, 2003). Similar findings were reported by Iskra-Golec, Folkard, Marek, and Noworel (1996), who found that Polish nurses working 12-hour workdays reported worse sleep quality and more chronic fatigue than nurses working 8-hour shifts did. Sleep opportunity, actual achieved sleep, and the quality of sleep are all affected by extended work shifts.

Adverse health and safety outcomes of extended work hours include increased rates of musculoskeletal disorders, needlestick injuries, work-related falls, and motor vehicle accidents (covered later in this chapter). All of these can be attributed to reduced vigilant attention, fatigue, and decreased neuromuscular fine motor control associated with sleep deficiency. Nurses often consider fatigue a normal part of the job, and may not make the association between successive sustained hours and later impaired health. Working without adequate sleep between shifts can lead to negative chronic health effects including CVD, metabolic syndrome, diabetes, obesity, decreased immune function, and increased cancer risk (Institute of Medicine [IOM], 2006).

The Institute of Medicine made specific hours-of-service recommendations about limits on nursing hours (IOM, 2004), recommending that nurses work no more than 12 hours per day and no more than 60 hours per week. The American Nurses' Association has two position statements related to maintaining alertness on the job. The first encourages nurses to obtain adequate rest and appear for work fully able to perform their job (American Nurses Association [ANA], 2006a). The second encourages employers to provide appropriate work schedules so that nurses can achieve adequate rest (ANA, 2006b). Both positions rely on the professionalism of the nurse to self-regulate sleep and fatigue risk, and given the evidence of sleep deficiency among 12-hour shift nurses neither position can be achieved using this scheduling paradigm. Sleep researchers in Australia are advocating the use of safety management systems rather than regulation of hours of work to manage worker fatigue, and recommend that each industry develop a fatigue-management code-of-practice to reduce this occupational hazard (Dawson & McCullough, 2005). However, the tools to implement such an approach (e.g., fitness for duty testing) are not widely available for commercial use and the best that can be done is to manage fatigue risk by limiting unsafe schedules using scheduling software based on biomathematical models of performance.

Early Start Times

Nurses in some specialties such as preoperative and surgical care have early start times. Commutes in heavy metropolitan traffic or long rural commutes can also produce sleep deficiencies that resemble early start times. Although there have been no nursing studies examining this scheduling pattern, two studies showed that sleepiness, and conversely alertness at work are affected by early start times. In a study of train operators, levels of sleepiness among workers with early start times were compared with those working later starting morning shifts (Ingre, Kecklund, Akerstedt, Soderstrom, & Kecklund, 2008). Individuals starting work prior to 4:30 AM achieved only 5 hours of sleep and there was a linear increase of 0.7 hours of sleep for every hour of delay in start time among those whose start times ranged from 4:30 AM to 9:00 AM. An experimental study where workers' morning start times were delaying by one hour showed significant improvements in alertness at work and increased duration of sleep prior to their shift (Rosa, Harma, Pulli, Mulder, & Nasman, 1996).

Shiftwork and Shift Rotation

Health care work is characterized by 24-hour operations. Regardless of whether night shifts are permanent or rotating, mandatory or voluntary, these workers get about 10 hour less sleep per week than day shift workers (Akerstedt, 2003) and poorer quality sleep. Portela, Rotenberg, and Waissmann (2004) found that nurses working at least five 12-hour night shifts in the two week prior had 1.5 times the odds for not enough time for rest and leisure compared to nurses working day shifts.

Circadian desynchronization during night shift work and switching back to nocturnal sleep on days off has been associated with complex changes in cardiovascular, metabolic and immune function. There is a large literature of epidemiologic and physiologic studies that describe the effect of sleep deficiency and circadian disruption on adverse health outcomes which is too large to include in this paper. We mention just a few studies here to demonstrate the magnitude of this effect. Kawachi et al.'s examination of incidence data from more than 79,000 nurses in the Nurses' Health Study showed a 51% increase in risk of coronary heart disease in nurses who remained on the night shift for 6 or more years (Kawachi et al., 1995). Cardiovascular effects of night shift include sympathetic activation and a failure to retain a normal blood pressure (BP) dip during sleep, with night shift nurses not returning to baseline BP when off-duty after a shift (Lo, Liau, Hwang, & Wang, 2008). In a 4-year longitudinal study, the cumulative incidence of metabolic syndrome among night shift health care workers was 9% compared to 1.8% for day shift workers (Pietroiusti et al., 2010). Night shift workers do not have an adequate dose of darkness to synthesize adequate melatonin, a strong natural anti-inflammatory hormone that is produced in dark conditions. The International Agency for Research on Cancer, a body of the World Health Organization, has classified shift work as a "probable" carcinogen, with suspected links to melatonin deficiency. Danish night shift workers who have developed breast cancer have been compensated by their employers as a result of this occupational link (Wise, 2009). Clearly, night shift workers have increased risk for chronic diseases as a result of working at night; however, there is little recognition of the occupational basis for these chronic illnesses among workers or employers.

Some nurses choose to work the night shift. Advantages include receiving higher wages than others who work in the same position during other shifts (Camerino et al., 2008) and working when fewer supervisors are present. Whether by choice or employer mandate, the health risks of night shift remain unchanged. Strategies to reduce the health risks of night shift work have received recent attention. Smith, Fogg, and Eastman (2009) recommend that night workers adopt a sleep pattern that is intermediate between day and night shift (e.g., sleep 2 a.m.–10 a.m. on days off) to reduce the circadian impact of switching from night to day shift, although this is not practical for 12-hour shift workers. Scott, Hofmeister, Rogness, and Rogers (2010b) recently piloted a multifaceted fatigue countermeasures program to improve the quantity and quality of nurses' sleep. The intervention included sleep education, strategic planned naps, adequate staffing with completely relieved breaks, and provision of appropriate schedules to reduce fatigue risk. They found that sleep duration improved by 30 or more minutes on average, subjective sleep quality improved at 12 weeks postintervention, and drowsiness at work was also reduced as planned naps were used. In this study, drowsy driving episodes decreased by 27% at 12 weeks. Employers and nurses will need to work together to protect the health of shift workers by using these fatigue reduction measures.

Safety Culture and Climate

Aspects of work organization, such as management models, resource allocation, staffing levels and work scheduling, and decision making have an important effect on the health and safety of the workforce. In health care, such "quality of worklife" factors may also be associated with a range of quality indicators and patient safety (Conklin, MacFarland, Kinnie-Steeves, & Chenger, 1990). Safety culture, defined as the underlying principles, norms, values and beliefs of an organization with respect to safety (Roberts, 1990; Schein, 1985) and safety climate, defined as employees shared perceptions regarding safety within their organization, are important aspects of work organization. The mechanism by which safety climate is thought to protect worker health and safety is through improved compliance with safe work practices (Clarke, 2006; DeJoy, 1996; Gershon, Karkashian, & Grosch, 2000; Oliver, Cheyne, Tomas, & Cox, 2002; Seo, Torabi, Blair, & Ellis, 2004; Zohar, 2000).

No consensus exists regarding the elements and metrics for measuring safety climate, but published scales generally include the dimensions of management commitment, communication, priority of safety, management support for safe work practice, work environment supportive of safety, job hindrances and feedback (Gershon et al., 2009).

Studies examining safety climate in a number of settings including the OR (Makary, Sexton, & Freischlag, 2006a, 2006b) and hospital labor and delivery (L&D; Sexton, Holzmueller, & Pronovost, 2006) have documented a wide range in safety climate scores measured across units, hospitals and disciplines. In L&D units in 44 hospitals in diverse regions of the U.S, good teamwork climate was associated with better information management at point of transitions and communication during shift change. Job satisfaction was associated with a "good team climate" among 96 general practices in six Australian states (Harris et al., 2007), as well as greater satisfaction by patients with their care (Proudfoot et al., 2007).

Stone and Gershon surveyed 837 RNs across 39 ICUs in 23 hospitals and found a significant inverse correlation between organizational climate and musculoskeletal injuries and with all types of nurse injuries combined. They also found that ICUs in hospitals that had attained Magnet® accreditation has lower rates of negative occupational health incidents (Stone & Gershon, 2009). A 1998 cross sectional survey of 2,287 medical-surgical unit nurses in 22 U.S. hospitals, reported that poor organizational climate and high workloads were associated with 50% to twofold increases in the likelihood of needlestick injuries and near-misses to hospital nurses (Clarke et al., 2002). More recently, Smith et al found that needlestick injuries were correlated with various aspects of safety culture in a large teaching hospital in Japan (Smith et al., 2010).

Teamwork and Communication
Health care trails other high-hazard, high consequence industries such as aviation and nuclear power generation, in their efforts to introduce concepts such as high reliability organization and crew resource management. These industries have reduced risk to their workforce and the public they serve by implementing measures to limit organizational failures, technical failures and human error. Among the myriad of system level failures cited in the Institute of Medicine (IOM) report, *To Err is Human*, improved teamwork and communication skills across health care disciplines stand out as essential to reducing medical errors, improving quality and transitioning into a new era of health care delivery (Kohn, Corrigan, & Donaldson, 2000). Interdisciplinary training is making its way into the health professions. This is improving discipline-specific knowledge and roles as well as communication about responsibility for patient care.

There has been a dramatic increase in research focusing on teamwork and patient safety since publication of *To Err is Human* (Kohn et al., 2000). By contrast, there is a dearth of research examining teamwork in relationship to nurse health and safety. Among the few studies that have examine poor teamwork, is the large European "NEXT" study. Nearly 40,000 nurses from 10 European countries participating in this study completed a baseline questionnaire to identify risk factors for violence in health care. Quality of teamwork was found to be a major predictor of violence risk, when controlling for other risk factors. Odds ratios for frequent violent episodes from patients/ relatives were 1.35 (95% CI 1.24–1.48) and 1.52 (85% CI 1.33–1.74) for those nurses who reported the quality of teamwork as medium and low, respectively (Estryn-Behar et al., 2008). A grounded theory approach was used by Trenoweth (2003) to understand mental health nurses assessment of risk in clinical crisis situations. Nurses reported that they perceived lower levels of risk when working in a skilled team.

CHEMICAL HAZARDS

Disinfectants (e.g., glutaraldehyde, ethylene oxide), waste gases (e.g., anesthetics), and hazardous drugs (e.g., chemotherapeutic medications) are just some of the myriad chemicals to which health care workers are exposed. It has been estimated that in the hospital setting, employees are exposed to an average of 300 chemicals (National Institute for Occupational Safety and Health [NIOSH], 1998, 2002). Among these substances are those that are known to cause adverse health effects and others for which insufficient or no testing has been completed.

Drugs are classified as hazardous if studies in animals or humans indicate that exposures to them have a potential for causing cancer, developmental or reproductive toxicity, or harm to organs (NIOSH, 2004). Health care workers handling a range of hazardous drugs given for therapeutic benefits may suffer from the well recognized side effects of patients receiving the drugs. Occupational exposure to hazardous drugs is associated with acute effects such as skin rashes (Krstev, Perunicic, & Vidakovic, 2003; McDiarmid & Egan, 1988; Valanis, Vollmer, Labuhn, & Glass, 1993); chronic effects including adverse reproductive events (Krstev et al., 2003; Valanis, Vollmer, Labuhn, & Glass, 1997) and possibly cancer (Skov et al. 1992). The International Agency for Research on Cancer (IARC) has classified at least 10 commonly used antineoplastics drugs or combination of these drugs as carcinogenic to humans, with an equal number listed as "probably" carcinogenic to humans primarily based on animal studies (IARC 2006). A significantly increased risk of leukemia has been reported among oncology nurses identified in the Danish cancer registry for the period 1943–1987 (Skov et al., 1992).

It is in the interest of health care workers and their employers to ensure that the safe handling guidelines established by OSHA are applied in their work setting. The guidelines (Occupational Safety and Health Administration [OSHA], 1986) include procedures for storing and handling these medications. Only trained individuals should prepare these drugs, and appropriate handling equipment used. Controlling workers' exposure to such airborne chemicals necessitates respiratory protection measures including the use of specially designed booths. The handling and disposal of body fluids of patients treated with hazardous drugs also creates exposure opportunities for a wide range of health care employees, including nurses, nurse aids, housekeeping and maintenance. Despite the fact that recommendations for safe handling of hazardous drugs have been available since 1986, 11 of 12 studies reported cyclosphosphamide in the urine of health care workers indicating that current safety practices are far from adequate (Sessink & Bos, 1999). More recent studies (Connor & McDiarmid, 2006) have documented drug contamination on work surfaces in pharmacies and patient treatment areas.

Chemicals are used in health care to clean and disinfect instruments and surfaces such as formaldehyde are carcinogens and also have been linked to occupational asthma cases among health care workers (Liss et al., 2003; McGregor, Bolt, Cogliano, & Richter-Reichhelm, 2006; Quinn, Fuller, Bello, & Galligan, 2006). While OSHA standards have sought to protect workers from hazardous gas sterilants such as ethylene oxide, much work to ensure individuals' safety remains. Leaks caused by poorly maintained distribution lines allow these gases to be released, where workers in central supply may inhale them. It is important to acknowledge that not only is ethylene oxide a carcinogen, neurotoxin, reproductive health hazard, and also linked with eye damage, but it is also extremely flammable (Steenland, Whelan, Deddens, Stayner, & Ward, 2003; Tompa et al., 2006).

Chemical exposure associated with the increased use of examination and surgical latex gloves in the early 1990s led to an epidemic of allergic reactions to natural rubber latex (NRL) among nurses and other health-care workers. The prevalence of latex allergy among health-care workers is estimated to be between five and 18%, with atopic workers at greater risk (Bousquet et al., 2006; Toraason et al., 2000). Reactions range from irritant (nonallergic) contact dermatitis to latex allergy (immediate hypersensitivity). Even very low levels of exposure can trigger life threatening allergic reactions in some sensitized individuals. In response to this epidemic, NIOSH published an "Alert" document in 1997 recommending that when protection from infectious agents is needed, powder-free low protein latex gloves be used (NIOSH, 1997). A systematic review of primary prevention of latex sensitization and occupational asthma found that substitution of powdered latex gloves with low protein powder-free NRL gloves or latex-free gloves benefited both workers' health and cost and human resource savings for employers (LaMontagne, Radi, Elder, Abramson, & Sim, 2006; Malerich, Wilson, & Mowad, 2008). It should be noted that, even though symptoms may resolve among previously sensitized workers with NRL avoidance therapy, detectable IgE indicate continued sensitization remains beyond five years, and thus continued avoidance of NRL is needed (Smith et al., 2007).

Health care workers can become exposed to anesthetic waste gases while conducting various job related tasks. Incomplete seals on airway instruments continue to expose anesthesiologist to nitrous oxide (Schebesta et al., 2010). While transferring patients to the recovery room, workers may inhale gases breathed out by patients. The exposure levels of gases are generally higher during anesthesia in children up to 10 years of age than in older patients (Meier, Jost, & Ruegger, 1995). When operating room scavenging systems are not regularly serviced, anesthetic agents remain in the air (Meier et al.).

The health care industry also has a significant impact on the global environment and in particular the communities surrounding health care facilities. Hazardous, solid and medical waste all contribute to air pollution and water contamination. Hospitals alone generate more than 2 million tons of waste annually (Health Care Without Harm [HCWH], 2007), with emissions of dioxins and mercury of particular concern (Environmental Protection Agency [EPA], 1997, 2001). Recent efforts at "greening" hospitals hold promise for reducing the current impact of the health care industry on the environment. Many of the largest on-site hospital incinerators have been shut down, and a growing number of hospitals have pledged to reduce toxic emissions, including their waste stream, and make purchasing decisions that will prevent pollution from dioxins, mercury and other toxic materials (Environmental Working Group, 1998).

INFECTIOUS DISEASES

Health care workers are occupationally exposed to a range of infectious diseases via direct contact with pathogens and through airborne and bloodborne transmission. Occupational transmission of airborne infectious diseases has been recognized since the 1950s, beginning with tuberculosis (TB), and later focusing on pertussis, varicella, measles, and rubella. Over the past decade, newly emergent organisms, such as those that cause severe acute respiratory syndrome (SARS) and H1N1 influenza have been the primary concern and a focus of research and therefore will be discussed in this chapter. The primary bloodborne pathogens of concern to health care workers continue to be human immunodeficiency virus (HIV), hepatitis B virus (HBV), and hepatitis C virus (HCV).

Traditionally, influenza viruses have been thought to spread from person to person primarily through large-particle respiratory droplet transmission. However, airborne transmission also occurs via small particle aerosols in the vicinity of the infectious individual, with the relative contribution of the different modes of influenza transmission unclear at this time (Tellier, 2009).

Between November 2002 and July 2003, 1,725 health care workers worldwide contracted SARS, a human respiratory disease caused by a novel corona virus. Health care workers comprised 20% of all reported probable cases worldwide (WHO, 2003). The disease appeared to be transmitted primarily by droplets and direct contact. In some hospitals, attack rates among health care workers were nearly 60%, primarily because of delayed recognition of SARS (Russi et al., 2009). Worldwide, SARS caused 774 deaths in 2002 and 2003, with a case fatality rate of 9.6%. Even when health care workers used personal protective equipment (PPE), some patient-care activities, such as intubation, were associated with increased risk of SARS transmission (Centers for Disease Control [CDC], 2009a).

In the spring of 2009, a novel H1N1 influenza virus, derived from swine, avian, and human strains, emerged and spread rapidly, primarily via droplet spread. In response, WHO declared a Phase 6 Pandemic. Through July 2009, the case-fatality rate of H1N1 influenza has been estimated to be below 0.1%. H1N1 has disproportionately affected children as well as adults below the age of 60 (the age of most health care workers). This is in stark contrast with seasonal flu from which the elderly and infirmed are at considerably greater risk of infection and related mortality and morbidity. The main hazard to health care workers occurs when patients acutely ill with H1N1 influenza are not promptly diagnosed, when they are not properly isolated, and when health care workers do not have available and/or use recommended PPE. Universal Respiratory Protection, which requires that symptomatic patients don surgical masks when entering a health care facility, would decrease the risk of transmission to health care workers (CDC, 2009b). To date, compliance with this guidance has been limited.

Although annual influenza vaccination is recommended for health care workers and is a high priority for reducing morbidity associated with influenza in health care settings, vaccination coverage level among health care worker is inadequate. Only 44.4% of health care workers received seasonal vaccination during the 2006–2007 season; coverage increased modestly (49%) during the 2007–2008 season (Fiore et al., 2010). Coverage levels during the 2009 pandemic were higher for seasonal vaccine, but remained low for the 2009 pandemic vaccine. By mid-January 2010, estimated vaccination coverage among health care workers was 37% for 2009 pandemic influenza A (H1N1) and 62% for seasonal influenza. Overall, 64% received either of these influenza vaccines, higher coverage than any previous season, but only 35% reported receiving both vaccines (Fiore et al., 2010).

Vaccination of health care workers has been associated with reduced work absenteeism (Elder, 1996; Lemaitre et al., 2009) and with fewer deaths among nursing home patients (Carman et al., 2000, Hayward et al., 2006; Lemaitre et al., 2009) and elderly hospitalized patients (Thomas, Jefferson, Demicheli, & Rivetti, 2006). Factors associated with a higher rate of influenza vaccination among workers include older age, being a hospital employee, having employer-provided health-care insurance, having had pneumococcal or hepatitis B vaccination in the past, or having visited a health-care professional during the preceding year. Worker who decline vaccination frequently express doubts about the risk for influenza and the need for vaccination and are concerned about vaccine effectiveness and side effects, and dislike injections (Ofstead, Tucker, Beebe, & Poland, 2008). Mandatory vaccinations, as practiced by a number of health care organizations during the 2009–2010 flu seasons, continues to be controversial, especially in the absence of compliance with all aspects of CDC's 2007 Guideline for Isolation Precautions.

HEALTH CONSEQUENCES

Nursing work can lead to acute or chronic health problems because of physical and psychosocial demands, work schedules, environmental hazards, and exposure to pathogens. It is beyond the scope of this chapter to fully document all of the health consequences that accrue from nurses' work as the physiologic processes underlying responses to work stress influence every body system. We have included four common work-related conditions: musculoskeletal disorders, gastrointestinal symptoms, burnout, and WFC.

Musculoskeletal Disorders

Musculoskeletal disorders (MSDs) are common among nurses, nurse's aides, and other health care workers worldwide. There are a plethora of cross-sectional prevalence studies that show that the 12-month prevalence of low back pain (45–76%) is much more prevalent that neck (28–60%), shoulder (35%), or knee pain (22%), however rates vary considerably depending on case definition (Bos, Krol, van der Star, & Groothoff, 2007; Solidaki et al., 2010; Tinubu, Mbada, Oyeyemi, & Fabunmi, 2010; Trinkoff, Lipscomb, Geiger-Brown, & Brady, 2002). Lifetime prevalence of any musculoskeletal symptom is quite high with 80–85% of nurses reporting at least one episode (Hignett, 1996; Tinubu et al., 2010). Many nurses have musculoskeletal pain at multiple sites (Solidaki et al., 2010). Both physical work demands and psychosocial demand such as job strain (high job demands coupled with low decision latitude over work) show a recurring association with MSDs in cross sectional studies (Josephson, Lagerstrom, Hagberg, & Wigaeus, 1997; Schoenfisch & Lipscomb, 2009; Trinkoff, Le, Geiger-Brown, Lipscomb, & Lang, 2006). When examined in one longitudinal study, longer duration (e.g., 12-hour shifts) and higher intensity of physical demands predicted incident MSDs over 15 months (Trinkoff, Le, et al., 2006). However, in the large European NEXT study, psychosocial risk factors were more strongly associated with disability from back injury then were physical demands or availability of lifting devices (Simon et al., 2008). Despite the inability of cross sectional studies to examine causative relationships between work-related risk factors and incident MSDs, we continue to see new studies being published using nonstandard case definitions, and using exposure measures that are not comparable to previous studies. Under-reporting of work-related injuries is common (Menzel, 2004) and reduces the usefulness of compensation claims to estimate the prevalence of these injuries.

Preventing MSDs is important to retain a healthy nursing workforce. Nurses that left jobs from multiple hospitals in Sweden over a three year period were surveyed to identify reasons for this change (Fochsen, Josephson, Hagberg, Toomingas, & Lagerstrom, 2006). These nurses often attributed their leaving to musculoskeletal problems (neck and shoulder were common) as well as working in situations where they had manual patient handling demands but limited access to lifting devices. In home care there are usually no such devices and the working conditions are not standardized, nor controllable by an organization. In a study of home care nurses (Horneij, Jensen, Holmstrom, & Ekdahl, 2004) low back pain, high strain work, and high perceived physical demands increased use of sick leave over 18 months prospectively for those who had not used sick leave in the previous 18 months. In addition to work-related consequences, Trinkoff et al. (2002) found that injured nurses often curtailed nonwork activities and recreation, reducing their quality of life. There is some promising work on measuring the mismatch between nurses' work ability and their work environment (Gilworth et al., 2007) that may increase knowledge about how to modify employment to prevent MSD-related nursing retention problems.

Extensive research involving task analysis and biomechanical evaluations of patient handling tasks has documented high levels of stress on caregivers when performing patient transfers and repositioning tasks. The use of portable or ceiling-mounted mechanical lifts significantly reduces the back compression force of the caregiver by approximately two-thirds when compared with manual methods (Anderson, 2001; Marras, Davis, Kirking, & Bertsche, 1999; Zhuang, Stobbe, Hsiao, Collins, & Hobbs, 1999). However, interventions to prevent MSDs continue to focus on changing nurses' knowledge (e.g., training in body mechanics) and own health behavior (e.g., physical exercise, proper shoes) rather than organizational level interventions (e.g., limiting work hours, "no lift" policies, ergonomic equipment readily available; Chiu & Wang, 2007; Yuan et al., 2009). Training in lifting techniques (e.g., "back school") were deemed ineffective based on a systematic review (Hignett, 2003). Primary preventive measures such as appropriate lifting devices are effective in reducing MSDs (Evanoff, Wolf, Aton, Canos, & Collins, 2003), but must be readily accessible and with management support for nurses to use them. The American Nurses' Association "Handle with Care" campaign promotes adoption of a zero-lift policy for nurses, and cites cost effectiveness data from three studies where workman's compensation injuries and lost workdays from injuries were reduced by more than half and the costs for investment in equipment were recouped in 3–4 years (Collins, Wolf, Bell, & Evanoff, 2004). There are some state-level regulations but no Federal regulations to support "no-lift" policies (Morse et al., 2008). Prevention of MSDs is particularly important now that hospitals are increasing their bariatric services including bariatric surgery (Muir & Archer-Heese, 2009).

Gastrointestinal Disturbances

Nurses working shift work and rotating shifts have a higher prevalence of gastrointestinal (GI) symptoms and disorders (reflux, gastritis, ulcer disease, irritable bowel, abdominal discomfort, use of antacids and proton-pump inhibitors) based on cross-sectional surveys of convenience samples (Bilski, 2006; Nojkov, Rubenstein, Chey, & Hoogerwerf, 2010; Sveinsdottir, 2006; Zhen Lu, Ann Gwee, & Yu Ho, 2006). This is not surprising, as all gastrointestinal functions are regulated by clock-genes that are misaligned when there is work-related circadian misalignment. These GI symptoms were more related to sleep deprivation associated with shift work, rather than the shift work itself in one study (Zhen Lu et al., 2006), but in a recent cross-sectional study of 399 nurses, this was not found to be the case. In this study, night shift nurses had a higher risk for irritable bowel syndrome, and rotating shift nurses showed more abdominal pain than day shift irrespective of sleep quality (Nojkov et al., 2010). Nurses attribute some of their poor daytime sleep after a night shift to GI complaints (Chan, 2009), thus the association between shift work, sleep deprivation and GI complaints may be bidirectional.

Another risk factor for gastrointestinal disease is infection with Helicobacter pylori. In most adults, colonization with this bacteria occurred during childhood, with 30–40% of adults showing evidence of colonization (van Mark, Spallek, Groneberg, Kessel, & Weiler, 2010). Nurses and other health care workers who work in endoscopy suites have higher rate of infection in 3 of 4 studies when compared to matched samples (Nojkov et al., 2010), with rate of infection increasing as the number of endoscopic procedures increased (Nishikawa et al., 1998) particularly over the first five years of working in this specialty in one study (Wang, Lu, & Wang, 1997), although another study contradicts these results (Chong et al., 1994). Because the transmission of H. pylori is human-human (fecal-oral), and because the prevalence of this bacterium is higher in low socioeconomic strata and increases with age, nurses working in settings with increased exposure risk from these populations must be vigilant. It has been postulated that these infections can be prevented by using appropriate infection control measures (Wang et al., 1997), but this has not been tested.

It has also been postulated that those colonized with H. pylori have a higher risk of progressing to gastritis or peptic ulcer disease if they work the night shift, although results have been inconsistent. A study of automotive workers (with schedules similar to nurses) showed that H. pylori was more prevalent in shift workers, but that clinical GI symptoms did not correlate with shift pattern (van Market al., 2010). However, in a sample of infected workers with dyspepsia who were assessed by endoscopy, the odds of duodenal ulcer were nearly four times higher in shift workers when compared with day workers (Pietroiusti et al., 2006), suggesting a stronger effect for shift work in a later stage of infection.

Nurses working the night shift sometimes take a meal break during their shift, and some report that food is hard to digest at night (Bilski, 2006). Night nurses display higher caffeine consumption, and often eat to preserve alertness rather than to counter hunger, as hunger is generally decreased at night (Lowden et al., 2001). Since institutional food services are nearly always closed at night they rely on vending machines or take-out foods from local all-night eateries. Their food choices are often unhealthful. Despite the Magnet® hospital move towards creating a 'healthy work environment' for nurses, night shift nurses do not have the same opportunities for healthful food that day nurses enjoy.

Burnout

Burnout is a phenomenon that has been extensively studied in the health and social assistance professions. The cause of burnout is well documented. This condition is caused by prolonged exposure to work-related stress (Dobson & Schnall, 2009). Mental health symptoms predominate including a sense of emotional depletion, loss of energy, cynicism, emotional distance from others at work, low productivity and a negative self-image. Burnout is not the same as clinical depression, but can precede depression if it is prolonged. There are more than one hundred international cross-sectional prevalence studies of burnout rates among nurses going back to the 1970s, some with fairly small samples, and usually using the Maslach Burnout Inventory as the measure of burnout. Point or 12-month prevalence rates varied widely, with 30–50% of nurses experiencing threshold symptoms in one or more of the Maslach subscales (emotional exhaustion, depersonalization, reduced sense of personal accomplishment). Because the studies are often segregated by type of nursing (e.g., ICU nurses, hemodialysis nurses, military nurses, etc.) there is an inference that the type of job stress inherent in that type of nursing is associated with the burnout, although in many studies the actual work stressors are not characterized or measured.

Cross-sectional nurses' burnout prediction studies focus on both macro-organizational and work unit job stressors. From a macro-organizational context, three types of work stress increased burnout among nurses in recent studies: adverse management practices and lack of supervisor skill (Pedrini et al., 2009), organizational restructuring and the effects of downsizing (Greenglass & Burke, 2002), and inadequate staffing levels (Garrett, 2008) which are under the control of the organization. There are many job stressors associated with burnout at the level of the actual work unit context of the nurse. These include adverse work schedules (working more than 8 hours per day, or working shift work; Lang, Pfister, & Siemens, 2010) and overtime, whether mandatory or voluntary (especially if feeling pressured to do so; Patrick & Lavery, 2007). Work overload, including high physical and mental demands, were also linked to burnout in nursing home nurses (van den Tooren & de Jonge, 2008), and ICU nurses (Embriaco, Papazian, Kentish-Barnes, Pochard, & Azoulay, 2007). Nurses who care for patients and families who present a high degree of emotional demand, or place the nurse in situations where there is conflict about how best to care for the patient are also at increased risk for burnout. Examples include military nurses who have a higher exposure to injured veterans from Afghanistan and Iraq wars (Lang et al., 2010), pediatric bone marrow transplant patients on units with high acuity (Gallagher & Gormley, 2009), and nursing home nurses where families have expectations for care that cannot be delivered (Abrahamson, Suitor, & Pillemer, 2009).

It can be argued that cross-sectional studies of burnout are suspect since the burned out state of the respondent could influence their appraisal of work stressors. We have been able to locate only one English language longitudinal study of nurses where predictors were assessed prior to incident cases of nurses' burnout. In a recent cohort of more than 1,300 Swedish nurses, higher level of personal empowerment at baseline was associated with higher burnout at one year, an unexpected finding (Hochwalter, 2008). The author explained this surprising result by reflecting that the empowerment measure examined psychological empowerment but did not measure actual structural empowerment (e.g., provision of resources on the job), and both empowerment and burnout appeared to be stable traits within subjects at baseline and 1 year.

There are consequences of nursing burnout to employers. The European NEXT study of more than 28,000 nurses in 10 countries demonstrate that nurses with high burnout scores had three times the risk of having high intent to leave their job in half of the countries where nurses were surveyed (Estryn-Behar et al., 2007). Sickness absence also has adverse economic consequences to the organization. In a qualitative study where nurses out on sick leave for two or more months due to burnout-related conditions showed that the primary factor influencing their sickness absence was the employer's devaluation of nurses and failing to include them in the process of decision making that directly affected their daily work (Billeter-Koponen & Freden, 2005). In addition to adverse consequences for employers, patients cared for by a nursing staff with high unit-aggregated nurse burnout scores were often less satisfied than those in hemodialysis facilities where nurses were more positive (Argentero, Dell'Olivo, & Ferretti, 2008).

Nurse studies were heavily represented in a review of 25 intervention studies where burnout prevention was the focus (Awa, Plaumann, & Walter, 2010). Of the 25 intervention trials only two were focused at changing the organization of work, 19 provided individual-level interventions, and the others combined these two modalities. Individual-level interventions were directed towards changing the worker's affective reaction to stress (psychotherapy, counseling), increasing their hardiness to cope with stress (cognitive behavioral training, communication skills, adaptive skill training), increasing their social support, or reducing the impact of stress by using relaxation exercises or recreation such as music making. In seven of the ten individual-level randomized controlled trials there was a significant decrease in burnout. The one organizational-level intervention that was conducted with nurses introduced primary nursing as the care delivery process, and this was not effective in reducing burnout. There were six intervention studies where organizational and individual level interventions were combined, and in three of these studies, burnout was decreased. The authors recommended these combined interventions, with better study design, longer follow up, and measures to reduce study dropout.

Work–Family Conflict

Occupational scientists have examined the organization of work and its effect on the home lives of workers. Allen, Herst, Bruck, and Sutton's (2000) model of WFC described the three main dimensions of this phenomenon. WFC influences work-related outcomes (job satisfaction, organizational commitment, intent to leave, absenteeism, job performance), nonwork related outcomes (marital and family satisfaction, family performance, life satisfaction), and worker stress-related outcomes (burnout, substance abuse, depression, somatic symptoms; Allen et al., 2000). The prevalence of WFC is quite high among nurses, with 50% of nurses reporting having work-related interference with family at least once a week (Grzywacz, Frone, Brewer, & Kovner, 2006). Although family life sometimes interferes with work, this was far less common (11%) in this prevalence study. In Allen's review, the relationship between increased WFC and decreased job satisfaction was robust. Sources of WFC were remarkably consistent among studies, including high levels of work demands, irregular work hours, pressure to work overtime, and inflexibility in work hours to accommodate child care needs (Fujimoto, Kotani, & Suzuki, 2008; Simon, Kümmerling, Hasselhorn, & Next-Study Group, 2004; Yildirim & Aycan, 2008).

Although WFC often influenced intent to leave, actual nurse retention was often not assessed in these studies. The exception is a longitudinal study by Brewer, Kovner, Greene, and Cheng (2009) where macro-contextual factors such as market area wages and benefits exerted significant influence on whether nurses actually remained in a nursing job. In this study WFC was a significant cross-sectional predictor of nurses' desire to quit and intent to leave their job within one year. However, when actual employment in nursing was measured one year later, market forces (higher wages and better benefits) were the significant predictor of whether nurses were retained in nursing. These authors point out that family-friendly work environments may attract and retain younger nurses with children under age 6 (for example, flexible hours, concierge services). The availability, quality and cost of childcare continue to be a source of WFC for employed mothers (Poms, Botsford, Kaplan, Buffardi, & O'Brien, 2009), which could also link market forces to job retention. Taken as a whole, these studies suggest that solutions for reducing WFC are under the control of the employer, and necessitate a reorganization of the work environment.

Aging Workforce

Health care workers continue to work to a later age than they have in prior years. Buerhaus, Staiger, and Auerbach, (2009) estimates that by 2012 nurses in their 50s are anticipated to comprise nearly one quarter of the RN population, with the average age of RNs projected to be 44.5 years. Older health care workers have strengths that they bring to the workforce. For example, older home care RNs were found to have more education, report less burnout, have greater confidence when working with demanding clients, and receive more respect from their peers (McPhaul & Lipscomb, 2009). Given these strengths, retaining such workers is advantageous. However, present working conditions and assignments should be modified to accommodate these workers and reduce the possibility of injury to staff and clients. The age-related decline in strength and increased joint pain make physical tasks such as lifting more difficult. Because of natural declines in vision and hearing certain working conditions such as insufficient lighting, excessive noise, and regular interruptions can contribute to fatigue, reduced focus, and medical errors. Kemmlert and Lundholm (1998) found that workers age 45 and older were more likely to experience slip, trip, and fall (STF) accidents than younger workers.

The effects of normal aging on endurance make excessive work more difficult. Older workers are being asked to perform in ways that exceed reasonable expectations when they are called to work night shifts, extended work shifts (e.g., 12-hour days), overtime hours or work many consecutive days without time off. Costa and DiMilia (2008) note that between the ages of 45–50, individuals experience greater intolerance of shift and night work. Compared to their younger counterparts, older workers have less efficient sleep which can contribute to fatigue, although they may appear to be less sleepy than younger workers during the night shift. Older workers often provide care for their sick, elderly or disabled loved ones at home, which reduces times for rest and recovery (Silverstein, 2008). These factors suggest the need to further investigate the relationship between age and increased injuries, the impact of shift work and patient safety.

SAFETY CONSEQUENCES

Work organization and policies and the physical work environment play important roles in keeping nurses safe during their work shift, and while driving home. This section of the chapter describes four common injury outcomes of nurses' work: needlestick injuries; slips, trips, and falls; workplace violence, and drowsy driving. Most organizations view these as isolated random incidents but the risk factors for each are well document, they are modifiable by making organizational changes, and there is evidence for effective intervention strategies. As these safety hazards can have career-ending or fatal consequences for nurses, we encourage health care employers to improve occupational surveillance and primary preventive measures to reduce nurses' risk for illness and injury.

Needlestick Injuries

Exposure to bloodborne pathogens through contact with contaminated sharps has lead to serious consequences among a large number of health care workers.

Each year, an estimated 600,000 to 800,000 needlestick injuries occur in the United States among these workers, 54% involving nurses. While these numbers already appear substantial, it is important to note that underreporting is estimated at 39–56% (Perry, Parker, & Jagger, 2001). This significant health risk has continued to impact workers following enactment of the Occupational Safety and Health Administration (OSHA) Bloodborne Pathogens (BBP) Standard of 1991 which required employers of health care workers to have exposure control plans. The subsequent Needlestick Safety and Prevention Act of 2001 sought to enforce greater compliance of the OSHA BBP Standard. Additionally, it required employers to regularly review their exposure control plans, record injuries, and discontinue use of dangerous, conventional needles and sharps devices (29 CRF 1910.1030; Lee, Botteman, Xanthakos, & Nicklasson, 2005; OSHA, 1991, 2001).

Nevertheless, health care workers continue to become exposed to bloodborne pathogens via needlestick and sharps injuries. Trinkoff, Le, Geiger-Brown, and Lipscomb's (2007) population-based longitudinal study of needlestick injuries reported the cumulative incidence of RN needlestick injuries was 16.3% over 15 months of follow up. Factors that predicted a needlestick included working 12-hour shifts, nonday shift hours and weekends, controlling for frequency of needle use. In this study, one-third of needle sticks occurred with safer-designed needles, so engineering controls have not solved this problem. These incidents have both physical and emotional consequences. Among the individuals affected, approximately 6–30% will develop Hepatitis B, 0.4–1.8% will develop Hepatitis C, and 0.25–0.4% will develop HIV (Centers for Disease Control and Prevention, 2003). Thankfully, under the BBP Standard the Hepatitis B vaccine is made available free of charge to health care workers; resulting in a dramatic reduction in HBV infections in health care workers; a rate lower than in the general population. Unfortunately, there is no such option for those exposed to Hepatitis C or HIV, which greatly underlines the importance of safeguarding these workers.

It is important to stress that these injuries can be dramatically reduced by discontinuing the use of conventional sharps. Prevention strategies should also entail the purchase and correct use of sharps devices with engineered injury-protection features, needleless devices and proper disposal containers. Post-exposure prophylaxis and counseling should be provided and all incidents should be logged and reviewed. Moreover, staff should be engaged in the selection of safety-engineered sharps devices, and help identify strategies for addressing barriers to reporting (Scharf, McPhaul, Trinkoff, & Lipscomb, 2009).

Drowsy Driving

Drowsy driving represents a risk to both nurses and to the public with whom they share the road. The National Highway Transportation Safety Board estimates that each year drowsy driving is responsible for more than 100,000 police-reported crashes, 71,000 injuries, 1,550 deaths and $12.5 billion in diminished productivity and property loss, although they acknowledge that this is an underestimate because of inconsistent police reporting methods (Moore, Kaprielian, & Auerbach, 2009). Two studies of nurses have examined self-reported drowsy driving using a daily log for four weeks of duty time (Dorrian et al., 2008; Scott et al., 2007). In Scott's study, nearly two thirds of nurses reported at least one drowsy driving episode during the four week measurement period, and a small number (3%) were drowsy after every shift. As expected, night shift nurses and nurses with shorter sleep before the shift had more difficulty than those working the day shift. Both studies confirmed that when nurses struggle to remain awake at work they have a higher likelihood of also being drowsy on the ride home (Dorrian et al., 2008; Scott et al., 2007). The best data on drowsy driving are from a study of 100 video-instrumented cars driven over 42,000 miles where drivers were continuously observed during naturalistic driving (Dingus et al., 2006). This study showed that 22% of all motor vehicle crashes, and 16% of near-crashes could be attributed to drowsy driving.

These data are instructive, since systematic data collection on drowsy driving motor vehicle crashes in many U.S. states is poor because police are not trained to assess and collect these data (National Sleep Foundation, 2008). In European nations and Australia, where crash reporting is more consistent, the estimate of drowsy driving as a cause of MVC is 10–30%. Drowsy driving accidents tend to be more severe as the driver fails to brake before the collision. The authors are aware of several instances of nurses being killed while driving home from work in single car, off the road accidents.

There are numerous drowsy driving studies that implicate work schedules with extended shifts (Robb, Sultana, Ameratunga, & Jackson, 2008), night shift (Rogers, Holmes, & Spencer, 2001; Stutts, Wilkins, Scott Osberg, & Vaughn, 2003), inadequate sleep prior to working (Gander, Marshall, Harris, & Reid, 2005; Philip & Akerstedt, 2006; Valent, Di Bartolomeo, Marchetti, Sbrojavacca, & Barbone, 2010). However, there are significant inter-individual differences in tolerance to sleep deprivation that can be traced to genetic polymorphisms (Czeisler, 2009) so some nurses may be less tolerant of sleep deprivation and thus have a greater risk for drowsy driving. Drivers with sleep disorders such as sleep apnea, narcolepsy, insomnia, and restless leg syndrome also have a higher risk for drowsy driving (Volna & Sonka, 2006).

In addition to work-related sleep deprivation, behavioral lifestyle choices can also increase the risk for drowsy driving (Papadakaki, Kontogiannis, Tzamalouka, Darviri, & Chliaoutakis, 2008), including "workaholism" and recreational activities. Specific work demands during the shift can increase fatigue and the risk of MVC with injuries. In a cohort of energy industry workers, the risk for crashes was increased for those with "nervously tiring work," sustained standing, and working in uncomfortable positions (Chiron, Bernard, Lafont, & Lagarde, 2008); all of these have also been described as stressors in nursing. Most drivers are aware of their sleepiness prior to crashing but that self-awareness does not deter them from continuing to drive drowsy (Nabi et al., 2007), and some nurses report having had several drowsy driving accidents during commutes home thus awareness does not translate into preventive behavior. Nurses are often aware of their drowsiness on the commute home, and take countermeasures to combat the urge to sleep. The most popular countermeasures were the least effective, including driving with the car window open, radio playing loud music, and least often, taking a rest (Vanlaar, Simpson, Mayhew, & Robertson, 2007). Caffeine is an effective countermeasure (De Valck & Cluydts, 2001; De Valck, De Groot, & Cluydts, 2003; De Valck, Quanten, Berckmans, & Cluydts, 2007), at least temporarily, but will disrupt subsequent sleep leaving the nurse even more sleep deprived upon returning for the next shift. Naps are also an effective countermeasure (Signal, Gander, Anderson, & Brash, 2009; Smith, Kilby, Jorgensen, & Douglas, 2007), however most nurses prefer to leave at the end of their work shift rather than napping briefly to avoid drowsy driving. In most institutions, planned napping during the work shift is not an option. A recent pilot intervention to reduce fatigue in nurses showed decreased drowsy driving by 27% 12 weeks postintervention and markedly decreased motor vehicle crashes (Scott, Hofmeister, Rogness, & Rogers, 2010a, 2010b). Even without driver awareness, employers can use fatigue risk management software to look for potential driving risks among employees based on their work schedules (Moore-Ede et al., 2004).

In addition to relying on nurses to avoid drowsy driving there are also engineering controls that can reduce the risk for MVAs and reduce the injuries incurred if there is a crash. Rumble strips have saved drivers from exiting the lane, and research demonstrates that these have a short-lived alerting effect (Anund, Kecklund, Vadeby, Hjalmdahl, & Akerstedt, 2008). Some automobile models are coming out with systems to detect drowsiness and alert the driver, although these are available only in high-end automobiles at present.

Slips, Trips, and Falls

One of the most common reasons for health care employee visits to the occupational health unit is injury from a slip, trip or fall (Bell et al., 2008; Drebit, Shajari, Alamgir, Yu, & Keen, 2010). These injuries comprise about one-fifth of nonfatal occupational injuries in the United States based on OSHA First Report logs reported to the BLS (2009), however many employees do not use the occupational health unit but rather their own personal medical care provider, thus this may be an underestimate. Among health care employers, hospitals have the highest rate of lost work-time injuries, which is three times greater than for other private industries (Bell et al., 2008). Because of the size of the nursing workforce, they have a large number of claims but their rate of claims (1 per 100 FTE) is lower than for hospital food service workers, custodial and housekeeping workers, and EMS ambulance workers (Bell et al., 2008). Community workers, such as home health nurses, also have a very high rate, which may be due to working in an uncontrolled environment in the home, as well as in rain and ice (Drebit et al., 2010). Many injuries are sprains, strains, and tears, however fractures are common in older workers, such as postmenopausal nurses with low body mass (Cherry et al., 2005). Wet floors, cluttered hallway, irregular surfaces, inadequate lighting and improper footwear are common precipitants of falls (Bell et al., 2008). Surgical areas such as laparoscopy suites have multiple exposed cords and tubing in a dimly lit environment, and are high risk areas for falls (Cappell, 2010). In order to prevent these events a comprehensive program should include inspection of the physical work environment as well as consideration of work organization factors such as rushing, fatigue, safety culture, and equipment decisions that increase the latent environment in which slips, trips and falls can occur (Bentley, 2008). A prevention program implemented in three hospitals over 3 years produced a decreased rate of slips, trips and falls among hospital workers, with pre-intervention rates of 1.67 per 100 FTE, falling to 0.76 per FTE for the three years following the intervention (Bell et al., 2008).

Workplace Violence

Incidents of workplace violence in health care are prevalent and at times fatal. Across all industries, violent acts and assaults were the second leading cause of occupational injury related death and the leading cause of occupational injury death among women, with approximately 564 deaths per year occurring between 2004 and 2008 (BLS, 2010). By comparison, 1.7 million incidents of nonfatal violence occurred annually each year from 1992 to 1996 according to data from the National Crime Victimization Survey (NCVS; Warchol, 1998). Six percent of these injuries required medical treatment and 44% of the 1.7 incidents were reported to law enforcement authorities. A more recent report from a nationally representative study found that 41.4% of workers reported acts of psychological aggression and 6% reporting incidents of physical aggression (Schat, Frone, & Kelloway, 2006). Twelve percent of the 1.7 million annual nonfatal incidents of workplace violence documented in the NCVS occurred in health care workers (Warchol, 1998). The highest incidence rate among medical personnel was seen among nurses; 22 incidents per 1,000 workers.

A framework for addressing workplace violence, first developed by California OSHA and later revised and published in the 2001 Report to the Nation on Workplace Violence, classifies the various types of violence by the relationship between the perpetrator and the worker victim (University of Iowa Injury Prevention Research Center, 2001):

- Type I (Criminal Intent): Results while a criminal activity (e.g., robbery) is being committed and the perpetrator has no legitimate relationship to the workplace.
- Type II (Customer/Client): The perpetrator is a customer or client at the workplace (e.g., health care patient) and becomes violent while being served by the worker.
- Type III (Worker-on-Worker): Employees or past employees of the workplace are the perpetrators in this case.
- Type IV (Personal Relationship): The perpetrator in this case usually has a personal relationship with an employee (e.g., domestic violence in the workplace).

While this section will focus on Type II (patient/client) violence, Type I (criminal intent) and Type III (co-worker) violence also occur in health care. Patient/client violence is a well-documented occupational hazard in health care (Lipscomb & Love, 1992; NIOSH, 2009; Warchol, 1998). In a study conducted by Bensley and colleagues (1997), 73% of psychiatric hospital staff participating reported experiencing minor injuries related to patient aggression within the past 12 months. Moreover, the incidence rate of assaults leading to minor injuries reported via a staff survey was 437 per 100 employees annually, which was far greater than the number of incidents reported through administrative channels Bensley, et al., 1997). There are various organizational, environmental, and personal factors associated with patient/client assaults. These include workplace security, understaffing, transporting patients, and patient history of violent behavior (NIOSH, 2002). In a 1999 study by Lee, Gerberich, Waller, Anderson, and McGovern, the presence of security guards was found to reduce assault rates among hospital nurses. Other characteristics such as a high patient/staff ratio were associated with higher rates of assault. Inadequate staffing was also correlated with greater incidents of patient violence in the 2005 National Survey of the Work and Health of Nurses, which was completed by 18,676 employed Canadian nurses. Other significant predictors of violence included working non-day shifts and having less experience (Shields & Wilkins, 2009). Among patient characteristics, having a history of violent behavior is a major risk factor for future violence. In a study by Drummond, Sparr, and Gordon (1989), "flagging" records of patients with a history of violent behavior reduced staff assaults by 91%. This is particularly important as many studies indicate that it is often the same, small number of patients who commit the majority of these violent acts (Hillbrand, Foster, & Spitz, 1996).

Prevention strategies for reducing workplace violence in health care often is limited to training to recognize cues and other signs of patient behavior and teaching techniques for defusing escalating behavior . In mental health settings, training regarding the management of violent patients is usually required. Among the few studies reviewing the effectiveness of these trainings, the results have been mixed. While no difference in nurses' confidence and safety was found post-training by Hurlebaus and Link (1997), Lehmann, Padilla, Clark, and Loucks (1983) noted greater confidence and knowledge among trained staff. Evidence of the need for and effectiveness of comprehensive workplace violence programming are beginning to be recognized. A number of states that have introduced legislation to mandate such programs, as they are effective in reducing violence.

OSHA's "Guidelines for Preventing Workplace Violence for Healthcare and Social Service Workers" (OSHA, 1986, 2004) recommend instituting health and safety programs which feature a comprehensive risk assessment, hazard prevention and control, post-incident response, and recording and evaluation of incidents. Studies have demonstrated the feasibility of implementing and maintaining these programs (Adamson, 2009; Lipscomb et al., 2006). Moreover, these programs have been associated with reduced risk for violence in psychiatric facilities (Lipscomb, 2006).

RECOMMENDATIONS FOR FUTURE RESEARCH

Our recommendations for future research and policy development address the need for different research methods to the study of health care worker health and safety as well as for approaches to better understand and ultimately modify organizational level factors associated with a range of hazardous working conditions. Although cross-sectional studies are a necessary beginning to establish the prevalence of a specific exposure or health outcome, this literature has far too many "dead ends" where valuable prevalence studies never led to longitudinal studies that could establish causal links between exposures and occupational health outcomes for nurses. We contend that without large sample multisite prospective cohort studies, the science falls short of its goal.

For studies of nurses working in hospitals, more attention should be paid to measuring unit level variation of work culture and work organization. Methods for cross-level analyses (individual-unit, unit-hospital) are well-developed and examination of these cross-level influences has the potential to shed new light on nurse retention, illness and injury. We contend that variables often aggregated to the hospital level actually reflect unit level processes where work culture is most influential. Magnet® level designation among health care institutions is based on a range of indicators of quality of the nurse practice environment. Research is needed to evaluate the sustainability of these desirable working conditions once Magnet status is achieved. More studies of home care and rural settings are necessary as these health care settings are underrepresented in the literature, and nurses working in these settings have unique health and safety risks that are largely undocumented.

National efforts to recruit more students into professional nursing have been successful on a number of levels. Research addressing the role of health and safety in the retention of these nurses is needed to assure an adequate stable future nursing workforce. Studies should include unit, hospital and macro-contextual variables as well as individual adverse exposures. The importance of such macro-context studies may become apparent as health care reform legislation is implemented, and rigorous evaluation research to assess the effect of these policy changes is needed.

We also support participatory action research methods as a highly ethical means of collecting occupational data and working with nurses and administrators to improve the quality of nurses' work life. Using this study design, nurses will have substantial input into the selection of hazard controls. Nurses and other direct care workers have critical job related expertise that should be drawn upon to inform control strategies for the prevention of exposure to hazardous working conditions. For example, the revised OSHA Bloodborne Pathogen standard of 2000 requires that front line nurses have input into the selection and testing of safer needle devices. Research, including demonstration projects, is needed to evaluate the impact of this element of the standard and interventions designed to enhance nurse input into decision making regarding improved safety.

A number of states have passed legislation mandating various health and safety provisions, including those addressing safe lifting, workplace violence prevention, safe staffing ratios. Policy research is needed to evaluate the impact of these laws on a range of worker and institution level outcomes. These policy research initiatives will benefit from cross-disciplinary teams of scientists, policy specialists, and communication experts to move scientific findings into actual workplace changes that benefit the health and safety of nurses, other health care providers and ultimately improve patient care.

ACKNOWLEDGMENT

The authors acknowledge Joan Kanner, MA, for her contribution to this manuscript.

REFERENCES

Abrahamson, K., Jill Suitor, J., & Pillemer, K. (2009). Conflict between nursing home staff and residents' families: Does it increase burnout? *Journal of Aging and Health*, 21(6), 895–912.

Adamson, A., Vincent, A., & Cundiff, J. (2009). Common ground, not a battle ground: Violence prevention at a detoxification facility. *Journal of Psychosocial Nursing and Mental Health Services*, 47(8), 28–35.

Akerstedt, T. (2003). Shift work and disturbed sleep/wakefulness. *Occupational Medicine (Oxford, England)*, 53(2), 89–94.

Allen, T. D., Herst, D. E., Bruck, C. S., & Sutton, M. (2000). Consequences associated with work-to-family conflict: A review and agenda for future research. *Journal of Occupational Health Psychology*, 5(2), 278–308.

American Nurses Association. (2006a). *Assuring patient safety: The employers' role in promoting healthy nursing work hours for registered nurses in all roles and settings*. Washington, DC: American Nurses Association. Retrieved from http://www.nursingworld.org/assurring safetyemployerps

American Nurses Association. (2006b). *Assuring patient safety: Registered nurses' responsibility in all roles and settings to guard against working when fatigued*. Washington, DC: American Nurses Association. Retrieved from http://www.nursingworld.org/assurringsafetynurseps

Anderson, B. T. (2001). Sudden movements of the spinal column during health-care work. *International Journal of Industrial Ergonomics*, 28(1), 47–53.

Anund, A., Kecklund, G., Vadeby, A., Hjälmdahl, M., & Akerstedt, T. (2008). The alerting effect of hitting a rumble strip–A simulator study with sleepy drivers. *Accident; Analysis and Prevention*, 40(6), 1970–1976.

Argentero, P., Dell'Olivo, B., & Ferretti, M. S. (2008). Staff burnout and patient satisfaction with the quality of dialysis care. *American Journal of Kidney Diseases: the Official Journal of the National Kidney Foundation*, 51(1), 80–92.

Awa, W. L., Plaumann, M., & Walter, U. (2010). Burnout prevention: A review of intervention programs. *Patient Education and Counseling*, 78(2), 184–190.

Bell, J. L., Collins, J. W., Wolf, L., Gronqvist, R., Chiou, S., Chang, W. R., . . . Evanoff, B. (2008). Evaluation of a comprehensive slip, trip and fall prevention programme for hospital employees. *Ergonomics*, 51(12), 1906–1925.

Bentley, T. (2009). The role of latent and active failures in workplace slips, trips and falls: An information processing approach. *Applied Ergonomics*, 40(2), 175–180.

Bensley, L., Nelson, N., Kaufman, J., Silverstein, B., Kalat, J., & Shields, J. W. (1997). Injuries due to assaults on psychiatric hospital employees in Washington State. *American Journal of Industrial Medicine*, 31(1), 92–99.

Billeter-Koponen, S., & Fredén, L. (2005). Long-term stress, burnout and patient-nurse relations: Qualitative interview study about nurses' experiences. *Scandinavian Journal of Caring Sciences*, 19(1), 20–27.

Bilski, B. (2006). [Influence of shift work on the diet and gastrointestinal complains among nurses. A pilot study]. *Medycyna Pracy*, 57(1), 15–19.

Boivin, D. B., Tremblay, G. M., & James, F. O. (2007). Working on atypical schedules. *Sleep Medicine*, 8(6), 578–589.

Bos, E., Krol, B., van der Star, L., & Groothoff, J. (2007). Risk factors and musculoskeletal complaints in non-specialized nurses, IC nurses, operation room nurses, and X-ray technologists. *International Archives of Occupational and Environmental Health*, 80(3), 198–206.

Bousquet, A., Flahault, O., Vandenplas, J., Ameille, J.J., Duron, C., Pecquet, K.,...Annesi-Maesano, I. (2006). Natural rubber latex allergy among health care workers: A systemic review of the evidence. *Journal of Allergy and Clinical Immunology*, 118, 447–454.

Brewer, C. S., Kovner, C. T., Greene, W., & Cheng, Y. (2009). Predictors of RNs' intent to work and work decisions 1 year later in a U.S. national sample. *International Journal of Nursing Studies*, 46(7), 940–956.

Buerhaus, P. I., Staiger, D. O., & Auerbach, D. I. (2009). *The future of the nursing workforce in the United States: Data, trends and implications*. Sudbury, MS: Jones and Bartlett Publishers.

Bureau of Labor Statistics. (2005). *Incidence rates for nonfatal occupational injuries and illnesses involving days away from work per 10,000 full-time workers by industry and selected parts of body affected by injury or illness, 2005, Table R8*. Retrieved from www.bls.gov/iif/oshwc/osh/case/ostb1664.pdf

Bureau of Labor Statistics. (2009). *Incident rates of nonfatal occupational injuries and illnesses by case type*. Retrieved from http://www.bls.gov/iif/oshwc/osh/os/ostb2071.pdf

Bureau of Labor Statistics. (2010). Fatality data are from the Census of Fatal Occupational Injuries, Factsheet issued July 14, 2010.

Calnan, D. (2000). Wainwright and S. Almond, Job strain, effort-reward imbalance and mental distress: A study of occupations in general medical practice. *Work & Stress*, 14, 297–311.

Camerino, D., Conway, P. M., Sartori, S., Campanini, P., Estryn-Béhar, M., van der Heijden, B. I., & Costa, G. (2008). Factors affecting work ability in day and shift-working nurses. *Chronobiology International*, 25(2), 425–442.

Cappell, M. S. (2010). Injury to endoscopic personnel from tripping over exposed cords, wires and tubing in the endoscopy suite: A preventable cause of potentially severe workplace injury. *Digestive Diseases & Sciences*, 55(4), 947–951.

Carman, W. F., Elder, A. G., Wallace, L. A., McAulay, K., Walker, A., Murray, G. D., & Stott, D. J. (2000). Effects of influenza vaccination of health-care workers on mortality of elderly people in long-term care. A randomised controlled trial. *Lancet*, 355(9198), 93–97.

Centers for Disease Control and Prevention/NIOSH. (1996). *Violence in the workplace—Risk factors and prevention strategies*. Retrieved from www.cdc.gov/niosh/violcont.html

Centers for Disease Control and Prevention/NIOSH. (2002). *Violence: Occupational hazards in hospitals (No. 2002-101)*: CDC: National Institute for Occupational Safety and Health.

Centers for Disease Control and Prevention. (2003). *Exposure to blood: What every health care worker needs to know*. Retrieved October 15, 2008, from www.cdc.gov/ncidod/dhqp/pdf/bbp/Exp_to_Blood.pdf

Centers for Disease Control and Prevention. (2009a). Interim results: Influenza A (H1N1) 2009 monovalent vaccination coverage—United States, October—December 2009. *MMWR*, 59, 44–48.

Centers for Disease Control and Prevention. (2009b). Novel influenza A (H1N1) virus infections among health-care personnel–United States, April-May, 2009. *MMWR*, 58, 641–645.

Centers for Disease Control and Prevention/NIOSH. (2009). *State of the Sector: Healthcare and social assistance identification of research opportunities for the next decade of NORA executive summary (No. 2009-138)*: CDC: National Institute for Occupational Safety and Health.

Chan, M. F. (2009). Factors associated with perceived sleep quality of nurses working on rotating shifts. *Journal of Clinical Nursing, 18*(2), 285–293.

Cherry, N., Parker, G., McNamee, R., Wall, S., Chen, Y., & Robinson, J. (2005). Falls and fractures in women at work. *Occupational Medicine (Oxford, England), 55*(4), 292–297.

Chiu, M. C., & Wang, M. J. (2007). Professional footwear evaluation for clinical nurses. *Applied Ergonomics, 38*(2), 133–141.

Chiron, M., Bernard, M., Lafont, S., & Lagarde, E. (2008). Tiring job and work related injury road crashes in the GAZEL cohort. *Accident; Analysis and Prevention, 40*(3), 1096–1104.

Chong, J., Marshall, B. J., Barkin, J. S., McCallum, R. W., Reiner, D. K., Hoffman, S. R., & O'Phelan, C. (1994). Occupational exposure to Helicobacter pylori for the endoscopy professional: A sera epidemiological study. *The American Journal of Gastroenterology, 89*(11), 1987–1992.

Clarke, S. (2006). The relationship between safety climate and safety performance: A meta-analytic review. *Journal of Occupational Health Psychology, 11*(4), 315–327.

Collins, J. W., Wolf, L., Bell, J., & Evanoff, B. (2004). An evaluation of a "best practices" musculoskeletal injury prevention program in nursing homes. *Injury Prevention: Journal of the International Society for Child and Adolescent Injury Prevention, 10*(4), 206–211.

Conklin, D., MacFarland, V., Kinnie-Steeves, A., & Chenger, P. (1990). Medication errors by nurses: Contributing factors. *AARN News Letter, 46*(1), 8–9.

Connor, T. H., & McDiarmid, M. A. (2006). Preventing occupational exposures to antineoplastic drugs in health care settings. *CA: A Cancer Journal for Clinicians, 56*(6), 354–365.

Costa, G., & Di Milia, L. (2008). Aging and shift work: A complex problem to face. *Chronobiology International, 25*(2), 165–181.

Czeisler, C. A. (2009). Medical and genetic differences in the adverse impact of sleep loss on performance: Ethical considerations for the medical profession. *Transactions of the American Clinical and Climatological Association, 120,* 249–285.

Dawson, D., & McCulloch, K. (2005). Managing fatigue: It's about sleep. *Sleep Medicine Reviews, 9*(5), 365–380.

DeJoy, D. M. (1996). Theoretical models of health behavior and workplace self-protection. *Journal of Safety Research, 27*(2), 61–72.

De Valck, E., & Cluydts, R. (2001). Slow-release caffeine as a countermeasure to driver sleepiness induced by partial sleep deprivation. *Journal of Sleep Research, 10*(3), 203–209.

De Valck, E., De Groot, E., & Cluydts, R. (2003). Effects of slow-release caffeine and a nap on driving simulator performance after partial sleep deprivation. *Perceptual and Motor Skills, 96*(1), 67–78.

De Valck, E., Quanten, S., Berckmans, D., & Cluydts, R. (2007). Simulator driving performance, subjective sleepiness and salivary cortisol in a fast-forward versus a slow-backward rotating shift system. *Scandinavian Journal of Work, Environment & Health, 33*(1), 51–57.

Dingus, T. A., Klauer, S. G., Neale, V. L., Petersen, A., Lee, S. E., Sudweeks, J.,...Knipling, R. R. (2006). *The 100-car naturalistic driving study; Phase II—Results of the 100-car field experiment.* Washington, DC: National Highway Traffic Safety Administration. DOT HS 31 810 593:1–352.

Dobson, M., & Schnall, P.L. (2009). From stress to distress: The impact of work on mental health. In P. L. Schnall, M. Dobson, & E. Rosskam (Eds.), *Unhealthy work: Causes, consequences, cures.* Amityville, NY: Baywood Publishing Company, Inc.

Dorrian, J., Tolley, C., Lamond, N., van den Heuvel, C., Pincombe, J., Rogers, A. E., & Drew, D. (2008). Sleep and errors in a group of Australian hospital nurses at work and during the commute. *Applied Ergonomics, 39*(5), 605–613.

Drebit, S., Shajari, S., Alamgir, H., Yu, S., & Keen, D. (2010). Occupational and environmental risk factors for falls among workers in the healthcare sector. *Ergonomics, 53*(4), 525–536.

Drummond, D. J., Sparr, L. F., & Gordon, G. H. (1989). Hospital violence reduction among high-risk patients. *JAMA: the Journal of the American Medical Association, 261*(17), 2531–2534.

Edéll-Gustafsson, U. M., Kritz, E. I., & Bogren, I. K. (2002). Self-reported sleep quality, strain and health in relation to perceived working conditions in females. *Scandinavian Journal of Caring Sciences, 16*(2), 179–187.

Elder, A. G., O'Donnell, B., McCruden, E. A., Symington, I. S., & Carman, W. F. (1996). Incidence and recall of influenza in a cohort of Glasgow healthcare workers during the 1993–4 epidemic: Results of serum testing and questionnaire. *BMJ (Clinical Research Ed.), 313*(7067), 1241–1242.

Embriaco, N., Papazian, L., Kentish-Barnes, N., Pochard, F., & Azoulay, E. (2007). Burnout syndrome among critical care healthcare workers. *Current Opinion in Critical Care, 13*(5), 482–488.

Environmental Protection Agency. (1997). *Mercury Study Report to Congress*, Vols. 1–8. Washington, DC: Office of Air Quality Planning and Standards and Office of Research and Development. Report no. EPA-452/R-97-005.

Environmental Protection Agency. (2001). *Water quality criterion for the protection of human health: Methylmercury.* Washington, DC: Office of Water. Report no. EPA-823-R-01-001.

Environmental Working Group. (1998). *An analysis of pollution prevention in America's top hospitals.* Retrieved from http://www.ewg.org/reports/greening

Estryn-Béhar, M., Van der Heijden, B. I., Oginska, H., Camerino, D., Le Nézet, O., Conway, P. M., ... Hasselhorn, H. M. (2007). The impact of social work environment, teamwork characteristics, burnout, and personal factors upon intent to leave among European nurses. *Medical Care, 45*(10), 939–950.

Evanoff, B., Wolf, L., Aton, E., Canos, J., & Collins, J. (2003). Reduction in injury rates in nursing personnel through introduction of mechanical lifts in the workplace. *American Journal of Industrial Medicine, 44*(5), 451–457.

Fiore, A. E., Uyeki, T. M., Broder, K., Finelli, L., Euler, G. L., Singleton, J. A., ... Cox, N. J. (2010). Prevention and control of influenza with vaccines: Recommendations of the Advisory Committee on Immunization Practices (ACIP), 2010. *MMWR, 59*(RR-8), 1–62.

Fochsen, G., Josephson, M., Hagberg, M., Toomingas, A., & Lagerström, M. (2006). Predictors of leaving nursing care: A longitudinal study among Swedish nursing personnel. *Occupational and Environmental Medicine, 63*(3), 198–201.

Fujimoto, T., Kotani, S., & Suzuki, R. (2008). Work-family conflict of nurses in Japan. *Journal of Clinical Nursing, 17*(24), 3286–3295.

Gallagher, R., & Gormley, D. K. (2009). Perceptions of stress, burnout, and support systems in pediatric bone marrow transplantation nursing. *Clinical Journal of Oncology Nursing, 13*(6), 681–685.

Gander, P. H., Marshall, N. S., Harris, R. B., & Reid, P. (2005). Sleep, sleepiness and motor vehicle accidents: A national survey. *Australian and New Zealand Journal of Public Health, 29*(1), 16–21.

Garrett, C. (2008). The effect of nurse staffing patterns on medical errors and nurse burnout. *AORN Journal, 87*(6), 1191–1204.

Geiger-Brown, J., Rogers, V. E., Trinkoff, A., Kane, R., & Scharf, S. (2010). *Sleep, sleepiness and neurobehavioral performance of sleep-deprived 12-hour shift nurses.* Unpublished manuscript.

Gershon, R. R., Karkashian, C. D., Grosch, J. W., Murphy, L. R., Escamilla-Cejudo, A., ... Martin, L. (2000). Hospital safety climate and its relationship with safe work practices and workplace exposure incidents. *American Journal of Infection Control, 28*(3), 211–221.

Gershon, R. R. M., DeJoy, D. M., Borwegen, B., Braun, B., Silverstein, B., ... Cullen, J. (2009). Health and safety culture. In *State of the sector: Healthcare and social assistance* (pp. 87–97). Atlanta, GA: CDC/NIOSH.

Gilworth, G., Bhakta, B., Eyres, S., Carey, A., Anne Chamberlain, M., & Tennant, A. (2007). Keeping nurses working: Development and psychometric testing of the Nurse-Work Instability Scale (Nurse-WIS). *Journal of Advanced Nursing, 57*(5), 543–551.

Greenglass, E. R., & Burke, R. J. (2002). Hospital restructuring and burnout. *Journal of Health and Human Services Administration, 25*(1), 89–114.

Grzywacz, J. G., Frone, M. R., Brewer, C. S., & Kovner, C. T. (2006). Quantifying work-family conflict among registered nurses. *Research in Nursing & Health, 29*(5), 414–426.

Harris, M. F., Proudfoot, J. G., Jayasinghe, U. W., Holton, C. H., Powell Davies, G. P., Amoroso, C. L.,... Beilby, J. J. (2007). Job satisfaction of staff and the team environment in Australian general practice. *The Medical Journal of Australia, 186*(11), 570–573.

Hayward, A. C., Harling, R., Wetten, S., Johnson, A. M., Munro, S., Smedley, J.,... Watson, J. M. (2006). Effectiveness of an influenza vaccine programme for care home staff to prevent death, morbidity, and health service use among residents: Cluster randomised controlled trial. *BMJ (Clinical Research Ed.), 333*(7581), 1241.

Health Care Without Harm [www.noharm.org/us/medicalwaste/issue]. Accessed date May 23, 2007.

Health Resources and Services Administration (HRSA). (2010). *The registered nurse population: Initial findings from the 2008 National Sample Survey of Registered Nurses.* Retrieved from http://bhpr.hrsa.gov/healthworkforce/rnsurvey/initialfindings2008.pdf

Heller, K. (1998). The 'petty pilfering of minutes' of what has happened to the length of the work day in Australia? *International Journal of Manpower, 19*(4), 266–280.

Hignett, S. (1996). Work-related back pain in nurses. *Journal of Advanced Nursing, 23*(6), 1238–1246.

Hignett, S. (2003). Intervention strategies to reduce musculoskeletal injuries associated with handling patients: A systematic review. *Occupational and Environmental Medicine, 60*(9), E6.

Hillbrand, M., Foster, H. G., & Spitz, R. T. (1996). Characteristics and cost of staff injuries in a forensic hospital. *Psychiatric Services (Washington, D.C.), 47*(10), 1123–1125.

Horneij, E. L., Jensen, I. B., Holmström, E. B., & Ekdahl, C. (2004). Sick leave among home-care personnel: A longitudinal study of risk factors. *BMC Musculoskeletal Disorders, 5*(1), 38.

Hochwalter, J. (2008). A longitudinal study of the relationship between empowerment and burnout among registered and assistant nurses. *Work, 30,* 343–352.

Hughes, R. G., & Rogers, A. E. (2004). Are you tired? *The American Journal of Nursing, 104*(3), 36–38.

Hurlebaus, A. E., & Link, S. (1997). The effects of an aggressive behavior management program on nurses' levels of knowledge, confidence, and safety. *Journal of Nursing Staff Development: JNSD, 13*(5), 260–265.

International Agency for Research on Cancer (IARC). (2006).Vanadium pentoxide. *IARC Monographs on the Evaluation of Carcinogenic Risks to Humans, 86,* 227–292.

Ingre, M., Kecklund, G., Akerstedt, T., Söderström, M., & Kecklund, L. (2008). Sleep length as a function of morning shift-start time in irregular shift schedules for train drivers: Self-rated health and individual differences. *Chronobiology International, 25*(2), 349–358.

Institute of Medicine. (2004). *Keeping patients safe: Transforming the work environment of nurses.* Washington, DC: National Academy Press.

Institute of Medicine. (2006). *Sleep disorders and sleep deprivation: An unmet public health problem.* H. R. Colten & B. M. Alteveogt (Eds.). Washington, DC: National Academies Press.

Iskra-Golec, I., Folkard, S., Marek, T., Noworel, C. (1996). Health, well-being and burnout of ICU nurses on 12- and 8- hour shifts. *Work & Stress, 10,* 251–256.

Johnson, J. V., & Hall, E. M. (1988). Job strain, work place social support, and cardiovascular disease: A cross-sectional study of a random sample of the Swedish working population. *American Journal of Public Health, 78*(10), 1336–1342.

Josephson, M., Lagerström, M., Hagberg, M., & Wigaeus Hjelm, E. (1997). Musculoskeletal symptoms and job strain among nursing personnel: A study over a three year period. *Occupational and Environmental Medicine, 54*(9), 681–685.

Josten, E. J., Ng A Tham, J. E., & Thierry, H. (2003). The effects of extended workdays on fatigue, health, performance and satisfaction in nursing. *Journal of Advanced Nursing, 44*(6), 643–652.

Karasek, R. A. (1979). Job demands, job decision latitude and mental strain. *Administrative Sciences Quarterly, 24,* 286–308.

Kemmlert, K., & Lundholm, L. 1998, Slips, trips and falls in different work groups with reference to age. *Safety Science, 28,* 59–75.

Kohn, L. T., Corrigan, J. M., Donaldson, M. S. (Eds.). (2000). *To err is human: Building a safer health system.* Washington, DC: National Academy Press.

Krstev, S., Perunicic, B., & Vidakovic, A. (2003). Work practice and some adverse health effects in nurses handling antineoplastic drugs. *La Medicina Del Lavoro, 94*(5), 432–439.

LaMontagne, A. D., Radi, S., Elder, D. S., Abramson, M. J., & Sim, M. (2006). Primary prevention of latex related sensitisation and occupational asthma: A systematic review. *Occupational and Environmental Medicine, 63*(5), 359–364.

Lang, G. M., Pfister, E. A., & Siemens, M. J. (2010). Nursing burnout: Cross-sectional study at a large Army hospital. *Military Medicine, 175*(6), 435–441.

Laschinger, H. K., Finegan, J., Shamian, J., & Almost, J. (2001). Testing Karasek's Demands-Control Model in restructured healthcare settings: Effects of job strain on staff nurses' quality of work life. *The Journal of Nursing Administration, 31*(5), 233–243.

Lee, J. M., Botteman, M. F., Xanthakos, N., & Nicklasson, L. (2005). Needlestick injuries in the United States. Epidemiologic, economic, and quality of life issues. *AAOHN Journal: Official Journal of the American Association of Occupational Health Nurses, 53*(3), 117–133.

Lee, S. S., Gerberich, S. G., Waller, L. A., Anderson, A., & McGovern, P. (1999). Work-related assault injuries among nurses. *Epidemiology (Cambridge, Mass.), 10*(6), 685–691.

Lehmann, L. S., Padilla, M., Clark, S., & Loucks, S. (1983). Training personnel in the prevention and management of violent behavior. *Hospital & Community Psychiatry, 34*(1), 40–43.

Lemaitre, M., Meret, T., Rothan-Tondeur, M., Belmin, J., Lejonc, J. L.,...Carrat, F. (2009). Effect of influenza vaccination of nursing home staff on mortality of residents: A cluster-randomized trial. *Journal of the American Geriatrics Society, 57*(9), 1580–1586.

Lipscomb, J. A., & Love, C. C. (1992). Violence toward health care workers: An emerging occupational hazard. *AAOHN Journal: Official Journal of the American Association of Occupational Health Nurses, 40*(5), 219–228.

Lipscomb, J., McPhaul, K., Rosen, J., Brown, J. G., Choi, M., Soeken, K.,...Porter, P. (2006). Violence prevention in the mental health setting: The New York state experience. *The Canadian Journal of Nursing Research = Revue Canadienne De Recherche En Sciences Infirmières, 38*(4), 96–117.

Liss, G. M., Tarlo, S. M., Doherty, J., Purdham, J., Greene, J., McCaskell, L., & Kerr, M. (2003). Physician diagnosed asthma, respiratory symptoms, and associations with workplace tasks among radiographers in Ontario, Canada. *Occupational and Environmental Medicine, 60*(4), 254–261.

Lo, S. H., Liau, C. S., Hwang, J. S., & Wang, J. D. (2008). Dynamic blood pressure changes and recovery under different work shifts in young women. *American Journal of Hypertension, 21*(7), 759–764.

Lowden, A., Holmbäck, U., Akerstedt, T., Forslund, A., Forslund, J., & Lennernäs, M. (2001). Time of day type of food–relation to mood and hunger during 24 hours of constant conditions. *Journal of Human Ergology, 30*(1–2), 381–386.

Makary, M. A., Sexton, J. B., Freischlag, J. A., Holzmueller, C. G., Millman, E. A., Rowen, L., & Pronovost, P. J. (2006). Operating room teamwork among physicians and nurses: Teamwork in the eye of the beholder. *Journal of the American College of Surgeons, 202*(5), 746–752.

Makary, M. A., Sexton, J. B., Freischlag, J. A., Millman, E. A., Pryor, D., Holzmueller, C., & Pronovost, P. J. (2006). Patient safety in surgery. *Annals of Surgery, 243*(5), 628–32; discussion 632.

Malerich, P. G., Wilson, M. L., & Mowad, C. M. (2008). The effect of a transition to powder-free latex gloves on workers' compensation claims for latex-related illness. *Dermatitis, 19*(6), 316–318.

Marmot, M., Siegrist, J., Theorell, T., & Feeney, A. (1999). Health and the psychosocial environment at work. In M. Marmot & R. G. Wilkinson (Eds.), *Social determinants of health* (pp. 105–131). Oxford, UK: Oxford University Press.

Marras, K. G., Davis, B. C., Kirking, B. C., & Bertsche, P. K. (1999). A comprehensive analysis of low-back disorder risk and spinal loading during the transferring and repositioning of patients using different techniques, *Ergonomics, 42,* 904–926.

McDiarmid, M., & Egan, T. (1988). Acute occupational exposure to antineoplastic agents. *Journal of Occupational Medicine, 30*(12), 984–987.

McGregor, D., Bolt, H., Cogliano, V., & Richter-Reichhelm, H. B. (2006). Formaldehyde and glutaraldehyde and nasal cytotoxicity: Case study within the context of the 2006 IPCS Human Framework for the Analysis of a cancer mode of action for humans. *Critical Reviews in Toxicology, 36*(10), 821–835.

McPhaul, K., & Lipscomb, J. A. (2009). *Healthy aging for a sustainable workforce.* Retrieved from http://www.soeh.org/pdf/AgingWorkersWorkshopReport_11%2009_Final.pdf

Meier, A., Jost, M., Rüegger, M., Knutti, R., & Schlatter, C. (1995). [Narcotic gas burden of personnel in pediatric anesthesia]. *Der Anaesthesist, 44*(3), 154–162.

Menzel, N. N. (2004). Back pain prevalence in nursing personnel: Measurement issues. *AAOHN Journal: Official Journal of the American Association of Occupational Health Nurses, 52*(2), 54–65.

Moore, R. T., Kaprielian, R., & Auerbach, J. (2009). *Asleep at the Wheel. Report of the Special Commission on Drowsy Driving.* Boston, MA: Massachusetts Department of Public Health.

Moore-Ede, M., Heitmann, A., Guttkuhn, R., Trutschel, U., Aguirre, A., & Croke, D. (2004). Circadian alertness simulator for fatigue risk assessment in transportation: Application to reduce frequency and severity of truck accidents. *Aviation, Space, and Environmental Medicine, 75*(3 Suppl.), A107–A118.

Morse, T., Fekieta, R., Rubenstein, H., Warren, N., Alexander, D., & Wawzyniecki, P. (2008). Doing the heavy lifting: Health care workers take back their backs. *New Solutions: a Journal of Environmental and Occupational Health Policy: NS, 18*(2), 207–219.

Muir, M., & Archer-Heese, G., (2009). Essentials of a Bariatric Patient Handling Program. *OJIN: The Online Journal of Issues in Nursing, 14*(1), 5.

Nabi, H., Rachid Salmi, L., Lafont, S., Chiron, M., Zins, M., & Lagarde, E. (2007). Attitudes associated with behavioral predictors of serious road traffic crashes: Results from the GAZEL cohort. *Injury Prevention: Journal of the International Society for Child and Adolescent Injury Prevention, 13*(1), 26–31.

National Institute for Occupational Safety and Health (NIOSH). (1997). *Alert: Preventing allergic reactions to latex in the workplace.* Cincinnati, OH: DHHS.

National Institute for Occupational Safety and Health (NIOSH). (1998). *Guidelines for protecting the safety and health of healthcare workers.* U.S. Department of Health and Human Services, Public Health Service, Centers for Disease Control and Prevention, National Institute for Occupational Safety and Health. DHHS (NIOSH) Publication No. 88–119.

National Institute for Occupational Safety and Health (NIOSH). (2002). Nonfatal Illness. In *Worker Health Chartbook, 2000.* Cincinnati, OH: U.S. Department of Health and Human Services,

Public Health Service, Centers for Disease Control and Prevention, National Institute for Occupational Safety and Health, DHHS (NIOSH) Publication No. 2002-120. Retrieved from www.cdc.gov/niosh/pdfs/2002-120.pdf

National Institute for Occupational Safety and Health (NIOSH). (2004). *Preventing occupational exposure to antineoplastic and other hazardous drugs in health care settings.* U.S. Department of Health and Human Services, Public Health Service, Centers for Disease Control and Prevention, National Institute for Occupational Safety and Health, DHHS (NIOSH) Publication No. 2004-165. Retrieved from http://www.cdc.gov/niosh/docs/2004-165/

National Sleep Foundation. (2008). *State of the States Report on Drowsy Driving.* Retrieved from http://drowsydriving.org/resources/2008-state-of-the-states-report-on-drowsy-driving/

Nishikawa, J., Kawai, H., Takahashi, A., Seki, T., Yoshikawa, N., Akita, Y., & Mitamura, K. (1998). Seroprevalence of immunoglobulin G antibodies against Helicobacter pylori among endoscopy personnel in Japan. *Gastrointestinal Endoscopy, 48*(3), 237–243.

Nojkov, B., Rubenstein, J. H., Chey, W. D., & Hoogerwerf, W. A. (2010). The impact of rotating shift work on the prevalence of irritable bowel syndrome in nurses. *The American Journal of Gastroenterology, 105*(4), 842–847.

Occupational Safety and Health Administration. (1986). *Work Practice Guidelines for personnel dealing with cytotoxic (antineoplastic) drugs.* US Dept. Labor, Instruction publication 8–1.1, Office of Occupational Medicine, Washington, DC.

Occupational Safety and Health Administration. (1991). *Bloodborne Pathogens Standard.* Washington, DC: U.S. Department of Labor.

Occupational and Safety Health Administration. (2001). *Needlestick Safety and Prevention Act.* Washington, DC: U.S. Department of Labor.

Occupational Safety and Health Administration. (2004). *Guidelines for preventing workplace violence for health care & social service workers* (No. OSHA 3148–01R 2004).

Ofstead, C. L., Tucker, S. J., Beebe, T. J., & Poland, G. A. (2008). Influenza vaccination among registered nurses: Information receipt, knowledge, and decision-making at an institution with a multifaceted educational program. *Infection Control and Hospital Epidemiology: the Official Journal of the Society of Hospital Epidemiologists of America, 29*(2), 99–106.

Oliver, A., Cheyne, A., Tomas, J.M., & Cox, S. (2002). The effects of organizational and individual factors on occupational accidents. *Journal of Occupational and Organizational Psychology, 75,* 473–488.

Papadakaki, M., Kontogiannis, T., Tzamalouka, G., Darviri, C., & Chliaoutakis, J. (2008). Exploring the effects of lifestyle, sleep factors and driving behaviors on sleep-related road risk: A study of Greek drivers. *Accident; Analysis and Prevention, 40*(6), 2029–2036.

Patrick, K., & Lavery, J. F. (2007). Burnout in nursing. *The Australian Journal of Advanced Nursing: a Quarterly Publication of the Royal Australian Nursing Federation, 24*(3), 43–48.

Pedrini, L., Magni, L. R., Giovannini, C., Panetta, V., Zacchi, V., Rossi, G., & Placentino, A. (2009). Burnout in nonhospital psychiatric residential facilities. *Psychiatric Services (Washington, D.C.), 60*(11), 1547–1551.

Perry, J., Parker, G., & Jagger, J. (2001). Percutaneous injuries in home healthcare settings. *Home Healthcare Nurse, 19*(6), 342–344.

Philip, P., & Akerstedt, T. (2006). Transport and industrial safety, how are they affected by sleepiness and sleep restriction? *Sleep Medicine Reviews, 10*(5), 347–356.

Pietroiusti, A., Forlini, A., Magrini, A., Galante, A., Coppeta, L., Gemma, G.,...Bergamaschi, A. (2006). Shift work increases the frequency of duodenal ulcer in H pylori infected workers. *Occupational and Environmental Medicine, 63*(11), 773–775.

Pietroiusti, A., Neri, A., Somma, G., Coppeta, L., Iavicoli, I., Bergamaschi, A., & Magrini, A. (2010). Incidence of metabolic syndrome among night-shift healthcare workers. *Occupational and Environmental Medicine, 67*(1), 54–57.

Poms, L. W., Botsford, W. E., Kaplan, S. A., Buffardi, L. C., & O'Brien, A. S. (2009). The economic impact of work and family issues: Child care satisfaction and financial considerations of employed mothers. *Journal of Occupational Health Psychology, 14*(4), 402–413.

Portela, L. F., Rotenberg, L., & Waissmann, W. (2004). Self-reported health and sleep complaints among nursing personnel working under 12 h night and day shifts. *Chronobiology International, 21*(6), 859–870.

Proudfoot, J., Jayasinghe, U. W., Holton, C., Grimm, J., Bubner, T., Amoroso, C.,...Harris, M. F. (2007). Team climate for innovation: What difference does it make in general practice? *International Journal for Quality in Health Care, 19*(3), 164–169.

Quinn, M. M., Fuller, T. P., Bello, A., & Galligan, C. J. (2006). Pollution prevention–occupational safety and health in hospitals: Alternatives and interventions. *Journal of Occupational and Environmental Hygiene, 3*(4), 182–93; quiz D45.

Robb, G., Sultana, S., Ameratunga, S., & Jackson, R. (2008). A systematic review of epidemiological studies investigating risk factors for work-related road traffic crashes and injuries. *Injury Prevention: Journal of the International Society for Child and Adolescent Injury Prevention, 14*(1), 51–58.

Roberts, K. H. (1990). Some characteristics of high reliability organizations. *Organanization Science, 1*, 160–177.

Rogers, A., Holmes, S., & Spencer, M. (2001). The effect of shiftwork on driving to and from work. *Journal of Human Ergology, 30*(1–2), 131–136.

Rosa, R. R., Härmä, M., Pulli, K., Mulder, M., & Näsman, O. (1996). Rescheduling a three shift system at a steel rolling mill: Effects of a one hour delay of shift starting times on sleep and alertness in younger and older workers. *Occupational and Environmental Medicine, 53*(10), 677–685.

Ruggiero, J. S. (2003). Correlates of fatigue in critical care nurses. *Research in Nursing & Health, 26*(6), 434–444.

Russi, M., Buchta, W. G., Swift, M., Budnick, L. D., Hodgson, M. J., Berube, D., & Kelafant, G. A. (2009). Guidance for Occupational Health Services in Medical Centers. *Journal of Occupational and Environmental Medicine / American College of Occupational and Environmental Medicine, 51*(11), 1e–18e.

Sauter, S. L., Brightwell, W. S., Colligan, M. J., Hurrell, J. J., Katz, T. M., LeGrande, D.E.,...Tetrick, L.E. (2002). *The changing organization of work and the safety and health of working people: Knowledge gaps and research directions.* DHHS (NIOSH) Publication No. 2002-116. Cincinnati, OH: Department of Health and Human Services, Public Health Service, Centers for Disease Control and Prevention, National Institute for Occupational Safety and Health.

Scharf, B. B., McPhaul, K. M., Trinkoff, A., & Lipscomb, J. (2009). Evaluation of home health care nurses' practice and their employers' policies related to bloodborne pathogens. *AAOHN Journal: Official Journal of the American Association of Occupational Health Nurses, 57*(7), 275–280.

Schebesta, K., Lorenz, V., Schebesta, E. M., Hörauf, K., Gruber, M., Kimberger, O., Chiari, A.,...Krafft, P. (2010). Exposure to anaesthetic trace gases during general anaesthesia: CobraPLA vs. LMA classic. *Acta Anaesthesiologica Scandinavica, 54*(7), 848–854.

Schein, E. H. (1985). *Organisational culture and leadership.* San Francisco, CA: Jossey-Bass.

Scott, L. D., Hofmeister, N., Rogness, N., & Rogers, A. E. (2010a). An interventional approach for patient and nurse safety: A fatigue countermeasures feasibility study. *Nursing Research, 59*(4), 250–258.

Scott, L. D., Hofmeister, N., Rogness, N., & Rogers, A. E. (2010b). Implementing a fatigue countermeasures program for nurses: A focus group analysis. *The Journal of Nursing Administration, 40*(5), 233–240.

Scott, L. D., Hwang, W. T., Rogers, A. E., Nysse, T., Dean, G. E., & Dinges, D. F. (2007). The relationship between nurse work schedules, sleep duration, and drowsy driving. *Sleep, 30*(12), 1801–1807.

Schoenfisch, A. L., & Lipscomb, H. J. (2009). Job characteristics and work organization factors associated with patient-handling injury among nursing personnel. *Work (Reading, Mass.), 33*(1), 117–128.

Seo, D. C., Torabi, M. R., Blair, E. H., & Ellis, N. T. (2004). A cross-validation of safety climate scale using confirmatory factor analytic approach. *Journal of Safety Research, 35*(4), 427–445.

Sessink, P. J., & Bos, R. P. (1999). Drugs hazardous to healthcare workers. Evaluation of methods for monitoring occupational exposure to cytostatic drugs. *Drug Safety: An International Journal of Medical Toxicology and Drug Experience, 20*(4), 347–359.

Sexton, J. B., Holzmueller, C. G., Pronovost, P. J., Thomas, E. J., McFerran, S., Nunes, J., . . . Fox, H. E. (2006). Variation in caregiver perceptions of teamwork climate in labor and delivery units. *Journal of Perinatology: Official Journal of the California Perinatal Association, 26*(8), 463–470.

Shields, M., & Wilkins, K. (2009). An update on mammography use in Canada. *Health Reports, 20*(3), 7–19.

Siegrist, J. (1996). Adverse health effects of high-effort/low-reward conditions. *Journal of Occupational Health Psychology, 1*(1), 27–41.

Siegrist, J. (2005). Social reciprocity and health: New scientific evidence and policy implications. *Psychoneuroendocrinology, 30*(10), 1033–1038.

Signal, T. L., Gander, P. H., Anderson, H., & Brash, S. (2009). Scheduled napping as a countermeasure to sleepiness in air traffic controllers. *Journal of Sleep Research, 18*(1), 11–19.

Silverstein, M. (2008). Meeting the challenges of an aging workforce. *American Journal of Industrial Medicine, 51*(4), 269–280.

Simon, M., Kümmerling, A., & Hasselhorn, H. M.; Next-Study Group. (2004). Work-home conflict in the European nursing profession. *International Journal of Occupational and Environmental Health, 10*(4), 384–391.

Simon, M., Tackenberg, P., Nienhaus, A., Estryn-Behar, M., Conway, P. M., & Hasselhorn, H. M. (2008). Back or neck-pain-related disability of nursing staff in hospitals, nursing homes and home care in seven countries—results from the European NEXT-Study. *International Journal of Nursing Studies, 45*(1), 24–34.

Skov, T., Maarup, B., Olsen, J., Rørth, M., Winthereik, H., & Lynge, E. (1992). Leukaemia and reproductive outcome among nurses handling antineoplastic drugs. *British Journal of Industrial Medicine, 49*(12), 855–861.

Smith, A. M., Amin, H. S., Biagini, R. E., Hamilton, R. G., Arif, S. A., Yeang, H. Y., & Bernstein, D. I. (2007). Percutaneous reactivity to natural rubber latex proteins persists in health-care workers following avoidance of natural rubber latex. *Clinical and Experimental Allergy: Journal of the British Society for Allergy and Clinical Immunology, 37*(9), 1349–1356.

Smith, M. R., Fogg, L. F., & Eastman, C. I. (2009). A compromise circadian phase position for permanent night work improves mood, fatigue, and performance. *Sleep, 32*(11), 1481–1489.

Smith, S. S., Kilby, S., Jorgensen, G., & Douglas, J. A. (2007). Napping and nightshift work: Effects of a short nap on psychomotor vigilance and subjective sleepiness in health workers. *Sleep and Biological Rhythms, 5*(2), 117–125.

Solidaki, E., Chatzi, L., Bitsios, P., Markatzi, I., Plana, E., Castro, F., Palmer, K., . . . Kogevinas, M. (2010). Work-related and psychological determinants of multisite musculoskeletal pain. *Scandinavian Journal of Work, Environment & Health, 36*(1), 54–61.

Steenland, K., Whelan, E., Deddens, J., Stayner, L., & Ward, E. (2003). Ethylene oxide and breast cancer incidence in a cohort study of 7576 women (United States). *Cancer Causes & Control: CCC, 14*(6), 531–539.

Stutts, J. C., Wilkins, J. W., Scott Osberg, J., & Vaughn, B. V. (2003). Driver risk factors for sleep-related crashes. *Accident; Analysis and Prevention, 35*(3), 321–331.

Sveinsdóttir, H. (2006). Self-assessed quality of sleep, occupational health, working environment, illness experience and job satisfaction of female nurses working different combination of shifts. *Scandinavian Journal of Caring Sciences, 20*(2), 229–237.

Tellier, R. (2009). Aerosol transmission of influenza A virus: A review of new studies. *Journal of the Royal Society, Interface / the Royal Society, 6*(Suppl. 6), S783–S790.

Thomas, R. E., Jefferson, T. O., Demicheli, V., & Rivetti, D. (2006). Influenza vaccination for health-care workers who work with elderly people in institutions: A systematic review. *The Lancet Infectious Diseases, 6*(5), 273–279.

Tinubu, B. M., Mbada, C. E., Oyeyemi, A. L., & Fabunmi, A. A. (2010). Work-related musculoskeletal disorders among nurses in Ibadan, South-west Nigeria: A cross-sectional survey. *BMC Musculoskeletal Disorders, 11,* 12.

Tompa, A., Jakab, M., Biró, A., Magyar, B., Fodor, Z., Klupp, T., & Major, J. (2006). Chemical safety and health conditions among Hungarian hospital nurses. *Annals of the New York Academy of Sciences, 1076,* 635–648.

Toraason, M., Sussman, G., Biagini, R., Meade, J., Beezhold, D., & Germolec, D. (2000). Latex allergy in the workplace. *Toxicological Sciences: An Official Journal of the Society of Toxicology, 58*(1), 5–14.

Trenoweth, S. (2003). Perceiving risk in dangerous situations: Risks of violence among mental health inpatients. *Journal of Advanced Nursing, 42*(3), 278–287.

Trinkoff, A., Geiger-Brown, J., Brady, B., Lipscomb, J., & Muntaner, C. (2006). How long and how much are nurses now working? *The American Journal of Nursing, 106*(4), 60–71, quiz 72.

Trinkoff, A. M., Le, R., Geiger-Brown, J., & Lipscomb, J. (2007). Work schedule, needle use, and needlestick injuries among registered nurses. *Infection Control and Hospital Epidemiology: the Official Journal of the Society of Hospital Epidemiologists of America, 28*(2), 156–164.

Trinkoff, A. M., Le, R., Geiger-Brown, J., Lipscomb, J., & Lang, G. (2006). Longitudinal relationship of work hours, mandatory overtime, and on-call to musculoskeletal problems in nurses. *American Journal of Industrial Medicine, 49*(11), 964–971.

Trinkoff, A. M., Lipscomb, J. A., Geiger-Brown, J., & Brady, B. (2002). Musculoskeletal problems of the neck, shoulder, and back and functional consequences in nurses. *American Journal of Industrial Medicine, 41*(3), 170–178.

Tucker, P., Barton, J., & Folkard, S. (1996). Comparison of eight and 12 hour shifts: Impacts on health, wellbeing, and alertness during the shift. *Occupational and Environmental Medicine, 53*(11), 767–772.

University of Iowa Injury Prevention Research Center (UIIPRC). (2001). *Workplace violence—A report to the nation.* Iowa City, IA: University of Iowa.

Valanis, B. G., Vollmer, W. M., Labuhn, K. T., & Glass, A. G. (1993). Acute symptoms associated with antineoplastic drug handling among nurses. *Cancer Nursing, 16*(4), 288–295.

Valanis, B., Vollmer, W., Labuhn, K., & Glass, A. (1997). Occupational exposure to antineoplastic agents and self-reported infertility among nurses and pharmacists. *Journal of Occupational and Environmental Medicine / American College of Occupational and Environmental Medicine, 39*(6), 574–580.

Valent, F., Di Bartolomeo, S., Marchetti, R., Sbrojavacca, R., & Barbone, F. (2010). A case-crossover study of sleep and work hours and the risk of road traffic accidents. *Sleep, 33*(3), 349–354.

van der Doef, M., & Maes, S. (1999). The job demand-control (-support) model and psychological well-being: A review of 20 years of empirical research. *Work and Stress, 13,* 87–114.

van den Tooren, M., & de Jonge, J. (2008). Managing job stress in nursing: What kind of resources do we need? *Journal of Advanced Nursing, 63*(1), 75–84.

Vanlaar, W., Simpson, H., Mayhew, D., & Robertson, R. (2007). *Fatigued and drowsy driving. Attitudes, concern and practices of Ontario drivers.* Ontario, Canada: Traffic Injury Research Foundation.

van Mark, A., Spallek, M., Groneberg, D. A., Kessel, R., & Weiler, S. W. (2010). Correlates shift work with increased risk of gastrointestinal complaints or frequency of gastritis or peptic ulcer in *H. pylori*-infected shift workers? *International Archives of Occupational and Environmental Health, 83*(4), 423–431.

Volná, J., & Sonka, K. (2006). Medical factors of falling asleep behind the wheel. *Prague Medical Report, 107*(3), 290–296.

Wang, G. L., Lu, Y. K., & Wang, L. (1997). [Prevention of Helicobacter pylori infections in gastroenterological nurses]. *Zhonghua Hu Li Za Zhi = Chinese Journal of Nursing, 32*(10), 562–564.

Warchol, G. (1998). *Workplace violence, 1992-96* (No. July 1998, NCJ 168634). Washington, DC: U.S. Department of Justice, Office of Justice Programs.

Wise, J. (2009). Danish night shift workers with breast cancer awarded compensation. *BMJ (Clinical Research Ed.), 338*, b1152.

World Health Organization. *Summary table of SARS cases by country, 1 November 2002–7 August 2003.* Retrieved from http://www.who.int/csr/sars/country/en/country2003_08_15.pdf

Yildirim, D., & Aycan, Z. (2008). Nurses' work demands and work-family conflict: A questionnaire survey. *International Journal of Nursing Studies, 45*(9), 1366–1378.

Yuan, S. C., Chou, M. C., Hwu, L. J., Chang, Y. O., Hsu, W. H., & Kuo, H. W. (2009). An intervention program to promote health-related physical fitness in nurses. *Journal of Clinical Nursing, 18*(10), 1404–1411.

Zhen Lu, W., Ann Gwee, K., & Yu Ho, K. (2006). Functional bowel disorders in rotating shift nurses may be related to sleep disturbances. *European Journal of Gastroenterology & Hepatology, 18*(6), 623–627.

Zhuang, Z., Stobbe, T. J., Hsiao, H., Collins, J. W., & Hobbs, G. R. (1999). Biomechanical evaluation of assistive devices for transferring residents. *Applied Ergonomics, 30*(4), 285–294.

Zohar, D. (2000). A group-level model of safety climate: Testing the effect of group climate on microaccidents in manufacturing jobs. *The Journal of Applied Psychology, 85*(4), 587–596.

CHAPTER 9

Magnetism and the Nursing Workforce

Patricia R. Messmer and Marian C. Turkel

ABSTRACT

The focus of this chapter is to highlight practice exemplars and research findings related to the five components of the new Magnet Model®. A brief overview of the historical development and professional evolution of the American Nurses Credentialing Center (ANCC) Magnet Recognition Program® is presented followed by a brief overview of the original fourteen forces of magnetism. Content related to empirical practice-based research framed under the components of transformational leadership; structural empowerment; exemplary professional practice; new knowledge, innovation, and improvement; and empirical outcomes is presented and discussed. The authors provide key findings from scholarly publications and describe how the findings contribute to the creation of work environments based on the tenets of magnetism. The chapter concludes with a brief over of the ANCC Pathway to Excellence Program®.

In her September 1980 Presidential address to the American Academy of Nursing (AAN), Linda Aiken articulated the scope of the nursing shortage; over 80% of American Hospitals do not have the adequate staffing with some 100,000 vacancies in hospital nursing positions, which is having a crippling effect on day-to-day operations (AAN, 1983; ANA, 2010 reissue). In order to identify ways to

© 2011 Springer Publishing Company
DOI: 10.1891/0739-6686.28.233

help solve this problem, the Governing Council of the AAN appointed a Task Force on Nursing Practice to examine the characteristics of systems facilitating professional practice in hospitals (McClure, Poulin, Sovie, & Wandelt, 2002). Selected AAN Fellows were asked to nominate potential Magnet hospitals that demonstrated success in recruiting and retaining professional nurses on their staffs (AAN, 1983; ANA, 2010 reissue).

Out of the 165 hospitals nominated, 46 were selected with 41 participating. Five of the nominated hospitals were unable to participate because of scheduling problems. A staff nurse representative along with the director of nursing engaged in separate group interviews and articulated their concepts of the conditions that made their hospital a good place to work. The 14 Forces of Magnetism evolved from this original Magnet Study. Aiken's (1994) study demonstrated lower Medicare mortality in Magnet Hospitals. Aiken, Havens, and Sloane's (2009) research documented that American Nurses Credentialing Center (ANCC) Magnet hospital designation is a valid marker of good nursing care. An associated energy is created in nurses of Magnet-designated facilities as a forum for nursing staff to showcase their work is created, resulting in a great deal of organizational pride (Horstman et al., 2006). The following is a brief overview of the original 14 Forces of Magnetism as defined by the ANCC (2005, 2008a, 2008b).

Force 1. Quality of Nursing Leadership: Knowledgeable, strong, risk-taking nurse leaders follow a well-articulated, strategic, and visionary philosophy in the day-to-day operations of the nursing services. Nursing leaders, at all levels of the organization, convey a strong sense of advocacy and support for the staff and for the patient. The results of quality leadership are evident in the nursing practice at the patient's side (ANCC Magnet Recognition Program, 2005). Drenkard (2005) indicated that the chief nurse officer (CNO)must be the role model for living the concepts in the Magnet Forces.

Force 2. Organizational Structure: Organizational structures are generally flat, rather than vertical, and decentralized decision-making prevails. The organizational structure is dynamic and responsive to change. Strong nursing representation is evident in the organizational committee structure. Executive-level nursing leaders serve at the executive level of the organization. The CNO typically reports directly to CNO. The organization has a functioning and productive system of shared decision-making (ANCC Magnet Recognition Program, 2005). Batcheller (2010) noted that the CNO's tenure is affected when there is a conflict with the chief executive officer and that the challenge nurse leaders face are to develop a competency model and roadmap in becoming transformational leaders.

Force 3. Management Style: Health care organization and nursing leaders create an environment supporting participation. Feedback is encouraged and valued and is incorporated from the staff at all levels of the organization. Nursing serving in leadership positions are visible, accessible, and committed to communicating effectively with staff (ANCC Magnet Recognition Program, 2005). Caroselli (2008) stressed that although the role of the chief nurse executive was complex, daunting, risk-laden, it provided unprecedented opportunities to influence the care of patents in a very broad context.

Force 4. Personnel Policies and Programs: Salaries and benefits are competitive. Creative and flexible staffing models that support a safe and healthy work environment are used. Personnel policies are created with direct care nurse involvement. Significant opportunities for professional growth exist in administrative and clinical tracks. Personnel policies and programs support professional nursing practice, work/life balance, and the delivery of quality care (ANCC Magnet Recognition Program, 2005). Laschinger, Finegan, Shamian, and Wilk (2001) identified that by linking structural empowerment with psychological empowerment, employees' emotional connectedness with the work setting were positively influenced. Jasovsky et al. (2005) reported on a cost-effective on-line system for collecting the demographic data for the Magnet monitoring reports.

Force 5. Professional Models of Care: There are models of care that give nurses the responsibility and authority for the provision of direct patient care. Nurses are accountable for their own practice as well as the coordination of care. The models of care (i.e., primary nursing, case management, family-centered, district, and holistic) provide for the continuity of care across the continuum. The models take into consideration patients' unique needs and provide skilled nurses and adequate resources to accomplish desired outcomes (ANCC Magnet Recognition Program, 2005). Wolf and Greenhouse (2007) believed that successful transformation and integration of a care delivery model into the DNA of the organization must be led by the CNO with unrelenting passion. The model should serve as the foundation for assessment, planning, organizing, job description, a reward and recognition system, recruitment, staff development and research.

Force 6. Quality of Care: Quality is the systematic driving force for nursing and the organization. Nurses serving in leadership positions are responsible for providing an environment that positively influences patient outcomes. There is a pervasive perception among nurses that they provide high-quality care to patients (ANCC Magnet Recognition Program, 2005). Magnet hospital nurses always rate the essential element of 'working with other nurses who are clinically competent" as "important" for quality of care and "present" in Magnet hospitals. Magnet hospital staff consider specialty certification, advanced education, and both formal and informal peer review as evidence of clinical competency (Kramer & Schmalenberg, 2004). Gawlinski (2007) stressed that outcome variables should be measured before (at baseline) and after the practice change. Measurement at these time points allows comparison and evaluation of the effects of practice change. The sustainability of the practice change can also be evaluated by measuring the process and outcome variables 6–12 months after implementation.

Force 7. Quality Improvement: The organization has structures and processes for the measurement if quality and programs for improving the quality of care and services within the organization (ANCC Magnet Recognition Program, 2005). Hinshaw (2006) reported that translating the Institute of Medicine's recommendations, *Keeping Patient Safe: Transforming the Work Environment of Nurses* into practice required an extensive collaboration among nurse administrators and nurse researchers to advance the quality of care. This was supported by Kramer and Schmalenberg (2005) who reported that the Magnet Recognition Program stimulated valuable and insightful research related to outcomes since staff nurses identified process/functions most essential to quality patient care.

Force 8. Consultation and Resources: The health care organization provides adequate resources, support, and opportunities for the utilization of experts, particularly advanced practice nurses. In addition, the organization promotes involvement of nurses in professional organizations and among peers in the community (ANCC Magnet Recognition Program, 2005). Evidence-based practice for advanced practice nurses incorporates critical thinking, accessing research resources, using evidence-based tools such as clinical practice guidelines and implementing the recommendations into clinical practice (Kleinpell & Gawlinski, 2005; Kleinpell, Gawlinski, & Burns, 2006).

Force 9. Autonomy: Autonomous nursing care is the ability of a nurse to assess and provide nursing actions as appropriate for patient care based on competence, professional expertise, and knowledge. The nurse is expected to practice autonomously, consistent with professional standards. Independent judgment is expected to be exercised within the context of their interdisciplinary and multidisciplinary approaches to patient/resident/client care (ANCC Magnet Recognition Program, 2005). Magnet hospitals have demonstrated better patient outcomes, safer patient care, increased autonomy and greater nurse satisfaction through mentoring programs (Fundeburk, 2008).

Force 10. Community and Health Care Organizations: Relationships are established within and among all types of health care organizations and the other community organizations to develop strong partnerships that support improved client outcomes and the health of the communities that they serve (ANCC Magnet Recognition Program, 2005). Collaboration among faculty, students and community partners contributes to learning opportunities while meeting the needs of communities (Sternas, O'Hare, Lehman, & Milligan, 1999).

Force 11. Nurses as Teachers: Professional nurses are involved in educational activities within the organization and community. Students from a variety of academic programs are welcomed and supported in the organization; contractual arrangements are mutually beneficial. There is a development and mentoring program for staff preceptors for all levels of students (including students, new graduates, experienced nurses, etc.). Staff members in all positions serve as faculty and preceptors for students from across academic programs. There is a patient education program that meets the diverse needs of patients in all of the care settings of the organization (ANCC Magnet Recognition Program, 2005). Walker, Urden, and Moody (2009) found that clinical nurse specialists most influenced the "Magnetic Forces" of "Nurses as Teachers," "Consultation and Resources," and Professional Development.

Force 12. Image of Nursing: The services provided by nurses are characterized as essential by other members of the health care team. Nurses are viewed as integral to the health care organization's ability to provide patient care. Nursing effectively influences system-wide processes (ANCC Magnet Recognition Program, 2005). For example, a diabetes resource group transformed diabetes care in a Magnet hospital improving glycemic management, thus enhancing the image of this multidisciplinary group (Gerard, Griffin, & Fitzpatrick, 2010).

Force 13. Interdisciplinary Relationships: Collaborative working relationships within and among the disciplines are valued. Mutual respect is based on the premise that all members of the health care team make essential and meaningful contributions in the achievement of clinical outcomes. Conflict management strategies are in place and are used effectively, when indicated (ANCC Magnet Recognition Program, 2005). Teamwork has a three-pronged approach of motivations, behaviors, and information flow with timely communication, flexible and adaptive coordination, and cohesive and reliable cooperation (Salas, Wilson, Murphy, King, & Salisbury, 2008).

Force 14. Professional Development: The health care organization values and supports the personal and professional growth and development of staff. In addition to quality orientation and in-service education addressed in Force 11, Nurses as Teachers, emphasis is placed on career development services. Programs that promote formal education, professional certification, and career development are evident. Competency-based clinical and leadership/management development is promoted and adequate human and fiscal resources for all professional development programs are provided (ANCC Magnet Recognition Program, 2005). Sherill and Roth (2007) described the capabilities and the role of the librarian along with library resources for facilities on the Magnet journey while Halfer (2009) discussed the outcomes of grant funding for a one-year pediatric RN internship for new graduates for achieving Magnet status.

MAGNET RECOGNITION PROGRAM OVERVIEW

In 1992, the Magnet Recognition Program® was assumed by the ANCC to recognize health care organizations that provided nursing excellence. The program also provided a vehicle for disseminating successful nursing practices and strategies. Recognizing quality patient care, nursing excellence, and innovations in professional practice, the Magnet Recognition Program® provided consumers with the ultimate benchmark to measure the quality of care that they can expect to receive.

When U.S. News & World Report publishes its annual showcase of "America's Best Hospitals," being an ANCC Magnet® organization contributes to the total score for quality of inpatient care. ANCC is one of only a few organizations providing outside data to the ranking methodology. In the 2010 listing, 8 of the top 10 (80%) medical centers featured in the prestigious Honor Roll are Magnet-recognized organizations. In the Children's Hospital Honor Roll, 6 of the top 8 (75%) hospitals were ANCC Magnet recognized (July 14, 2010). As of November 20, 2010, there are 378 Magnet designated facilities (www.anccnursecredialing.org).

The Magnet Recognition Program is based on quality indicators and standards of nursing practice as defined in the newly revised 3rd edition of the *ANA Nursing Administration: Scope & Standards of Practice* (2009). The Scope and Standards for nurse administrators and other "foundational documents" form the base upon which the Magnet environment was built. The Magnet designation process includes the appraisal of qualitative factors in nursing. These factors, referred to as "Forces of Magnetism," were first identified through the AAN's research conducted in 1983 (American Nurses Credentialing Center *Magnet Recognition Program®: Application Manual: Recognizing Nursing Excellence*).

The full expression of whether the Forces embody a professional environment is dependent on a strong visionary nursing leader who advocates and supports on-going professional development and excellence in nursing practice. As a result, the reputation and standards of the nursing profession are elevated. Magnet designation is considered the hallmark of nursing excellence; research has validated that the ANCC Magnet designation has a profound positive effect on nursing practice and patient care (Wolf, Triolo, & Reid Ponte, 2008).

In 2007, the Magnet Recognition Program undertook a statistical analysis of the 164 sources if evidence and reduced the 164 sources into 88, resulting in an alternative framework for grouping the criteria (Morgan, 2009). The new Model adopted in October 2009, has an overarching theme of Global Issues in Nursing and Health Care with five components (1) Transformational Leadership;

(2) Structural Empowerment; (3) Exemplary Professional Practice; (4) New Knowledge, Innovation and Improvement; and (5) Empirical Outcomes.

Drenkard (2009) and Wolf, Triolo, and Ponte (2008) described the new Magnet model and unveiled the ANCC Magnet Commission's vision that "Magnet organizations will serve as the font of knowledge and expertise for the delivery of nursing care globally." Drenkard subsequently (2010) outlined the business case for facilities on the Magnet® journey. The CNO needs to understand the data and articulate the potential for nursing excellence that results in decreased costs, improved productivity and improved health care outcomes. This strategy should positively affect how the CNO advocates for the level of support to engage in the process of participating in the Magnet Recognition Program. The ultimate outcome is improving costs through increasing nursing satisfaction, patient satisfaction and clinical outcomes.

Interestingly, the findings of Ulrich, Buerhaus, Donelan, Norman, and Dittus (2007) indicated that registered nurses in hospitals applying for Magnet recognition perceived better outcomes on certain factors than registered nurses employed in a Magnet-designated hospital. The significance of this finding is that nursing leadership should not become complacent once the hospital receives the Magnet recognition (Ulrich et al., 2007). Trinkoff and colleagues (2010) indicated that working in a Magnet-designated facility does not necessarily mean that nurses perceive working conditions, although working conditions have been found to be major factors in nurse retention.

TRANSFORMATIONAL LEADERSHIP

The new Magnet model re-emphasizes the importance of using a leadership style known as transformational leadership, which may create turbulence and involve atypical approaches to solutions. However, transformational leadership has been shown to be particularly effective in turbulent and uncertain environments (Adams, Erikson, Jones, & Paulo, 2009; Habel & Sherman, 2010). Transformational leaders have vision and influence; clinical knowledge and strong expertise relating to professional practice; and lead people when the need arises to be proactive in meeting the challenges and opportunities of the future.

The engagement and futuristic thinking of the nursing staff create a practice community that positions the entire organization to take full advantage of any current or emergent changes or innovations on the health care horizon (Meredith, Cohen, & Raia, 2010). Identifying and measuring success within the CNO population has proven complex and challenging for nurse executive educators, policy makers, practitioners, and researchers (Adams et al., 2009).

The CNO and the senior leadership team need to work in collaboration and as full partners to create a strategic vision for the future based on evidence, research and values. If workflow or physical redesign is in the strategic plan, it needs to include the foundation for a new health care facility and the framework for the post occupancy evaluation (Stichler, 2010). A systematic approach based on innovation must be developed within the environment to create that vision and enlighten the organization as to why change is necessary. At the same time, on-going transparent communication to every department asking how they intend to achieve and sustain that change is integral to stabilization and the creation of new ideas and innovation. Transformational leaders listen, challenge, influence and affirm as the organization evolves or undergoes work transition. Timely feedback and positive action for identified areas or opportunity reassure the nurses that their voices have been heard, and contribute to a culture of autonomy (Sharkey, Meeks-Sjostrom, & Baird, 2009).

Quality of nursing leadership includes competency, skill and educational level at all levels, measurement of nurse satisfaction is measured and involvement of nurses at all levels in decision-making. Of Kramer, Schmalenberg, and Maguire's (2010) structures and leadership practices essential for a Magnet (healthy) environment, the most instrumental was nurse managers who shared their power; requested evidence to make autonomous decisions; held staff accountable in positive, constructive ways for decision making; promoted group cohesion and teamwork and resolved conflicts constructively. Direct care nurses involved in formal and informal work groups are inspired to identify and make differences in their complex adaptive health care environment (Lacey, Teasley, & Cox, 2009; Upenicks & Sitterding, 2008). Nurse Managers need to empower nurses, provide support, create opportunities for nurses to increase their competencies, and reward and advance staff nurse autonomy (Kramer & Schmalenberg, 2003). There needs to be a high level of commitment and congruence between mission, vision, values, philosophy and strategic plan (Whitaker, 2009) and the management styles requires effective horizontal and verbal communication (Espinoza, Lopez, & Stonestreet, 2009).

The CNO should be visionary and influence others toward achievement of goal with open communication. Visibility and accessibility of the CNO reflects an evidence-based approach for the transformative nurse executive practice (Jost & Rich, 2010). Tagnesi, Dumont, and Rawlinson (2009) stressed that the CNO's rounding on all shifts and units help to maintain the pulse of the workforce and the pressing issues, thus improving communication and patient safety. Porter-O'Grady (2009) claims that, the pursuit of change and the creation of culture of innovation will certainly not be an option for the foreseeable future. Several instruments are available to evaluate the workplace (Berndt,

Parsons, Paper, & Browne, 2009). Weston (2009) reported that the Veterans Administration facilities measure RN's perceptions of the professional practice that contributes to enhanced nurse satisfaction, providing areas of focus for nurse executives.

STRUCTURAL EMPOWERMENT

Structural empowerment can be defined as a strong professional practice flourishing, encompassing, accessing and redesigning the nursing practice environment. Eaton-Spiva et al. (2010) described a project that provided a framework for current an on-going evaluation of the practice environment. The mission, vision, and values come to life to achieve outcomes important to the organization. Strong relationships and partnerships are developed with community organizations, volunteer activities and professional organizations. Porter, Kolcaba, McNulty, and Fitzpatrick (2010) reported a unique nursing labor management partnership, demonstrating the positive effect of nursing labor management partnership on nurse turnover and satisfaction.

There is collaboration with community-based organizations with high quality outcomes resulting from networking with nursing and developing sustainable partnerships. Fiscal resources are used to support community activities. Ballard (2010) advocates providing refresher education on the self-governance structure and implementing a nurse manager support group to share successes and role modeling. This helps build a strong self-governance structure. Kowalik and Yoder (2010) discussed a concept analysis of decisional involvement that is intended to distinguish decision-making, the act of deciding, from participation in decisional involvement, making a choice to participate in a process. The authors indicate that since there is a gap between which decisions staff nurses are actually involved in and which decisions they prefer to be involved in making, future research should be conducted to examine the variables causing this gap, followed by interventions tested to address these issues.

The image of nursing is enhanced when the CNO exerts influence on strategic planning and decision-making at the highest level. Nursing needs to receive recognition throughout the organization, including cash rewards of the senior leadership team (Stroth, 2010).

Professional development, a continuous learning environment, is evident as nurses are encouraged to grow as professionals and adequate fiscal and human resources are allocated (Cooper, 2009). Covell (2009) stated that evidence related to the impact of continuing professional development activities on patient and organizational outcomes provides administration with empirical support for decision making related to the allocation of funding for the nurses at the bedside. Cimiotti and colleagues (2005) indicated that nurses from Magnet hospitals have a positive perception of nursing competence in their work environment. The high scores related to a positive perception of nursing competence were positively correlated with high levels of professional certification on the Perceived Work Environment (PWE) instrument. Management needs to be foster and support excellence through development of clinical competence, leadership capability and support for national specialty certification (Bryne, Schroeter, & Mower, 2010; DeCampli, Kirby, & Baldwin, 2010; McDonald, Tulai-McGuinness, Madigan, & Shively, 2010). Sherman and Pross (2010) developed future leaders to build and sustain health work environments at the unit level.

EXEMPLARY PROFESSIONAL PRACTICE

There should be an understanding of the role of nursing with advancement of the role in the care delivery system and the relationship to patient, families, communities, and the interdisciplinary team. There needs to be an application of new knowledge and evidence with professional practice environments creating empowerment and engagement in the workplace that lead to optimal care (Fasoli, 2010). Professional models of care define and promote the professional role and incorporate evidence-based practice. Several models included Family-Centered Care, Benner's Novice to Expert, King's Theory of Goal Attainment and Watson's Theory of Human Caring or Primary Nursing (Jost, Bonnel, Chacko, & Parkinson, 2010). Buerhaus, Donelan, DesRoches, and Hess (2009) indicated that hospital CNOs and nurse managers should focus on reducing threats to physical and mental safety, promoting a blame-free culture, increasing respect for nurses, and improving RN involvement in decisions that affect unit operations and patient care.

Regardless of the practice model selected, a common language needs to be developed that showcases the major themes of the practice model. The practice model needs to be integrated into the language of the organization, and play a prominent role in nursing practice (Storey, Linden, & Fischer, 2008). An example is the O'Rourke Patient Care Model; a unifying mental picture that ties together the health workplace attributes with a professional model of practice that create and sustains the desired healthy workplace (Cornett & O'Rourke, 2009).

Staffing systems incorporate, patient needs, staff member skills sets and staff mix (Gordon, Buchanan, & Bretherton, 2008). Kramer and Schmalenberg (2005) found that more effective staffing structures were enabled by attention to factors identified by staff, partially influenced by scores on the on the Perception of Adequacy Staffing (PES) scale. Hickey, Gauvreau, Conner,

Sporing, and Jenkins (2010) described the relationship of nurse staffing skill mix and Magnet® Recognition to instructional volume and mortality for congenital heart surgery.

Consultation and resources include internal and external resources such as the hospital medical library (Sherwill-Navarro & Roth, 2007). Another example is using advanced practice nurses for their consultative vote. There has been continued growth in number and diversity of advanced practice nurses in academic health science centers as well as other facilities. This requires the availability of mechanisms for centralized administrative oversight and professional support of these populations (Ackerman, Mick, & Witzel, 2010). The Clinical Nurse Specialist (CNS) role is vital to attaining and maintaining Magnet Recognition; individuals in this role serve as consultants, resources and teachers and help lead professional development activities (Walker et al., 2009).

Participation in professional nursing organizations and participation community organizations is encouraged. Autonomy involves adherence with national professional nursing standards. Keys (2009) notes that autonomy requires that all nurses are able to practice without interference in their scope of practice. Policies and procedures shape the practice of nursing with access to appropriate literature and databases.

Peer review must be in place at all levels. Nurses as teachers include orientation, mentoring, patient and family education, clinical and leadership development, and scholarly initiatives. The University of Pittsburgh has online modules (Preceptorship: The Bridge Between Knowledge and Practice) that systemizes the process of training preceptors to ensure a more uniform experience for both preceptor and the student (Burns & Northcut, 2009).

Interdisciplinary relationships include committee and taskforces. Patient care documentation supports interdisciplinary decision-making. Teamwork is essential in interdisciplinary care teams; teamwork processes are vital within nursing teams and should be evaluated (Kalish, Lee, & Salas, 2010; Kalish, Weaver, & Salas, 2009; Parsons, Clark, & Cornett, 2007). Since positive nurse-physician relationships are essential to a Magnet organization, one should read 20,000 nurses tell their stories (Schmalenberg & Kramer, 2009).

NEW KNOWLEDGE, INNOVATION, AND IMPROVEMENT
Magnet organizations are ethically and professionally compelled to contribute to new knowledge, innovation and quality improvements. This component includes new models of care, application of existing evidence, new evidence and visible contributions to nursing science (ANCC Magnet Recognition Program, 2008). Conducting research generates new knowledge, and Evidence-based Practice

(EBP) integrates new knowledge into practice but requires dissimilar resources and processes (Reigle et al., 2008).

Achieving quality outcomes, best practices, and nursing excellence requires dissemination of new knowledge. Translating research into practice advances professional nursing practice, provides patients with care that is evidence based and fosters an environment grounded in the ANCC Magnet Recognition Program components (Atkinson, Turkel, & Cashy, 2008). Dols, Bullard, and Gembol (2010) believe that leaders maintain high levels of staff nurse motivation by disseminating findings through presentations and publications, and recognizing and celebrating these accomplishments; the best motivator for change is the implementation of a practice change based on research conducted at the facility. In addition, nurse executives can learn effective strategies for creating or refining nurse research programs by discussing the barriers and challenges with all levels of nursing staff (Weirbach, Glick, Fletcher, Rowlands, & Lyder, 2010).

Nurse researchers, executives and professionals must collaborate and share successes, lessons learned and insights in real time if nursing is to reduce the long lag time between innovation and adoption (Simpson, 2009). Knowledge management (KM) can serve as a framework for identifying, organizing, analyzing and translating knowledge into practice. KM has been applied in the development of clinical decision support systems to translate clinical practice guidelines into nursing practice (Anderson & Willson, 2009). Knowledge networks (KNs) are leadership tools that can increase social capital and innovation in organizations. Electronic or online KNs can maximize efficiency and effectiveness of communications and collaboration (MacPhee, Suryaprakash, & Jackson, 2009).

The quality improvement program should have a comprehensive plan that assesses, analyzes, and evaluates clinical and operational process and outcomes. There is ongoing monitoring, evaluation, and improvement of nurse-sensitive outcomes. There are clinical and operational indicators that are benchmarked with external entities. Cornell, Riodan, and Herrin-Griffith (2010) reported that a number of significant differences in the time spent on a variety of activities, but the duration and frequency of nurse activities were not drastically altered by the additional technology.

Anderson, Mokracek, and Lindy (2009) found the success of the Best Practice Council was attributed to clear directions, an aggressive timeline, and a short-term commitment required of team members who remained focused and on track. Jurkovich, Karpiuk, and King (2010) provided examples of perioperative excellence to attain Magnet recognition. Kane and Preze (2009) describe the nurses' perceptions of subspecialization in pediatric cardiac intensive care unit and quality outcomes.

Beal, Riley, and Lancaster (2008) and Riley, Beal, and Lancaster's (2008) work provided new insights into key elements essential for the development of scholarly practice, embracing scholarly nursing practice while balancing care giving with professional development. The participants believed others saw them as knowledgeable, approachable, receptive to teaching, and genuinely interested in the learning of others. Messmer and Gonzalez (2006) created a culture for promoting nursing research and clinical scholarship while Messmer, Jones, and Rosillo (2002) used nursing research projects to meet Magnet recognition program standards.

Turkel, Reidinger, Ferket, and Reno (2005) created a model for the integration of evidence-based practice and nursing research as part of the journey toward achieving Magnet recognition. Implementation of this model created a culture of scholarly inquiry for the registered professional nurse. An outcome of this initiative was the development of a nursing research fellowship for direct care registered nurses within the same organization (Turkel, Ferket, Reidinger, & Beatty, 2008). When the organization received the original Magnet designation and subsequent redesignation, the research fellowship received an exemplar from the appraisers. The success of these initiatives resulted in the creation of the Chicagoland Research Consortium, where 17 hospitals in the area collaborate and network around the areas of education, evidence-based practice and nursing research (Ferket, Reidinger, & Turkel, 2007).

Strout, Lancaster, and Schultz (2009) described a clinical Scholars Model as a grassroots approach to develop a cadre of clinical nurses with the EPB and research skills. Wise (2009) viewed the evidence-based practice committee as the mechanism that encourages nurses to guide their clinical practice and make recommendations. Simpson (2010) showed how engaged nurses could lead the way to improved outcomes through technology.

EMPIRICAL OUTCOMES

Outcomes need to be categorized in terms of clinical outcomes related to nursing, workforce outcomes, patient and consumer outcomes, and organizational outcomes. Quantitative national benchmarks should be established. Valey, Aiken, Sloane, Clarke, and Vargas' (2004) findings reinforce the need for change in the workforce that reduces nurses' high levels of job burnout and risk of turnover while maintaining patients' satisfaction with their care. Kalish (2010) found that the difference in perceptions between registered nurses and nursing assistants for missed nursing care pointed to a lack of teamwork in the form of closed-looped communications, inadequate leadership, team orientation, trust, and shared values. Clark (2009) stresses that training health staff in teamwork basics establishes a healthier workplace and creates the conditions for safer patient care provision. The Report Card of Nursing must demonstrate excellence.

The quality infrastructure system needs to promote, support and improve patient safety. Armstrong, Laschinger, and Wong (2009) demonstrated an important link between the quality and nature of a hospital nurses' work environment and the level of the patient safety climate in those same environments. A unit-based leadership model involving an attending physician, nurse leaders, and a quality specialist, collaborating on relevant and shared issues resulted in a decrease in hospital-acquired infections (Jost & Rich, 2010). Bacon and Mark (2010) demonstrated that work engagement and availability of support services had a significant impact on patient satisfaction. Albanese and colleagues (2010) engaged clinical nurses in quality and performance improvement activities. The implementation of the "Present on Admission Indicators" delegated responsibility to charge nurses to design and implement strategies for early recognition of suboptimal patient outcomes from care received at other facilities.

Meredith, Cohen, and Raia (2010) found that the best approach to engaging direct care registered nurses in evidence-based practice was their EBP fellowship, a 3–6 month part-time position for a staff nurse to research a nursing service priority. Their Transforming Care at the Bedside (TCAB) work was so successful that it was adopted by all the acute-care inpatient staff. An example was establishing Pyxis supply centers on inpatient units and installing two profile Pyxis medication dispensing towers on larger nursing units that resulted in expedient, convenient, and safe medication administration. Perez, Batcheller, and Chapell (2009) found that when participating in TACB, change takes time and perseverance, but is more likely to be successful due to frontline involvement. Stefanck (2008) recommended having a medication-dispensing machine in each patient room after participating in the TACB multi-site study.

There must be an integration of the American Nurses' Association Code of Ethics and Patient Bill of Rights guiding clinical decision making (Fowler, 2008). When research and evidence-based practice initiatives are incorporated into clinical operations process, nurses perceive they provide high quality of care with outcomes documented. One example of this integration could be palliative care with the goal to add life to the child's life not years to the child's life (Palliative Care for Children, AAP position paper, 2000).

Berndt et al. (2009) developed a tool to evaluate a healthy workplace index. Anderson, Manno, O'Connor, and Gallagher (2010) used a national database of nursing quality indicators data to study excellence in nursing leadership.

ANCC PATHWAY TO EXCELLENCE®

Not all facilities have the financial or human resources to pursue the Magnet journey. However, health care facilities that want to demonstrate their excellent nursing environments have another option—the ANCC Pathway to Excellence® designation (AMN Healthcare, Inc. and Nursezone.com, October 2009). In 2003, the Texas Nurses Association (TNA) began work to positively affect nurse retention by improving the workplace for nurses and established the Texas Nurse-Friendly™ Program for small/rural hospitals. The program was partially funded with a five-year grant from the U.S. Health Resources and Services Administration (HRSA). The goal of this program was to improve both the quality of patient care and professional satisfaction of nurses working in small and rural hospitals in Texas. The first Nurse-Friendly hospitals were designated in May 2005.

The ANCC Pathway to Excellence® credential is granted to health care organizations that create work environments where nurses can flourish. The designation supports the professional satisfaction of nurses and identifies best places to work. To earn Pathway to Excellence status, an organization must integrate specific Pathway to Excellence standards into its operating policies, procedures, and management practices. Confirmation of the essential Pathway to Excellence elements is obtained through written documentation and an online nurse survey whereas the confirmation of the Magnet Recognition standards is obtained through written documentation and a comprehensive site visit (ANCC Pathway to Excellence Program brochure, 2008).

REFERENCES

Ackerman, M. H., Mick, D., & Witzel, P. (2010). Creating an organizational model to support advanced practice. *Journal of Nursing Administration, 40*(2), 63–68.

Adams, J. M., Erikson, J. I., Jones, D. A., & Paulo, L. (2009). An evidence-based structure for transformative nurse executive practice: The model of the interrelationship of leadership, environments, and outcomes. *Nursing Administration Quarterly, 33*(4), 280–287.

Aiken, L. H., Havens, D. S., & Sloane, D. M. (2009). The Magnet nursing services recognition program. *Journal of Nursing Administration, 39*(7/8), S5–S14.

Aiken, L. H., Smith, H. L., & Lake, E. T. (1994). Lower medicare mortality among a set of hospitals known for good nursing care. *Medical Care, 32*(8), 771–787.

Albanese, M. P., Evans, D. A., Schantz, C. A., Bowen, M., Disbot, M., Moffa, J. S., . . . Polomano, R. C. (2010). Engaging clinical nurses in quality and performance improvement activities. *Nursing Administration Quarterly, 34*(3), 226–243.

Anderson, J. A., & Willson. (2009). Knowledge management: Organizing nursing care knowledge. *Critcal Care Nursing Quarterly, 32*(1), 1–9.

American Nurses Credentialing Center. (2005). *Magnet Recognition Program®: Application Manual* Silver Springs, MD: ANCC.

American Nurses Credentialing Center. (2008a). *Magnet Recognition Program®: Application Manual: Recognizing Nursing Excellence.* Silver Springs, MD: ANCC.

American Nurses Credentialing Center. (2008b). *Pathway to Excellence Program*™ brochure. Silver Springs, MD: ANCC.

Anderson, B. J., Manno, M., O'Connor, P., & Gallagher, E. (2010). Listening to nursing leaders. *Journal of Nursing Administration, 40*(4), 182–187.

Anderson, J. J., Mokracek, M., & Lindy, C. N. (2009). A nursing quality program driven by evidence-based practice. *Nursing Clinics of North America, 44*(1), 83–91.

Armstrong, K., Laschinger, H., & Wong, C. (2009). Workplace empowerment and Magnet hospital characteristics as predictors of patient safety climate. *Journal of Nursing Care Quality, 24*(1), 55–62.

Atkinson, M., Turkel, M., & Cashy, J. (2008). Overcoming barriers to research in a magnet community hospital. *Journal of Nursing Care Quality, 23*(4), 362–368,

Bacon, C. T., & Mark, B. (2010). Organizational effects on patient satisfaction in hospital medical-surgical units. *Journal of Nursing Administration, 39*(5), 220–227.

Ballard, N. (2010). Factors associated with success and breakdown of shared governance. *Journal of Nursing Administration, 40*(10), 411–416

Batcheller, J. (2010). Chief nursing officer: An analysis of the literature. *Nursing Clinics of North America, 45*(1), 11–31.

Beal, J. A., Riley, K. M., & Lancaster, D. R. (2008). Essential elements of an optimal clinical practice environment. *Journal of Nursing Administration, 38*(11), 488–493.

Berndt, A. E., Parsons, M. L., Paper, B., & Browne, J. A. (2009). Preliminary evaluation of the healthy workplace index. *Critical Care Nursing Quarterly, 32*(4), 335–344.

Bryne, S., & Mower, J. (2010). Perioperative specialty certification: The CNOR as evidence for Magnet excellence, *AORN, 91*(5), 618–621.

Buerhaus, P. I., Donelan, K., DesRoches, C., & Hess, T. (2009). Still making process to improve the hospital workplace? Results from the 2008 National Survey of registered nurses. *Nursing Economics, 27*(5), 289–301.

Burns, H. K., & Northcut, T. (2009). Supporting preceptors: A three-pronged approach for success. *The Journal of Continuing Education, 40*(11), 509–513.

Caroselli, C. (2008). The system chief nurse executive: More than sum of the parts. *Nursing Administration Quarterly, 32*(3), 247–252.

Cimiotti, J. P., Quinlan, P. M., Larson, E. L. Pastor, D. K., Lin, S. X., Stone, P. W. (2005). The Magnet process and the perceived work environment of nurses. *Nursing Research, 54*(6), 384–390.

Clark, P. R. (2009). Teamwork: Building healthier workplaces and providing safer care patient care. *Critical Care Nursing Quarterly, 32*(3), 221–231.

Cooper, E. (2009). Creating a culture of professional development: A milestone pathway tool for RNs. *Journal of Continuing Education in Nursing, 40*(11), 501–508.

Cornell, P., Riodan, M., & Herrin-Griffith, D. (2010). Transforming nursing workflow, Part 2. *Journal of Nursing Administration, 40*(10), 432–439.

Cornett. P. A., & O'Rourke, M. A. (2009). Building organizational capacity for a healthy work environment through role-based professional practice. *Critical Care Nursing Quarterly, 32*(3), 208–220.

Covell, C. L. (2009). Outcomes achieved from organizational investment in nursing continuing professional development. *Journal of Nursing Administration, 39*(10), 438–443.

DeCampli, P., Kirby, K. K., & Baldwin, C. (2010). Beyond the classroom to coaching: Preparing new nurse managers. *Critical Care Nursing Quarterly, 33*(2), 132–137.

Dols, J., Bullard, K., & Gembol, L. (2010). Setting a nursing research agenda. *Journal of Nursing Administration, 40*(5), 201–204.

Drenkard, K. (2009). The Magnet program. *Journal of Nursing Administration, 39*(7/8), 1–2.

Drenkard, K. (2010). The business case for Magnet®. *Journal of Nursing Administration, 40*(6), 263–269.

Drenkard, K. N. (2005). Sustaining Magnet: Keeping the forces alive. *Nursing Administration Quarterly, 29*(3), 214–222.

Eaton-Spiva, L. A., Buitrago, P., Trotter, L., Macy, A., Lariscy, M., & Johnson, D. (2010). Assessing and redesigning the nursing practice environment. *Journal of Nursing Administration, 40*(1), 36–42.

Espinoza, D. C., Lopez, A., & Stonestreet, J. S. (2009). The pivotal role of the nurse manager in healthy workplaces. *Critical Care Nursing Quarterly, 32*(4), 327–334.

Fasoli, D. (2010). The culture of nursing engagement: A historical perspective. *Nursing Administration Quarterly, 34*(1), 18–29.

Ferket, K., Reidinger, G., & Turkel, M. (March 2007). Achieving Magnet status: How research collaboration among nurses from different hospitals leads to Magnet success. *American Nurse Today,* 15–16.

Fowler, M. D. M. (Ed). (2008). *Guide to the code of ethics for nurses: interpretation and application.* Silver Spring, MD: American Nurses Association.

Fundeburk, A. (2008). Mentoring: The retention factor in the acute care setting. *Journal for Nurses in Staff Development, 24*(3), E1–E5.

Gawlinski, A. (2007). Evidence-base practice changes: Measuring the outcome. *AACN Advanced Critical Care, 18*(3), 320–322.

Gerard, S. O., Griffin, M. Q., & Fitzpatrick, J. (2010). Advancing quality diabetes education through evidence and innovation. *Journal of Nursing Care Quality, 25*(2), 160–167.

Gordon, S., Buchanan, J., & Bretherton, T. (2008). *Safety in numbers: nurse-to-patient ratios and the future of health care.* Ithaca, NY: Cornell University Press.

Habel, M., & Sherman, R. O. (October 11, 2010). Transformational leadership. *West Nurse.com,* 54–58.

Halfer, D. (2009). Supporting nursing professional development: A Magnet hospital. *Journal for Nurses in Staff Development, 25*(3), 135–140.

Hinshaw, A. S. (2006). Keeping patients safe: A collaboration among nurses administrators and researchers. *Nursing Administration Quarterly, 30*(4), 309–320.

Hickey, P., Gauvreau, K., Conner, J., Sporing, E., & Jenkins, K. (2010). The relationship of nurse staffing skill mix and Magnet® Recognition to instructional volume and mortality for congenital heart surgery. *Journal of Nursing Administration, 40*(5), 226–232.

Horstman, P. L., Bennett, C., Daniels, C., Fanning, M., Grimm, E., & Withrow, M. L. (2006). The road to Magnet one magnificent journey. *Journal of Nursing Care Quality, 21*(3), 206–209.

Jasovsky D. S., Dorman, L., Geisler, L., Douglas, P., Befnard, A., & Kleber, E. (2005). Magnet demographic data; Creating a system to streamline the process. *Journal of Nursing Administration, 35*(11), 490–496.

Jost, S. G., Bonnel, M., Chacko, S. J., & Parkinson, D. L. (2010). Integrated primary nursing: A care delivery model for the 21st century knowledge worker. *Nursing Administration Quarterly, 34* (3), 208–216.

Jost, S. G., & Rich, V. L. (2010). Transformation of a nursing culture through actualization of a nursing professional practice model. *Nursing Administration Quarterly, 34*(1), 30–40.

Jurkovich, P., Karpiuk, K., & King, C. (2010). Magnet recognition: Examples of perioperative excellence. *AORN Journal, 91*(2), 292–299.

Kalish, B., Lee, H., & Salas, E. (2010). The development and testing of the nursing teamwork survey. *Nursing Research, 59*(1), 42–50.

Kalish, B., Weaver, S. J., & Salas, E. (2009). What does nursing teamwork look like? A qualitative study. *Journal of Nursing Care Quality, 24,* 298–307.

Kalish, B. J. (2010). Nurse and nurse assistant perceptions of missed nursing care. *Journal of Nursing Administration, 39*(11), 485–493.

Kane, J. M., & Preze, E. (2009). Nurses' perceptions of subspecialization in pediatric cardiac intensive care unit. *Journal of Nursing Care Quality, 24*(1), 354–361.

Keys, Y. (2009). Perspective on autonomy. *Journal of Nursing Administration, 39*(9), 357–359.

Kleinpell, R. M., & Gawlinski, A. (2005). Assessing outcomes in advanced practice: The use of quality indicators and evidence-based practice. *AACN Clinical Issues, 16*(1), 43–57.

Kleinpell, R. M., Gawlinski, A., & Burns, S. (2006). Searching and critiquing literature essential for acute care NPS. *The Nurse Practitioner, 31*(8), 12–13.

Kowalik, S. A., & Yoder, L. H. (2010). A concept analysis of decisional involvement. *Nursing Administration Quarterly, 34*(3), 259–267.

Kramer, M., & Schmalenberg, C. (2004). Essentials of a magnetic work environment Part 1 *Nursing 2005, 34*(6), 50–54.

Kramer, M., & Schmalenberg, C. (2005). Revising the essentials of magnetism tool: There is more to adequate staffing than numbers. *Journal of Nursing Administration, 35*(4), 188–198.

Kramer, M., Schmalenberg, C., & Maguire, P. (2010). Nine structures and leadership practices essential for a Magnetic (healthy) environment. *Journal of Nursing Administration, 34*(1), 4–17.

Kramer, M., & Schmalenberg, C. E. (2003). Magnet hospital staff nurses describe clinical autonomy. *Nursing Outlook, 51*(1), 13–19.

Kramer, M., & Schmalenberg, C. E. (2005). Best quality patient care: A historical perspective on Magnet hospitals. *Nursing Administration Quarterly, 29*(3), 275–287.

Lacey, S. R., Teasley, S. R., & Cox, K. S. (2009). Differences between pediatric registered nurses' perception of organizational support, intent to stay, workload and overall satisfaction and years employed as a nurse in Magnet and Non-Magnet pediatric hospitals: Implications for administrators. *Nursing Administration Quarterly, 33*(1), 6–13.

Laschinger, H. K. S., Finegan, J., Shamian, J., & Wilk, P. (2001). Impact of structural and psychological empowerment on job strain in nursing work settings. *Journal of Nursing Administration, 31*(5), 260–272.

MacPhee, M., Suryaprakash, N., & Jackson, C. (2009). Online knowledge networking: What leaders need to know. *Journal of Nursing Administration, 39*(10), 415–422.

McDonald, S., Tulai-McGuinness, S., Madigan, E. A., & Shively, M. (2010). Relationship between staff nurse involvement in organizational structures and perception of empowerment. *Critical Care Nursing Quarterly, 33*(2),148–162.

Meredith, E. K., Cohen, E., & Raia, L. V. (2010). Transformational leadership: Application of magnet's new outcomes. *Nursing Clinics of North America, 45*(1), 49–64.

Messmer, P., Jones, S. G., & Rosillo, C. (2002). Using nursing research projects to meet Magnet recognition program standards. *Journal of Nursing Administration, 3*(10), 538–543.

Messmer, P. R., & Gonzalez, J. (2006). Creating a culture for promoting nursing research and clinical scholarship. In P. Yoder-Wise & K. Kowalski (Eds.), *Leading and managing: Nursing administration for the future* (Chap. 15, pp. 295–303). New York, NY: Mosby-Elsevier.

Morgan, S. H. (2009). The Magnet Model as a framework for excellence. *Journal of Nursing Care Quality, 24*(2), 105–108.

Parsons, M. L., Clark, P., & Cornett, P. A. (2007). Team behavioral norms: A shared vision for a healthy patient care workplace. *Critical Care Nursing Q, 30*(3), 213–218

Perez, C. Q., Viney, M., Batcheller, J., & Chapell, C. (2009). Spreading TCAB across network hospitals. *American Journal of Nursing, 109*(11), 46–49.

Porter, C., Kolcaba, K., McNulty, R., & Fitzpatrick, J. J. (2010). The effect of a nursing labor management partnership on nurse turnover and satisfaction. *Journal of Nursing Administration, 40*(5), 205–210.

Porter-O'Grady, T. (2009). Creating a context for excellence and innovation: comparing chief nurse executive leadership practices in Magnet and non-Magnet hospitals. *Nursing Administration Quarterly, 33*(3), 198–204.

Projected supply, demand and shortages of registered nurses: US Department and Health Services Health Resources and Services Administration Bureau of Health Professions. National Center for Health Workforce Analysis. July, 2002.

Reigle, B. S., Stevens, K. P., Belcher, J. V., Huth, M. M., McGuire, F., Mals, D., & Volz, T. (2008). Evidence-based practice and the road to magnet status. *Journal of Nursing Administration, 38*(2), 97–102.

Riley, J., Beal, J. A., & Lancaster, D. (2008). Scholarly nursing practice from the perspective of experienced nurses. *Journal of Advanced Nursing, 61*(4), 425–435.

Salas, E., Wilson, K. A., Murphy, C. E., King, H., & Salisbury, M. (2008, June). Communicating, coordinating and cooperating when lives depend on it: Tip for teamwork. *The Joint Commission Journal on Quality and Patient Safety, 34*(6), 333–341.

Schlmalenberg, C., & Kramer, M. (2009). Nurse-physician relationships in hospitals: 20,000 nurses tell their story. *Critical Care Nurse, 29*(1), 74–83.

Sharkey, K., Meeks-Sjostrom, D., & Baird, M. (2009). Challenges in sustaining excellence over time. *Nursing Administration Quarterly, 33*(2), 142–147.

Sherman, R., & Pross, E. (2010). Growing future leaders to build and sustain health work environments at the unit level. *The Online Journal of Issues in Nursing, www.nursingworld.org*

Sherwill-Navarro, P., & Roth, K. L. (2007). Magnet hospitals/magnetic libraries—the hospital medical library: A resource for achieving magnet status. *Journal of Hospital Librarianship, 7*(3), 21–31.

Simpson, R. L. (2009). Innovations in transforming organizations. *Nursing Administration Quarterly, 33*(3), 268–272

Simpson, R. L. (2010). Engaged nurses lead way to improved outcomes via technology. *Nursing Administration Quarterly, 54* (3), 268–273.

Stefanck, A. L. (2008). Transforming care at the bedside. *American Journal of Nursing, 108*(10), 27–29.

Sternas, K. A., O'Hare, O., Lehman, K., & Milligan, R. (1999). Nursing and medical student teaming for service learning in partnership with the community: An emerging holistic model for interdisciplinary education and practice. *Holistic Nursing Practice, 13*(2), 66–77.

Stichler, J. F. (2010). Predesign and postoccupancy evaluation. *Journal of Nursing Administration, 40*(2), 49–52,

Storey, S., Linden, E., & Fisher, M. L. (2008). Showcasing leadership exemplars to propel professional practice model implementation. *Journal of Nursing Administration, 38*(3), 138–141.

Stroth, C. (2010). Job embeddedness as a nurse retention strategy for rural hospitals. *Journal of Nursing Administration, 40*(1), 32–35.

Strout, T. D., Lancaster, K., & Schultz, A. A. (2009). Development and implementation of an inductive model for evidence-based practice: A grassroots approach for building evidence-based practice capacity in staff nurses. *Nursing Clinics of North America, 44*(1), 94–102.

Tagnesi, K., Dumont, C., & Rawlinson, C. (2009), The CNO: Challenges and opportunities on the journey to excellence. *Nursing Administration Quarterly, 35*(2), 159–167.

Texas Nurses Association. (2005, April-May). *TNA Designee First Nurse Friendly Hospitals Texas Nursing, 8.*

Trinkoff, A. M., Johantgen, M., Storr, C. L., Han, K., Liang, Y., Guises, A. P., & Hopkinson, S. (2010). A comparison of working conditions among nurse in Magnet and non-Magnet hospitals. *Journal of Nursing Administration, 40*(7/8), 309–319.

Turkel, M., Ferket, K., Reidinger, G., & Beatty, D. (2008). Building a nursing research fellowship in a community hospital. *Nursing Economics, 26*(1), 26–34.

Turkel, M., Reidinger, G., Ferket, K., & Reno, K. (2005). An essential component of the Magnet journey: Fostering an environment for evidence-based practice and nursing research. *Nursing Administration Quarterly, 29*(3), 254–262.

Ulrich, B. T., Buerhas, P. I., Donelan, K., Norman, L., & Dittus, R. (2007). Magnet status and registered nurse views of the work environment and nursing as a career. *JONA, 379(5),* 221–220.

Upenicks, V. V., & Sitterding, M. (2008). Achieving Magnet redesignation: A framework for cultural change. *Journal of Nursing Administration, 38*(10), 419–428.

Valey, D. C., Aiken, L. H., Sloane, D. M., Clarke, S. P., & Vargas, D. (2004). Nurse burnout and patient satisfaction. *Medical Care, 42*(2), 11-57–11-64

Walker, J. A., Urden, L. D., & Moody, R. (2009). The role of the CNS in achieving and maintaining Magnet status. *Journal of Nursing Administration, 39*(12), 515–523.

Weirbach, F. D., Glick, D. F., Fletcher, K., Rowlands, A., & Lyder, C. H. (2010). Nursing research and participant recruitment organizational challenges and strategies. *Journal of Nursing Administration, 40*(1), 43–48.

Weston, M. (2009). Managing and facilitating innovation and nurse satisfaction *Nursing Administration Quarterly, 33*(4), 329–334.

Whitaker, C. (2009). A chief nursing officer's perspective. *AORN Journal, 89*(4), 745–748.

Wise, N. J. (2009). Maintaining Magnet status: Establishing an evidence-based practice committee. *AORN Journal, 90*(2), 205–213.

Wolf, F., Triolo, P., & Reid Ponte, P. (2008). Magnet recognition program: The next generation. *Journal of Nursing Administration, 38*(4), 200–204.

CHAPTER 10

Standardized Nursing Languages

Essential for the Nursing Workforce

Dorothy Jones, Margaret Lunney, Gail Keenan, and Sue Moorhead

If we cannot name it, we cannot control it, practice it, research it, teach it, finance it, or put it into public policy.

Clark and Lang, 1991

ABSTRACT

The evolution of standardized nursing languages (SNLs) has been occurring for more than four decades. The importance of this work continues to be acknowledged as an effective strategy to delineate professional nursing practice. In today's health care environment, the demand to deliver cost-effective, safe, quality patient care is an essential mandate embedded in all health reform policies. Communicating the contributions of professional nursing practice to other nurses, health providers, and other members of the health care team requires the articulation of nursing's focus of concern and responses to these concerns to improve patient outcomes. The visibility of the electronic health record (EHR) in practice settings has accelerated the need for nursing to communicate its practice within the structure of the electronic format. The integration of SNLs into the patient record offers nurses an opportunity to describe the focus of their

© 2011 Springer Publishing Company
DOI: 10.1891/0739-6686.28.253

practice through the identification of nursing diagnosis, interventions and outcomes (IOM, 2010). Continued development, testing, and refinement of SNLs offers nursing an accurate and reliable way to use data elements across populations and settings to communicate nursing practice, enable nursing administrators and leaders in health care to delineate needed resources, cost out nursing care with greater precision, and design new models of care that reflect nurse-patient ratios and patient acuity that are data driven (Pesut & Herman, 1998). The continued use of nursing languages and acceleration of nursing research using this data can provide the needed evidence to help link nursing knowledge to evidence-driven, cost-effective, quality outcomes that more accurately reflect nursing's impact on patient care as well as the health care system of which they are a part. The evaluation of research to support the development, use, and continued refinement of nursing language is critical to research and the transformation of patient care by nurses on a global level.

STANDARDIZED NURSING LANGUAGES: ESSENTIAL FOR THE NURSING WORKFORCE

The development and use of standardized nursing languages (SNLs) are essential for the nursing workforce because discipline-focused languages, also referred to as data sets, nomenclatures, classifications, taxonomies, and terminologies, provide names for the clinical phenomena of concern to the nursing profession (refer to Table 10.1). Such names are needed to communicate and collaborate within the disciplines and with others, that is, patients, families, and system-wide stakeholders (Hayakawa & Hayakawa, 1990; Rutherford, 2008). The process of naming clinical phenomena (e.g., nursing diagnoses, nursing interventions, and patient outcomes) enables advancement of the profession as a discipline and a science through research and knowledge development (Avant, 1990; Gordon, 1994). By definition, one of the most important characteristics of a profession is a unique body of knowledge that defines the foundations of practice for members (Greenwood, 1957).

Smith and McCarthy (2010) state "the body of knowledge of the professional discipline distinguishes its practice, differentiates it from technical practice, and is comprised of the philosophies, ethics, theories, research, and art of the discipline" (p. 44). Continued progression of the nursing discipline is constantly needed to link the contribution of nursing knowledge to the achievement of high quality, cost-effective nursing care. The goal of SNLs is to name the phenomena of nursing concern so that locally, nationally, and internationally, nurses have access to the labels, definitions, and descriptions of clinical phenomena for communication with patients and others (Baernholdt & Lang, 2003).

TABLE 10.1

Terms, Definitions, and Standardized Languages

Term	Definition
ANA Core Criteria (nursing language criteria and definitions)	Support practice, clinically useful and unambiguous; systematic method of development, documented testing, and continued refinement, maintained on a regular basis. These criteria need to be present in all data sets, terminologies, or classifications
Class	A group, division, category, or set used to categorize or classify information
Classification	A way to arrange items (e.g., defining characteristics) based on relationships and assignment of names (e.g., interventions and outcomes) to groups of items
Data Set	Grouping of identified elements of particular interest within a context
Domain	The most abstract term in a taxonomy (e.g., functional domain)
Nomenclature	Terms that can be combined to represent more complex concepts; informed by preestablished rules
Taxonomy	Organization of concepts based on similarities into a conceptual framework
Terminology	Words for a concept or the vocabulary used to communicate a concept

Source: Adapted from Dochterman and Jones, 2003.

Consistency of communicating the content of nursing science through use of SNLs: (a) contributes to patient safety and other quality-based goals, (b) meets the requirements for participation in electronic health records (EHRs), (c) promotes greater autonomy and control of nursing practice, and (d) provides the clinical data for nurse administrators to meet many workforce goals. Patient safety and other quality-based goals are achieved through the aggregation, analysis, and interpretation of clinical data (Institute for Healthcare Improvement, n.d.; Institute of Medicine, 2000, 2003, 2004, 2010; Joint Commission, 2008). Using the standardized labels of nursing diagnoses, interventions and outcomes enables the establishment of databases to determine the nursing phenomena of concern, and isolate the interventions needed to help patients with specific problems (and identify those that do not) to achieve specific outcomes (Dochterman et al., 2005; Jenny, 1995). From such data, evidence-based and cost-effective quality care can be planned and implemented (Faster Cures, 2006).

The international growth of the electronic health record (EHR) has provided increased need for SNLs to communicate care. Implementation of EHRs requires use of standardized terms and the standard terms should be national and international in order to develop benchmarks and compare quality across localities. The integration of SNLs into patient documentation helps to foster nursing autonomy and control over clinical phenomena of concern that are clearly delineated and communicated to the public, other disciplines, and health care systems. In addition, nurse administrators will have access to needed clinical data to achieve optimum staffing patterns, address issues of patient acuity, cost out nursing care more accurately, attain desired patient outcomes in a timely manner, and describe professional practice to stakeholders (Lyon, 1990).

The purposes of this chapter are to identify the SNLs for clinical practice, describe the existing research support for SNLs, describe the methodologies that can be used for ongoing development, relate existing and future research to evidenced-based nursing, and explain the importance of nursing languages to the nursing workforce.

SNLs FOR CLINICAL PRACTICE

The SNLs for clinical practice have been developing since 1973 with the start of the organization that is now known as NANDA International (NANDA-I). In this section, the existing SNLs will be described, the research support for SNLs will be reviewed, and the relation of SNLs to evidenced-based nursing will be explained.

Existing SNLs

The initial call to address the development of SNLs occurred at the *First Task Force to Name and Classify Nursing* Diagnosis, in St. Louis, MO, in 1973. At that meeting, Gebbie and Lavin charged 100 invited nurse experts from the United States and Canada to develop and classify the health problems that are within the domain of nursing (Gebbie & Lavin, 1975). The meeting was guided by the need to increase the visibility of nursing in patient care, identify the names for computer files to record and organize nursing data, assign costs to nursing care, and link the judgments and decisions of nurses to actions and outcomes

The organization held the second conference in 1975, the third conference in 1978, and biannually since then. In 1982, the organization name was changed to the North American Nursing Diagnosis Association (NANDA). In 2002, it was decided that this name no longer applied because of the extensive involvement of nurses from many countries. In 2002, the name of North American Nursing Diagnosis Association was changed to NANDA International (I). The most recent meeting of NANDA-I, and first meeting external to the United States, was held in Madrid, Spain in May 2010.

Since 1973 to the present, a number of data sets, terminologies, and classifications have emerged in different ways. NANDA-I is a membership-driven group with committee structures (Kritek, 1978; Martin, 2005; Saba, 1997; Saba & Taylor, 2007), for example, the Taxonomy and Diagnosis Development Committees, working to maintain the NANDA-I taxonomy. The developers of the Nursing Interventions Classification (NIC) and the Nursing Outcomes Classification (NOC) were NANDA-I members but developed NIC and NOC with funding from the National Institutes of Health, using large research teams based at the University of Iowa (Bulechek, Butcher, & Dochterman, 2008; Johnson, Maas, & Moorhead, 1997–2002; Moorhead, Johnson, Maas, & Swanson, 2008). The University of Iowa continues to support maintenance of NIC and NOC at the Center for Nursing Classification and Clinical Effectiveness (CNCCE, n.d.).

The Omaha System and the Clinical Care Classification (CCC) were originated by community health nurses based on the perceived need for SNLs in home health care nursing (Martin & Scheet, 1992; Saba, 1997). Both classifications have since evolved for use in other settings including academic nurse-managed centers and nursing education (Canham, Mao, Yoder, Connolly, & Dietz, 2008; Feeg, Saba, & Feeg, 2008). These languages continue to evolve, for example, the Omaha System holds regular meetings and conferences to advance this model. In the last few years, the CCC was made available free in the reference database, SNOMED–CT. The Perioperative Nursing Data Set was developed and is promoted by the Association of Operating Room Nurses for specific use in perioperative nursing (e.g., Westendorf, 2007). The SNLs of were first developed and disseminated in the United States and Canada. Today, they are used internationally in countries such as Japan, Spain, and France.

International Classification of Nursing Practice

International Classification of Nursing Practice (ICNP) is described as a unified language system. It is an information tool that describes nursing practice within health information systems (ICN, 2007). It has been under development, and exposed to testing and translation since 1990; ICNP is described as an information tool that is able to articulate the nursing practice. The ICNP framework contains data elements that represent nursing practice in health information systems (Hyeoun-Ae, Hardiker, Bartz, & Coenen, 2005).

The ICN began work on the development of ICNP in 1990. Over the years, versions of ICNP were developed and tested. The data can be used by clinicians, researchers and administrators to describe nursing practice and the contributions of the discipline to patient care. The current version of ICNP is considered an effective resource to measure quality nursing care and is useful for research (Rotegaard, 2009; Simpson, 2007; Warren & Coenen, 1998). ICNP has several centers to continue refinement of the language including Deutschsprachiege ICNP, for German speaking group users, The Research Center for Nursing Practice (Australian Capital Territory and the University of Canberra) and the Chilean Center for ICNP Research and Development. There have been research studies conducted across cross-cultures using ICNP. These include cross mapping studies, validation studies and computer data base analysis (Dykes et al., 2009).

American Nurses Association—Nursing Practice Information and Infrastructure

In 2006, the American Nurses Association's (ANA *Committee on Nursing Practice Information and Infrastructure* developed a web site to update nurses on the SNLs and documentation. There are currently 13 nursing data sets, nomenclatures and classification systems approved by ANA for use in EHRs. Five terminology sets of nursing languages that include diagnoses, interventions and outcomes are included in the ANA approved list (ANA, 2006; Anderson, Keenan, & Jones, 2009). These are the (a) CCC, (b) ICNP, (c) combination of NANDA-I, the NIC, and the NOC, (d) Omaha System, and (e) Perioperative Nursing Data Set. Table 10.2 provides a list of ANA approved classifications, terminologies and data sets).

Within each of these five classification systems, the concepts common to professional nursing are addressed. These include, for example, self care, anxiety, fear, mobility, sleep, nutrition, constipation, skin breakdown, stress, coping, and self management of illnesses (e.g., NANDA-I, 2009). The current versions of NANDA-I, NIC, and NOC (NNN) taxonomies contain 1,147 research-based labels, definitions, and descriptions. Extensive numbers of research studies and position papers can be found related to these concepts in the Proceedings of Conferences in groups like NANDA-I since 1973 (NANDA-I Archives Boston College at burns.library@bc.edu NIC and NOC; e.g., Carroll-Johnson, 1990). The development of SNOMED RT is designed to create a reference terminology to allow for the use of multiple languages in a standardized format within EHR. Within SNOMED RT, all of the ANA approved languages can be mapped to accommodate NNN as well as other terminologies (refer to Table 10.2).

NANDA-I, NIC, and NOC

Over the years, conferences focusing on the combined work of NNN have been held nationally. NNN are the largest group of language developers within

TABLE 10.2

ANA Approved Standardized Languages

- North American Nursing Diagnosis Association–Taxonomy II—classifies nursing diagnosis (NANDA-I)
- *Nursing Intervention Classification (NIC)–Taxonomy*, 4th ed.—classifies nursing interventions
- *Nursing Outcomes Classification (NOC)–Taxonomy*, 4th ed.—classifies patient outcomes
- Gordon's Eleven Function Health Patterns
- Home Health Care Classification's (HCCC) classifies specific nursing diagnosis, interventions and outcomes (Homecare)
- Omaha system's structure classifies specific nursing diagnosis, interventions, and outcomes
- Patient Care Data Set (PCDS; Ozbolt)
- Perioperative Data Set (PNDS) classifies specific nursing diagnosis, interventions and outcomes (Perioperative care)
- International Classification of Nursing Practice (ICNP) classifies specific nursing diagnosis, interventions and outcomes (ICN)
- SNOMED RT (Systemized Nomenclature of Medicine clinical terms) reference terminology to cross map multiple classifications, etc.
- Clinical LOINC—Logical Observation Identifiers Names and Codes
- Nursing Minimum data Sets—NMDS Delaney, C. 2006
- NMMDS—Nursing Management Minimum Data Sets

North America, focusing on the expansion of the Classification of nursing diagnosis, nursing interventions and nursing outcomes, respectively. The goal of these meetings has been to explore further terminology development, especially around the development of a common structure for the three languages, and research methodologies. The availability of a common structure was thought to critical to the increased use of SNLs, articulation of the content and focus of nursing, future development of databases for advanced research, support prediction of staffing patterns and workload, and isolating costs associated with patient acuity and complexity.

In 2001, leaders from NNN received funding from the National Library of Medicine (R13LMO7243) to develop, implement and evaluate a project that supported "the assumptions underlying the languages of nursing diagnosis, interventions and outcomes; examine the existing taxonomic structures (NNN), and prepare the first draft of a common structure that united diagnosis, interventions and outcomes (Dochterman & Jones, 2003). A desired framework or *Desiderata* (Dochterman & Jones, 2007) was identified to guide development of a new organizing structure. Guidelines for the new language NNN structure included: (a) simplicity of structure that was theory neutral, (b) parsimony of groups, (c) clear language, (d) distinct definitions of diagnoses, interventions, and outcomes, and (e) useful to other disciplines to communicate with nursing.

The Proposed NNN Classification

The proposed NNN classification consisted of four domains and 28 classes and met the guidelines for a desired structure. The proposed structure allows for the placement of the three languages in the same domains and classes. Currently, NNN are working with this common structure with the hope that, over time, and with modification a unified structure for organizing nursing diagnoses, interventions, and outcomes could be realized. Kautz, Kuiper, Pesut, and Williams (2006) studied the use of NNN in a BSN program and found inconsistencies in the use of terminology by faculty and students. The authors recommended that faculty and students could benefit from using NNN throughout the curriculum to insure consistency in communicating and documenting nursing practice and to prepare nurses for the 21st century (e.g., Johnson et al. 2006).

Impact of SNLs

From the beginning, the goal of developing SNLs was to reflect and build upon nursing knowledge. Nursing has an established body of knowledge that has experienced accelerated growth in the past 45 years. Knowledge development, including the growth of grand, mid-range and practice-based theories, has reflected the philosophical underpinnings of the discipline. The core of nursing knowledge is relationships, that is, the nurse-patient, family, and community relationships. The SNLs capture these interactions by articulating the phenomena of concern that embody the knowledge and focus of the discipline (Jones, 2007).

Development of the existing SNLs reflects the social contract of nurses with society, as described in the Social Policy Statement (ANA, 2004) and the Nurse Practice Acts of many states in the United States, for example, New York State. The New York State Nurse Practice Act of 1972 states that nurses diagnose and treat human responses. Today, in conjunction with the social policy statement, most of the SNLs reflect that nurses address health promotion, risks or threats to health, and responses of individuals and groups to illness.

The SNLs link disciplinary knowledge to the delivery of care and offer nurses standardized approaches for describing their practice. The labels for nursing diagnoses, interventions, and patient outcomes are defined and described so that the meaning of the terms are as clear as possible to all those who use the labels. The structures used to organize SNLs are designed to create systems that are easily communicated and usable. For example, frameworks such as Gordon's functional Health Patterns have been used to organize nursing diagnosis. Table 10.1 provides a list of ANA approved nursing data sets, classifications and terminologies.

RESEARCH AND SNLs

The significant research support for use of SNLs provides strong evidence for nurse leaders to select SNLs for clinical practice (Gordon, 1987). In a bibliometric study of the CINAHL database to map the existing knowledge of SNLs, Anderson et al. (2009) searched for all types of literature sources, including books, chapters, journal articles, dissertations, brief reports, and abstracts, from 1982 to 2006 for the five terminology sets approved by ANA. A total of 1,140 unique items were identified and classified to one terminology set or another. The results were that the terminology set of NNN had the most extensive literature support (n = 879 of 1,140 sources; Anderson et al., 2009). The research support for standardized nursing diagnoses, nursing interventions, nursing-sensitive patient outcomes, and for combining NNN will be reviewed.

Research Support and Standardized Nursing Diagnoses

Since the beginning of NANDA-I in 1973, the Committee that accepts new diagnoses and changes in previously approved diagnoses has expected research studies to be submitted as one of the bases for diagnosis submissions. Diagnoses are only included on the approved list when there is sufficient research and literature support for the concept (NANDA-I, 2009).

In 1989, NANDA-I held a conference to explore the research methods being used and to propose methods for support of the inclusion of SNLs in the EHR (Carroll-Johnson, 1990). The topics that were explored included methods of validation, and other types of qualitative (Mc Farlane, 1990) quantitative, and integrative methods (Kim, 1990; Gordon, 1979; Schroeder, 1990). Many of the studies at that time were descriptive studies (Ferhing, 1986, 1987) and included concept analyses, diagnostic content and construct validity, frequency studies, and inter-rater reliability studies. Few studies reached predictive validity or focused on statistical methodologies, such as regression analyses. It was determined that instruments need to be developed that reflect the content and concepts of the discipline so that more rigorous investigations can be conducted.

The types of studies to develop knowledge of nursing diagnoses vary widely, are still mostly descriptive, and a large number of the studies presented at the 2010 AENTDE/NANDA-I conference in Madrid, Spain used experimental designs (e.g., Paans, Serrmeus, Nieweg, & Van Der Schano, 2010, May). A Pub med literature search of research studies in the last decade, year 2000 to 2010, revealed 162 published research studies that focused on, or included, nursing diagnoses from NANDA-I and other terminologies such as the ICNP or the PNDS. From the beginning of nursing diagnosis knowledge development, a strong focus has been on validating the existence of specific nursing diagnoses, defining characteristics, and risk factors in specific populations.

The content and construct validity of individual nursing diagnoses for use with specific populations have been established by nurses worldwide. The number of studies available is too extensive to identify, especially considering the many nursing organizations besides NANDA-I that focus on advancement of nursing diagnosis knowledge, for example, the Japan Society of Nursing Diagnosis, the Association of Common European Nursing Diagnoses, Interventions, and Outcomes (ACENDIO), the Brazilian Nursing Diagnosis Association, and the Spanish Nursing Diagnosis Society (AENTDE). Each of these organizations conduct annual or biannual conferences in which nursing diagnosis studies are presented and many are later published in a wide variety of international literature sources. For example, 674 papers and posters were presented at the May 2010 AENTDE-NANDA-I conference in Madrid, most of which were research.

Descriptive studies established the content and construct validity of the concepts that represent nurses' diagnoses, that is, the responses or experiences of people to health problems and life processes (NANDA-I, 2009). An example is a clinical study in two hospitals of patients ($n = 76$) who experienced one or more of the three respiratory diagnoses, Ineffective Breathing Pattern, Ineffective Airway Clearance, and Impaired Gas Exchange (Carlson-Catalano et al., 1998). The data collection instrument showed good validity and reliability, including both interrater and intrarater reliability. The findings and conclusions of the study were presented to the NANDA Diagnosis Review Committee and were used for refinement of these three diagnoses.

In a comprehensive review of the validation studies reported in Pub med and CINAHL databases, Berger (2008) noted that most of the identified studies were quantitative using nurse validation and clinical validation methods. Berger concluded that additional studies are needed for many diagnoses. For 72 diagnoses, at least one validation study was noted. For 59 diagnoses, one to four studies were found. For 84 diagnoses, no studies were found, but studies must have been done because submitters of new diagnoses are expected to submit research studies to NANDA-I with new diagnoses. Studies may have been conducted that were not published or were not traced in Berger's systematic review. Clinical methodologies, which are preferred for validation of diagnoses (Carlson-Catalano

& Lunney, 1995), were used with 50 studies analyzed by Berger. The need for additional studies using multivariate methods such as magnitude estimation scaling, Q sorting, factor analysis, and discriminate analysis were noted.

Naming Interventions, Research

A classification focused on nursing interventions is needed to provide consistent terms and definitions for the treatments nurses provide. The NIC provides guidelines for the selection of nursing interventions by nurses (Bulechek et al., 2008). This activity is a critical part of the clinical reasoning process that nurses use to select diagnoses, interventions and outcomes. Six factors are important to consider when choosing an intervention. First, selection of a nursing intervention for a particular nursing diagnosis is greatly influenced by the outcome the nurse is attempting to achieve. This requires the nurse to communicate with the patient and family members and to consider the time frame in which care is delivered. Outcomes provide the criteria to judge whether the nursing intervention is improving the status of the patient on a particular outcome. Second, the nurse chooses outcomes and interventions based on the characteristic of the nursing diagnosis. The intervention should target the etiological factors to eliminate or reduce the problem. In some cases, this is not possible so the nurse chooses an intervention to address the symptoms the patient is experiencing. The third factor for choosing an intervention is the research base of the intervention. This helps the nurse determine how effective the intervention has been in similar situations and with certain populations of patients. The fourth consideration focuses on the feasibility of providing an intervention. This includes factors such as the cost of providing the intervention, time for implementation, and how the intervention fits the total plan of care for all providers. The fifth factor to consider is the acceptability of the intervention to the patient. This must take into consideration the values, beliefs, religion and culture of the patient. The final factor is the capability of the nurse. This involves the nurse knowing the scientific rationale for the intervention, having the necessary skills (psychomotor and interpersonal) and the ability to function in the health care setting in which the intervention is performed (Bulechek et al., 2008). The selection of the right intervention based on these factors improves the quality of care provided to patients. Each intervention has a list of suggested activities that nurses can select to customize the intervention based on the needs of the patient. Any safety issue must be addressed in the plan of care and the selection of nursing interventions.

At the organizational level, the NIC has been used to measure nurse competency on specific interventions. Nolan (1998) describes how one organization used NIC to address competency validation on nursing interventions provided frequently in their organization. Nolan (1998, p. 27) defines competency as "an individual's *actual performance* in a particular situation. It describes how well an individual integrates knowledge, skill, attitudes and behavior in delivering care according to expectations. Competency is a complex phenomenon, and requires and evaluation of the employee's ability to meet job expectations and subsequent continuous effective care for assigned patients (del Bueno, 2001). This competency assessment, according to Nolan (1998), is based on the organization being able to identify the most frequent interventions (also diagnoses and outcomes) performed in the organization as a whole and for each individual unit so that education and testing of competency can be relevant to practice patterns. This knowledge informs nurses planning orientation for new employees as well as continuing education programs. Educational sessions can include clinical reasoning case studies focused on intervention selection to improve nurse's skills in this area. The frequently used nursing interventions need to be validated over time since changes in practice impact care delivery and because patient needs change when new medical treatments are introduced by other disciplines. Ongoing data at the organization and unit level is needed to address nurse competency and its impact on quality care and safety issues in any organization across health care settings. The classification has domains focused on safety and the health system to assist nurses in identifying interventions to ensure quality care and safety part of the plan of care.

SNLs and Measuring Outcomes

The NOC is essential to capturing the effectiveness of nursing interventions performed for identified nursing diagnoses. NOC provides standardized terms and definitions to identify patient outcomes. In the past, nurses have relied on goal statements to evaluate care. These were specific to the patient and difficult to compare across patient populations and settings. The NOC outcomes are designed to facilitate comparison of outcomes for populations of patients that nurses treat in a variety of settings and across settings as the patient moves across the continuum of care. The measurement scale(s) identified for each outcome in the classification allow nurses to measure the outcome prior to providing interventions and at selected times such as when the condition of the patient changes suddenly, at the end of a shift, prior to transfer to another unit, and at discharge. Nurses selecting outcomes must contemplate several factors as they select the best options. These factors include the type of health concern, the nursing, medical, and health problems that patient is encountering, the characteristics of the patient, patient resources, patient preferences, patient capacities and their treatment potential (Moorhead, Johnson, Maas, & Swanson, 2008). Clinical evaluation of the measurement scales in NOC was completed for 169 of the outcomes in the 2nd edition of NOC (Moorhead, Johnson, & Maas, 2004; Ruland & Bakken, 2003). The scales were found to be reliable and were able to capture changes in patient status even for short hospitalizations in acute care setting. This study also made it clear that holding an outcome rating steady over time for elderly patients in long-term care facilities was important in the assessment of quality care in these settings. Nurses need clinically useful tools to measure the day-to-day care of patients. Outcomes measurement is important to communicate the quality of care provided to patients, to system administrators and to the public policy makers (Jenkins, 1985).

Many organizations have focused their attention on the measurement of outcomes for "never events" such as falls, pressure ulcers, and urinary tract infections. NOC provides a systematic way to measure patient focused outcomes that measure the positive effects of nursing interventions and depict the results of interventions that prevent adverse events. The outcomes can be measured post intervention to identify the effectiveness of the plan of care. The response of the patient may be dramatic such as moving a rating from "1" to "5" or show incremental change over time. The benefits of using NOC outcomes is that both the patient and the provider can measure the effects of interventions and nurses can follow trends in specific outcomes with a population of patients they frequently treat.

Research Support for Linking NNN

In previous decades, studies focused on NNN as distinct and separate languages. Increasingly, studies are being conducted that test the value of using the three languages together, for example, Muller-Staub, Needham, Odenbriet, Lavin, and Achterberg (2006a, 2006b, 2007, 2008). When these three languages were studied separately, the types of studies and the focus of research differed. In the past, studies of NANDA-I diagnoses mainly focused on the one or more individual diagnoses of interest to specific members; studies of NIC and NOC have been larger studies of the two systems, in contrast to individual concepts within the systems. Research from Switzerland, Sweden, The Netherlands, and the United States support the combining of NNN.

In a pretest-posttest design, Muller-Staub et al. (2007) studied the effects of an educational intervention on the quality of documentation and effect on patient outcomes with nurses of 12 wards in a Swiss hospital. The educational intervention included how to implement nursing diagnoses, nursing interventions, and nursing-sensitive patient outcomes. Before and after the educational intervention, two sets of 36 randomly selected patient records were judged for quality, using the valid and reliable instrument, Quality of Nursing Diagnoses, Interventions and Outcomes (Q-DIO; Muller-Staub et al., 2010). Before the educational intervention, the mean score on quality of nursing diagnoses was .92 (SD = 0.41); one year after the intervention the mean score was 3.50

(SD = 0.55; p < .0001). Similarly, for identification of nursing interventions and patient outcomes, the mean scores were significantly higher one year after the education of nurses.

In a pretest–posttest study of nursing process documentation after a year-long education effort in a large hospital system (50 inpatient wards and 30 outpatient clinics), documentation improved in nursing assessment ($p \leq .05$), nursing diagnosis ($p \leq .01$), and nursing interventions ($p \leq .01$; Thoroddsen & Enfors, 2007). The SNLs of NANDA-I and the NIC were used to teach and document nursing diagnoses of human responses and nursing interventions. Patient outcomes were not taught using SNLs and it was the only aspect of the nursing process that did not improve with education.

The accuracy of six aspects of nurses' documentation was studied in a random sample of 10 medical centers of the Netherlands selected from 94 centers (Paans, Sermeus, Nieweg, & van der Schans, 2010b). Patient records (n = 341) were assessed by two independent trained reviewers using the D-Catch instrument to measure accuracy of the (a) record structure, (b) admission documentation, (c) diagnosis documentation, (d) intervention documentation, (e) progress and outcome evaluation, and (f) legibility. The results were that "28% contained all of the nursing process stages, 34% were more or less structured according to the nursing process stages and 38% were not structured at all according to these stages" (p. 4). The investigators conclude that EHRs should support nurses in their accuracy of documentation by providing guidelines and logically structured systems.

Consensus validation studies using action research methods were conducted with staff nurses for them to identify the nursing diagnoses, interventions, and outcomes that are relevant for specific populations served in hospitals, long-term care, ambulatory settings, and end-of-life care (Carlson, 2006; Lunney, McCaffrey, & Umbro, 2010; Lunney, McGuire, Endozo, & McIntosh-Waddy, 2010; Lunney, Parker, Fiore, Cavendish, & Pulcini, 2004; Minthorn & Lunney, in press). One of the purposes of the study design was to reduce the complexity of using NNN in clinical units that serve patients with specific types of health problems. Carlson (2006, 2010) developed the Total Consensus Method to achieve 100% consensus among experienced nurses of the specific terms to be used in standards of care and in the front screens of an EHR. This method was used for nurses to identify the terms that would be included in an Electronic Nursing Documentation System (ENDS) used by military nurses who specialize in care of persons with latent tuberculosis infection (Carlson, 2010).

In a study to identify the nursing diagnoses, nursing interventions, and patient outcomes that are relevant for adults with traumatic brain injury (TBI), "29 nursing diagnoses, each with 3–11 NIC interventions, and 1–13 NOC outcomes were identified as relevant to the TBI population served by nurses in the facility" (Lunney, McGuire, et al., 2010, p. 163).

A hospital-based study reported that nurses who provide care for adults with diabetes, 17 nursing diagnoses, each with 7–19 NIC interventions (N = 78) and 4–14 NOC outcomes (N = 76) were identified as relevant for adults with diabetes (Minthorn & Lunney, in press). This consensus validation method shows great promise for nurses in health care units to select the relevant terms for specific types of patient care from the 1,147 concepts in NNN.

Decision Support and NNN

The next generation of studies to support use of NNN will be those that test decision support systems (e.g., Carlson, 2010; Keenan, Tschannen, & Ford, 2010; Odenbreit, 2010; O'Neill, Dluhy, & Chin, 2005; O'Neill, Dulhy, Hansen, & Ryan, 2006). Carlson tested the ENDS in two army military settings, one in Hawaii and one in Texas (N = 13 nurses). The purposes were to capture the value of nursing care, especially by identifying patient care outcomes that were positively affected by nurses using the ENDS, provide standards of practice to guide nursing care, provide data for resource management, develop a reliable patient acuity index, and identify a revenue generation method. The ENDS performed as expected. The results included that the nurses used the nursing diagnoses for a majority of patients, the linked NIC interventions were used to address the nursing diagnoses, the linked NOC outcomes that resulted from the nursing interventions were rated, and the time it took for nursing interventions was identified. A majority of scores on the patient outcomes after nursing interventions were significantly higher than the baseline scores, demonstrating the positive effects of nursing diagnoses and interventions.

The HANDS documentation system (also discussed later in the chapter) uses NNN to be interoperable on technical, semantic, and process levels, to support continuity of care through data and information that are gathered in the same way, always available and easily accessible, in a consistent format, and retain the same meaning for those who use it (Keenan et al., 2010, May; Keenan, Tschannen, & Wesly, 2008; Keenan, Yakel, & Tschannen, 2008). With a decade of research data, it has been established that the HANDS system is cost effectively maintained and sustained over time, automatically generates new evidence from the data collected, and delivers data immediately back to the point of care.

The WiCareDoc expert system uses 26 questions to help nurses identify the best terms for use in clinical practice, for example, it reminds nurses to evaluate hypothetic diagnoses and proposes interventions and outcomes based on diagnoses (Odenbreit, 2010). The WiCareDoc was developed and tested in Switzerland; these types of expert systems are also being developed by nurses in other countries, for example, Spain, Brazil, and Japan.

SNLs and Evidence-Based Nursing

The visibility of the concept of evidence-based practice (EBP) serves as an important opportunity for nursing language development, utilization, and subsequent evaluation. The demand for EBP offers nurses opportunities to use the best research literature available, including the research on SNLs, to inform clinical decisions and decide on treatments and outcomes (Melynk & Fineout-Overholt, 2005). The best available evidence suggests that SNLs should be used in clinical practice and in EHRs (Kautz & Horn, 2008). The use of SNLs within EHRs gives nurses opportunities to ask research questions that can be answered using existing local databases (e.g., Dochterman et al., 2005).

At a follow-up meeting of the Institute of Medicine (2004), the group stressed the need for improved documentation around five chronic health problems to improve quality, cost-effective, high-quality patient care. Problems included diabetes, acute pain, heart failure and asthma. The report addressed the need for better measurements of patient-centered outcomes, standardized systems for disseminating information and sharing of EBPs that promoted self-management and led to the development of new models of care that could be costed out more accurately (Swan, Lang, & McGinley, 2004). Evidence contained in using SNLs consistently in nursing documentation can help make this goal a reality and promote the expansion of research driven nursing care.

Seven levels of evidence were identified in the literature, ranging from the highest level, that is, systematic reviews of randomized control trials, to the lowest level of evidence, which is that of expert opinion (Melynk & Fineout-Overholt, 2005). While the research on SNLs continues to grow, there is more work needed. It is essential that nurses continue to build research around the development, implementation, and evaluation of the SNLs and integrate the languages into EHRs. It is only when large data bases are available with standardized languages that we can test, refine and evaluate the languages, and identify predictive models that accurately link patient care elements with cost and staffing demands. Table 10.3 links the evidence available and links it with levels of evidence as proposed by nurse researchers.

SNLs, NURSING ADMINISTRATION, AND EHRs

The use of SNLs offer nurse executives and administrators an effective way to account for the complex demands of the work environment, while creating a professional practice environment that clearly communicates practice, decreases staff burdens, optimizes patients' experiences, and enhances satisfaction for nurses, patients, and families (Ebright, Patterson, Chalko, & Render, 2003). The

TABLE 10.3

Levels of Evidence and SNL Research

Level of Evidence	SNL Research
Level 1: Evidence from systematic review meta-analysis of all relevant control trials or evidence-based practice guidelines based upon RCTs	None identified
Level 2: Evidence obtained from at least one well-designed randomized clinical trial (RCT)	Studies of teaching SNLs and accuracy of nursing diagnoses (Levin, Lunney, & Krainovich-Miller, 2004; Mueller-Staub et al., 2007; Paans et al., 2010, May) and accuracy of documentation (Paans et al., 2010b)
Level 3: Evidence obtained from well controlled clinical trials without randomization (quasi experimental)	Studies of the effect of teaching critical thinking (e.g., Cruz et al., 2009), and of implementing policy (e.g., Thoroddsen & Enfors, 2007)
Level 4: Evidence from nonexperimental studies, for example, case control or cohort studies	Extensive numbers of nonexperimental studies (e.g., del Bueno, 2005; Gordon, 1987; Sparks, 1990). Measurement (Hoskins, 1989; Kim, 1990)
Level 5: Evidence from systematic reviews of descriptive/qualitative studies	Epidemiological studies on occurrence or frequency (e.g., Schroeder, 1990); testing and refinement, and some systematic reviews related to generation of diagnoses
Level 6: Evidence from single descriptive/qualitative studies	Many studies that focused on populations or groups to identify high frequency or commonly occurring nursing diagnoses. The literature continues to report these studies: Flanagan and Jones (2009), Jeffries, Cox, et al. (2010, in press), Gordon, 1987, Gordon and Sweeney (1979) Fehring's validation model (1987) to estimate content and construct validity of the concepts (Whitley, 1996)
Level 7: Evidence from opinion of authority or experts	Much of early development used expert opinion (e.g., Gebbie & Lavin, 1975), including Delphi methods, for concept development, testing, and refinement

importance of SNLs to the nursing workforce relates to the value and opportunities that can be derived from clear communication of nursing phenomena. Clear communication using standardized terms for nursing care enables the storage of data on nursing care in EHRs, contributes to improved quality and patient safety, improves the efficiency and effectiveness of care, and enables the autonomy and control of professional practice for nursing to grow as a profession and science.

Storage of Nursing Data in Electronic Health Records

Internationally, all paper-based health records will be replaced by an EHR in standardized formats that include multiple aspects of patient care currently recorded in other formats. In each health care setting, for example, primary care, acute care, ambulatory care, and so forth (HIMSS, 2010; Institute of Medicine [IOM], 2003b; National Committee on Vital and Health Statistics [NCVHS], 2010; Olsson, Lymberts, & Whitehouse, 2004), data will be communicated using prescribed formats to local, regional, national and international levels. In EHRs, the majority of patient care is recorded by using standard terminology, that is, file names that health providers use to store similar information (IOM, 2003b). Without standardized file names, the specific types of health care data could not be identified, aggregated, analyzed, or compared.

The goal of EHRs is to be able to describe the care that is being provided, to communicate that care to others, that is, interoperability, and to decide whether or not patient care meets the benchmarks for quality-based care, that is, meaningful use (IOM, 2003b; NCVHS, 2010). For nursing care to be visible in EHRs, nurses must use file names that depict nursing, not the file names of medicine, psychiatry and other health care disciplines. These ANA-approved SNLs provide the standardized file names to be used to communicate nursing care in EHRs.

Visibility of nursing in EHRs will enable nurses and others to identify the care being provided, and to analyze the quality of care (Lunney, Delaney, Duffy, Moorhead, & Welton, 2005; Westra, Delaney, Konicek, & Keenan, 2008). Paans, Sermeus, Nieweg, and Van Der Schans (2009, 2010a, 2010b) used SNLs and a measurement schema to determine the accuracy of documentation in patient records. Nursing care quality can only be improved when it is described and compared to benchmarks for quality. For example, the identification of acute pain and provision of appropriate interventions can be examined for whether nursing care meets the standards promulgated by the American Pain Society (2000). Previous studies have shown that there is variance in nursing diagnoses and interventions for pain (McCaffrey & Ferrell, 1997; Puntillo, Neighbor, O'Neill, & Nixon, 2003).

In addition, nurses' use of SNLs in the EHR will help to increase the visibility of nursing practice and enhance the continued growth of concepts essential to the discipline (Dochterman & Jones, 2007). Researchers will have a rich data base to test and refine nursing diagnoses, interventions, and outcomes and guide the development of predictive models to inform staffing and identify costs (Dochterman & Jones, 2003).

Improved Quality and Patient Safety

Improved quality and patient safety is expected with clear communication of nurses' data interpretations or diagnoses, nursing interventions, and patient outcomes. The phenomena that nurses address are complex and diverse (Clancy, Delaney, Morrison, & Gunn, 2006; Potter et al., 2004, 2005), making it a significant challenge to select the most appropriate diagnoses, interventions, and outcomes. In addition, the possibilities within human behavior and ways to help people improve their health are so numerous for nurses (1,147 concepts) that nurses are not likely to recall the most appropriate concepts. The availability of SNLs decreases nurses' cognitive demand (Ferrario, 2003) and makes it possible to select the terms that best apply in a particular situation so that high quality care can be achieved and communicated.

With the complexity of understanding and communicating human responses and experiences related to health problems and life processes, accurate interpretations of patient data are extremely difficult to achieve (Lunney, 2008a). Variance in accuracy is expected, whether or not nurses' name their data interpretations using a language of nursing diagnosis. Such variance has been substantiated in numerous studies (see Table 10.4). The risk of low accuracy is related to three broad categories identified by two nurse theorists, Margery Gordon (1994) and Doris Carnevali (Carnevali & Thomas, 1993): the nature of the diagnostic task, the situational context, and the diagnostician (Table 10.4). The SNLs that include possible diagnoses, or data interpretations, offer nurses the labels, definitions, and defining characteristics to consider and validate with patients in partnership models of care (Lunney, 2009c). In each study noted in Table 10.4, it was clear that data interpretations and, thus accuracy of nurses' diagnoses, varied widely. In studies that used the Lunney scoring method (e.g., Lunney, 1992; Lunney et al., 1997; Spies et al., 1994), nurses were scored on seven levels of the accuracy scale, from low (−1) to high (+5).

The use of SNLs in the EHR can lead to better communication of information within, between, and among disciplines. Increased accuracy of the language, improved decision making, and better documentation can help decrease errors, target problems, provide more accurate measures of quality and isolate factors that increase patient risk.

TABLE 10.4

Selected Studies that Show Variance in Nurses' Data Interpretations Based on Three
Categories of Factors That Influence Data Interpretations or Diagnoses

Categories and Researchers	Factors	Significant Findings
Situational Context		
Gordon, 1980	Time constraints	When information was deliberately restricted to no more than 12 units of info, subjects were more accurate (88%) than with unlimited information (48%; $p =.001$).
Cianfrani, 1984		Increased time to diagnose was associated with lower accuracy.
Tanner et al., 1987		Increased time to diagnose was associated with lower accuracy.
Lenz et al., 1986	Role in the health care system	Differences in interpretations of data were associated with CNS preparation or role.
Hasegawa et al., 2007	Diagnostic decision making responsibility	In a national survey of Japanese nurses ($N = 376$, 85% response rate), those who reported diagnostic responsibility demonstrated significantly higher competence in specific parts of the task case studies.
Nature of the Diagnostic Task		
Matthews & Gaul, 1979	Task complexity	With two case studies (CS), there was an inverse relationship between diagnostic ability and complexity of the CS (significance not mentioned, validity & reliability of the cases not established).
Corcoran, 1986	Task complexity	Complexity influenced planning interventions for cancer pain (diagnosis of cancer pain was implied).
Hughes & Young, 1990	Task complexity	Three CS were used with increasing task complexity ($n = 101$ nurses). Task complexity was associated with less consistency in decision making. Decision making varied with each task; Decision making was task specific.

TABLE 10.4

Selected Studies that Show Variance in Nurses' Data Interpretations Based on Three
Categories of Factors That Influence Data Interpretations or Diagnoses   (Continued)

Categories and Researchers	Factors	Significant Findings
Gordon, 1980	Task complexity	Subjects did better when information was limited (see above); unlimited amount of data was assoc with continuation of predictive hypothesis testing.
Cianfrani, 1984	Amount of data	With high amounts of data, accuracy decreased with 1 of the 3 CS ($p = .001$). There was an increase in errors with 2 of the 3 CS ($p = .02; p = .001$) and an increase in time with 2 of the 3 CS ($p = .005; p = .05$). More problems were hypothesized with 2 of the 3 CS ($p = .05; p = .01$).
	Relevance of data	Accuracy decreased with low relevance data for all 3 CS ($p < .0000$). There was an increase in errors with low relevance data with 2 of the 3 CS ($p = .04; p = .000$).
Hicks, Merritt, & Elstein, 2003	Task complexity	31% of critical care nurses ($N = 54$) from 3 hospitals demonstrated consistency of intervention decision making (diagnosis was implied) with a low complexity task; only 11% demonstrated consistent decision making with a high complexity task.
Diagnostician: Education		
Aspinall, 1976		Mean number of correct diagnoses out of 12
	Masters	4
	BS degree	3.93
	Associate (AAS)	3.35
	Diploma (DIP)	3.23
		Significant difference between BS and AD ($p < .05$) and between BS and Dip ($p < .01$).
Matthews & Gaul, 1979	Masters students	% stated correct diagnosis ($p < .008$) 62 (Explanation: more use of negative & positive cues)
	Baccalaureate students	50% who listed task diagnosis (estimated from bar graph)

(Continued)

TABLE 10.4

*Selected Studies that Show Variance in Nurses' Data Interpretations Based on Three
Categories of Factors That Influence Data Interpretations or Diagnoses   (Continued)*

Categories and Researchers	Factors	Significant Findings
Craig, 1986	Masters students	82 (had been taught the diagnostic process) 35 (no previous nursing, 1st year) 30 (entered as nurses, 1st year) 45 (entered as nurses, 2nd year) 42 (generic); 49 (RN)
	Baccalaureate students	46 (with internship); 46 (without internship)
	Diploma students	52 (with one year experience)
Konno et al., 2000	Diploma graduates College education Technical education	With a written CS, nurses with college education were more accurate than nurses with technical education. 91% had never learned nursing diagnosis so differences were related to other factors.
Lunney, 1992	Continuing education	BS nurses (n =86) who reported having additional education on nursing diagnosis after graduation were more accurate with 3 written CSs than nurses who reported that they had no additional education ($p < .05$).
Lunney et al., 1997	Continuing education	Nurses ($n = 62$) who reported having additional education on nursing diagnosis after graduation were more accurate with actual cases than nurses who reported they had no additional education.
Mueller-Staub et al.,2007	Continuing education	In a pretest-posttest study of nurses from 6 randomly selected wards of a Swiss hospital, the quality of patient records showed significant improvement in formulating nursing diagnoses ($p < .0001$).
Cruz, Pimenta, & Lunney, 2009	Continuing education (CE)	A 16-hour CE course on critical thinking for clinical judgment was offered to experienced nurses ($N = 39$); a pretest–posttest design was used to measure the effects. Accuracy of diagnosis improved with case study one ($p = .008$), case study two ($p = .042$) and overall ($p = .001$).

TABLE 10.4

Selected Studies that Show Variance in Nurses' Data Interpretations Based on Three
Categories of Factors That Influence Data Interpretations or Diagnoses   (Continued)

Categories and Researchers	Factors	Significant Findings
Hasegawa et al., 2007	Knowledge of nursing diagnosis definitions	Those nurses who scored higher on the test of nursing diagnosis definitions demonstrated higher accuracy with the two case studies.

Diagnostician: Use of Teaching Aids

Aspinall, 1979	Decisions trees List of problems No teaching aid	Three groups (gp), matched for education & experience, one experimental, two controls, t tests done, p < .001
		Experimental gp; $m = 3.8$; highest possible score = 6 Control gp; $m = 2.567$ Control gp; $m = 1.667$
Craig, 1986	Taught the diagnosis process	82% listed task diagnosis ($p < .001$) 7 other groups (see above) ranged from 30% to 56%
Tanner, 1982	Not taught Taught hypothesis testing	No significance between pre and post test; One explanation: Scoring of accuracy did not allow for variations in statements.
Thiele et al., 1986	Computer simulation	Junior and senior sts improved in cue recognition, cue sorting/linking, & clinical decision making with computer simulation ($p < .05$).
Fredette & O'Neill, 1987	5 hours didactic content on diagnostic process	2 studies, experimental & control gps. 1st study-experimental gp identified more diagnoses 2nd study-exp gp did better overall in diagnosing a case study & in written papers, did better in two categories
Pinnell et al., 1992, & Spies et al., 1994	20-hour course on nursing process with 4 hours on diagnostic reasoning	Average pre-course accuracy ($n = 73$ nurses) was 2.6 on Lunney's 7 point scale; after the course accuracy improved to n average of 3.1 ($p < .05$).

(Continued)

TABLE 10.4

*Selected Studies that Show Variance in Nurses' Data Interpretations Based on Three
Categories of Factors That Influence Data Interpretations or Diagnoses*   (Continued)

Categories and Researchers	Factors	Significant Findings
Lasater & Nielson, 2009	Concept-based learning	The intervention group ($n = 15$ students) who were taught using a concept-based approach scored statistically higher ($p \leq .05$) than the control group students ($n = 13$) on four types of clinical judgment, including data interpretation.
Paans et al., 2010, May	Education about the PES system	In a randomized factorial design study with four groups, knowledge of the PES system was significantly related to accuracy of nursing diagnoses.
Diagnostician: Nursing Experience		
Aspinall, 1976	Below 10 years	Greater number of correct diagnoses
	Over 10 years	Fewer number of correct diagnoses
Aspinall, 1979	Below 2 years	Scored highest; doubled score with decisions trees
	2–10 years	Scored lowest; profited least with decision trees
	Over 10 years	Scored low; profited most with decision trees
Tanner et al., 1987	Junior students ($n = 15$)	Positive association of gp status & accuracy ($p < .05$)
	Senior students ($n = 13$)	Generally, no difference between gps in 4 categories of data acquisition.
Westfall et al., 1986	Nurses ($n = 15$) Same population/ study as Tanner et al.	Experienced nurses generated more complex hypotheses than either group of students ($p = .03$).
Holden & Klingner, 1988	Students 1st semester juniors Last semester seniors Parents (juniors & seniors)	Task was to diagnose why an infant was crying (teething). Experienced gp (nurses and parents) asked for more information than inexperienced gp ($p < .05$). Experienced gp was more likely to ask for valid and reliable cue on 1st choice than inexperienced gp ($p < .01$). The experience of parenting was associated with 100% accuracy.

TABLE 10.4

Selected Studies that Show Variance in Nurses' Data Interpretations Based on Three Categories of Factors That Influence Data Interpretations or Diagnoses   (*Continued*)

Categories and Researchers	Factors	Significant Findings
Konno et al., 1999, 2000	Experienced nurses Years of experience	Experienced nurses were less accurate than students. There was no difference in accuracy by years of experience.
Junnola et al., 2002	Perceptions of influence of experience	90% of nurse participants ($N = 107$) said that professional experience influenced their identification of problems in an oncology case simulation
delBueno, 2005	Years of Experience	With 10 years of competency data from more than 30,000 nurses, it showed that ability to use clinical judgment for identification of patients' problems in 3 case simulations varied widely, with new nurses significantly worse than experienced nurses
Hasegawa et al., 2007	Years of Experience	Years of nursing experience was associated with higher diagnostic competency in all three measures of competency ($p \leq .05$). Only 35% ($n = 131$) of 376 nurses met all three levels of competency.
Diagnostician: Cognitive Strategies		
Gordon, 1980	Hypothesis generation	Number of hypotheses generated is not as important as the correct one being considered early in the task. Cessation of this strategy in the first half of the task was associated with accuracy.
	Predictive hypothesis testing Specific hypothesis testing	Use of this strategy in the second half of the task was associated with accuracy. Number of hypotheses generated is not as important as "correct" one being considered early in the task
Tanner, 1982	Hypothesis generation	Even when hypotheses are generated, they were not necessarily tested.

(*Continued*)

TABLE 10.4

Selected Studies that Show Variance in Nurses' Data Interpretations Based on Three Categories of Factors That Influence Data Interpretations or Diagnoses (Continued)

Categories and Researchers	Factors	Significant Findings
	Hypothesis testing Activation of early hypotheses	In one of the 3 CS (videotapes & hospital records), more experienced nurses activated early hypotheses (73%) than junior (27%) or senior students (38%) (*p* = .029).
Tanner et al., 1987	Question relevance	For 1 of the 3 CS, experienced nurses asked more relevant questions than students (*p* = .022).
	# of hypotheses # of questions	No difference among 3 gps with different levels of education and experience.
Matthews & Gaul, 1979	Types of cues used	Use of both negative and positive cues specific to the case was associated with accuracy; supports Gordon's results re: hypothesis testing
Thiele et al., 1991	Cue selection-relevant or nonrelevant	In a perioperative simulation, the pattern of cue selection of 86 junior sts was 68–85% accurate for relevant cues but also, with overselection, there was 50–60% selection of nonrelevant cues. 72% selected accurate diagnoses & 72% selected appropriate Nursing interventions; also 50–60% selected inaccurate diagnoses and inappropriate interventions.
Brannon & Carson, 2003	Representative Heuristic	Both nurses and student nurses (*N* = 182) dismissed the appropriate physical diagnoses when situational variables such as loss of job were included, showing that the representative heuristic was being used.
Ferrario, 2003	Four types of heuristics	With a national random sample of experienced (*n* = 173) and inexperienced (*n* = 46) emergency room nurses (*n* = 173) judged cases by causal factors significantly more often than inexperienced nurses (*n* = 46).

TABLE 10.4

Selected Studies that Show Variance in Nurses' Data Interpretations Based on Three
Categories of Factors That Influence Data Interpretations or Diagnoses (Continued)

Categories and Researchers	Factors	Significant Findings
Junnola et al., 2002	Information Acquisition	With a computer-based oncology case simulation, the four most important problems were mentioned by 65% of nurses ($N = 107$). Information acquisition in general was associated with identification of problems ($p \leq .05$).
Paans et al. 2010, May	Critical thinking Disposition	In a randomized study with four groups, truth-seeking and open-mindedness were positively related to accuracy of nursing diagnoses.
Diagnostician: Cognitive Abilities		
Gordon, 1980	Inferential ability	No relationship with accuracy using the results from the Graduate record Exam & Miller Analogies Test.
Matthews & Gaul, 1979	Critical thinking	No relationship between nursing diagnosis and critical thinking, as measured by the Watson-Glaser critical thinking appraisal.
Lunney, 1992	Divergent production of semantic units (Fluency)	Three valid and reliable case studies were used. Scores were low on the tests of divergent thinking. Accuracy was positively related to fluency with CS 2 ($p = .002$)
	Divergent production of semantic classes (Flexibility)	Accuracy was positively related to flexibility with CS 2 ($p = .03$). Accuracy was positively related to elaboration with CS 2 ($p = .03$) and CS 3 ($p = .03$).
	Divergent production of semantic implications (Elaboration)	Divergent thinking is probably more relevant to actual cases than written cases with defined amounts of data.
Paans et al., 2010, May	Analysis & Inference	In a randomized study with four groups, analysis and inference, as measured by the health sciences reasoning test were positively related to accuracy of nursing diagnoses.

Improved Effectiveness SNLs and Efficiency of Care

Improvement in effectiveness and efficiency is expected because the languages offer common meanings that are available to all users. When everyone uses the same defined terms, the messages about patient care are clearer, which improves effectiveness and efficiency. After the initial time period of getting used to an EHR, documentation takes less time because the standard terms can be clicked from a list, rather than writing extensive narrative reports. In a 36 hospital time and motion study (N = 767 nurses), it was shown that nurses spend a large majority of their time on documentation (35.3%; Hendrich, Chow, Skierczynski, & Lu, 2008), leaving them too little time to spend on direct patient care. The time needed for documentation needs to be reduced.

Effectiveness and efficiency are facilitated with measurement of nursing workload; the SNLs are invaluable for developing methods of measurement (e.g., Amundsen, 2010; Baumberger, Buchmann, Gilles, Kuster, & Lehmann, 2010; Palese, De Silvestre, Valoppi, & Tomietto, 2009). Both NANDA-I and the NIC are being used for workload measurement.

With growing attention being paid to identifying the cost-benefit ratio of nursing care, it has become critical to include SNLs in EHRs. In testimony provided by all language developers to the National Committee on Health and Vital Statistics in 2000 on the use of standardized languages, developers were asked to provide updated information related to the use of SNLs. All of the nursing developers provided information about the historical development of each language. The response by Insurers and other third party payers was that SNLs needed to be used on a national level. They noted that when nurses can agree on the language of choice opportunities cost out and negotiate reimbursement will be available. This position advanced the work of NNN and SNOWMED RT. With an adequate amount of clinical data that can be generated through use of SNLs, third party reimbursement for nursing care is a possibility for the future.

Autonomy and Control of the Profession and Science of Nursing

Autonomy is perceived to be a central attribute of a profession. When nurses practice autonomously using SNLs, they engage in the generation of diagnoses and interventions that are grounded in nursing's unique body of knowledge, have actions that are self-controlled, and do not require authorization by others (Lyons, 1990). As far back as 1969, Abdellah said, "Fundamental to the development of nursing science is the nurse's ability to make a nursing diagnosis and prescribe nurse actions or strategies that will result in specific responses in the patient" (1969, p. 390). Without SNLs, the voice of nursing is silent and professional autonomy is threatened (Lyons 1990).

In a study of the influence of SNLs on nurses' autonomy, Mrayyan (2005) concluded that it was important for nurses to use SNLs with each patient encounter in order to foster professional autonomy and clarify nurses' control over their practice. The author viewed the use of SNLs as an effective way to promote professional unity and role clarity within professional practice environments. Without the use of SNLs, communication of disciplinary knowledge is compromised and data to conduct research and advance the discipline are reduced or eliminated. In addition, the absence of SNLs in the workplace renders nursing decisions arbitrary and unscientific (Warren, Welton and Halloran, 2005).

WORKFORCE AND STANDARDIZED NURSING TERMINOLOGIES

Establishing and justifying nursing workforce targets requires the ability to continuously assess the impact of nurses' numbers and various roles on health care and patient outcomes. Without a clear strategy for demonstrating the impact of nursing care, there is no way to systematically and continuously improve care, justify effective staffing patterns, and promote cost-effective care. Prior to the development of nursing terminologies, it was virtually impossible to capture nursing's contribution in ways that would allow for a quantitative assessment of the impact of nursing care. The absence of meaningful data to characterize nursing's contribution has stifled the profession's ability to make credible workforce projections that are clearly linked to achieving specified outcomes.

The creation and availability of standardized nursing terminologies provide the basic building blocks needed to assess nurses' impact on health care and patient outcomes. Capturing nursing diagnoses, outcomes, and interventions with standardized terminologies in electronic documentation (EHRs) now make it possible to retrieve information about the focus and type of nursing care provided and the impact of it. The terminologies, though necessary, are not sufficient. If each EHR vendor system and each organization that uses the EHR independently adapt the standardized terminologies to meet unique vendor and organization specifications, the potential for evaluating the impact of nursing is lost or, at best, severely compromised. This "tweaking" is currently the rule rather than the exception and takes place variously at the user interface level, database architecture level, and training level. As a result of the "tweaking" the data captured using nursing terminologies is not reliable and valid and therefore not useful as evidence to characterize nursing practice.

HANDS Research Team

Needed is a common means to integrate the nursing terminologies into the EHRs that assures the reliability and validity of nursing data for use in accurately characterizing the nursing workforce's impact on health care and patient outcomes.

This has been the goal of the HANDS research team for over a decade. Since 1996, a team of researchers has engaged engaged in numerous rounds of development and testing of what is now a web-based dynamic care plan documentation and handoff communication system. The HANDS utilizes the standardized nursing terminologies of NANDAI, NOC, and NIC to represent nursing diagnoses, outcomes, and interventions respectively. The HANDS can be connected to any EHR and utilized as the coordination of care or care planning component (Dunn-Lopez & Keenan, 2010; Keenan, 2004–2008; Keenan, Falan, Heath, & Treder, 2003a; Keenan, Stocker, Barakauskas, Johnson, Maas, Moorhead, & Reed, 2003b; Keenan, Stocker, Barkauskas, Treder, & Heath, 2003c; Keenan, Stocker, Barkauskas, Treder, & Heath, 2003d; Keenan, Barkauskas, Johnson, Maas, Moorhead, Reed, 2003e; Keenan, Stocker, Geo-Thomas, Soporkar, Barkauskas, & Lee, 2002; Keenan & Yakel, 2005). The HANDS achieves the three levels of interoperability recommended for full interoperability by Health Level 7s EHR Interoperability Work Group (2007) to ensure data captured using HANDS is valid and reliable across all systems that use HANDS. The three levels of interoperability include semantic, technical, and process.

Semantic interoperability involves ensuring the meaning of the terms remains the same across users. Technical interoperability is achieved through use of a single standardized user interface and database structure. Process interoperability is achieved through adherence to the standardized training modules and same rules of use in practice (e.g., update at every formal nursing handoff; use of plan of plan of care to organize communication during formal handoffs).

In a recently AHRQ funded multi-site study (R01 HS015054–01, 2004–2008), HANDS was implemented and tested in four different types of hospitals in a total of eight diverse medical surgical units where 39,322 episodes of care were captured (episode = admission to discharge from a single unit) over a 2-year period (4 units participated for 1 year and 4 units participated for 2 years; see Table 10.5). Quota sampling was used to ensure broad representation of medical-surgical unit types and organizations. All units selected were required to meet the study readiness criteria, which included adequate staffing and agreement to use HANDS fully as directed to document the plan (an admission, update, or discharge) and use it to communicate about care at every formal handoff. The main aims of the study were to determine if interoperability could be maintained on all three levels across all units and to evaluate user satisfaction with HANDS and the standardized terminologies. Mixed methods were used to assess the aims and the results provided solid evidence that these three levels of interoperability can be achieved and maintained across very diverse settings. Also, nurses found HANDS significantly more useful than previous methods of care planning ($p \leq .01$) and were more satisfied with

TABLE 10.5

All EOL Episodes and Those with NANDA: Pain Diagnoses

Hospital	Unit	Unit Type	Total No. Episodes of Care	Total No. EOL Episodes	% EOL Episodes	No. EOL Episodes With Pain	% Pain Out of EOL Episodes
LCH1	1	General Medical	5,451	189	3.5	72	38.1
LCH1	2	Medical ICU	1,065	163	15.0	69	42.3
LCH1	3	Gerontology	9,046	519	5.7	113	21.8
UH	4	Cardiac Surgical	6,061	51	0.8	33	64.7
UH	5	Neuro Surgical	8,119	97	1.2	65	67.0
LCH2	6	Medical Gerontology	1,557	116	7.5	71	61.2
LCH2	7	General Medical	3,276	156	4.8	104	66.7
SCH	8	Medical Surgical	4,747	134	2.8	69	51.5
Total			39,322	1,425	3.6	596	41.8

Number of EOL patients as a percentage of all patients and the number of EOL patients with pain diagnosis as a percentage of all EOL patients in the HANDS database from 2C05 to 2007.

LCH1, large community hospital 1; UH, university hospital; LCH2, large community hospital 2; SCH, small community hospital, all in the Midwest.

NANDAI, NOC, and NIC after one to two years of use compared to that perceptions measured at baseline ($p \leq .01$).

The results of the AHRQ study, published in detail elsewhere (Keenan, 2009; Keenan et al., 2008), provide solid evidence that it is not only possible but also feasible to implement and maintain a single and universally useful plan of care system (interoperable on three levels) that utilizes NANDAI, NIC, and NOC across diverse care settings. These findings are powerful indicators that valid and reliable nursing care dare data can be generated with an electronically supported plan of care system that has been carefully designed and tested to meet both user and secondary stakeholder needs. The data collected with HANDS not only includes the nursing diagnoses, outcomes, interventions and changes in the across episodes but also other patient and nurse demographic information and nursing workload. The data gathered through routine documentation thus is automatically available to support day to day care as well as multiple secondary uses.

Secondary Uses of HANDS

The focus of the HANDS team at the University of Illinois is currently being directed toward demonstrating how the valid and reliable data captured in a system like HANDS can be used for multiple secondary purposes that can eventually support workforce policy. For the past year, the HANDS team has been conducting two pilot studies, with the help of three engineering teams at UIC (statistical, data mining, and usability). One of the studies has focused on understanding "Pain" management in end-of-life patients through use of a variety of statistical and data mining techniques and translating the evidence into prototype decision support alerts that will soon be tested. We were able to quickly isolate the end-of-life episodes ($n = 1,425$) in our anonymized database from the AHRQ study through pulling patient episodes of care that included one or more of the following criteria (1) NOC outcome: Comfortable Death; (2) NOC outcome: Dignified Life Closure; (3) NIC intervention: Dying Care; (4) Discharged to hospice medical facility; (5) Discharged to hospice home care; or (6) Expired (see Table 10.5). Our preliminary findings indicate that pain management at end of life is significantly below desirable levels in our "representative set" of acute care units and that certain constellations of nursing interventions are associated with better pain outcomes. These preliminary findings are soon to be published elsewhere.

Data gathered in the above reported AHRQ study is also being used for our second pilot. This pilot is focused on nurse related characteristics. Specifically, we are examining the impact of shift length and number of unique nurses per episode of care (continuity) on expected patient outcomes. Again, we are able to ask and answer these important workforce related questions precisely because this is data that was automatically picked up as nurses used the HANDS plan of care system to describe and monitor care across time. The findings for this pilot are also expected to be published soon elsewhere.

In summary, in this section we briefly explained why standardized terminologies are necessary but not sufficient to generate reliable and valid evidence to address nursing workforce issues and what is need to fill the gaps. A description of the more than 10-year research trajectory of the HANDS team, now located at the University of Illinois Chicago, was presented as an exemplar of how standardized nursing terminologies can be successfully implemented to generate valid and reliable nursing data to support policy around work force issues. The pilot studies, currently underway were also briefly described. These presentations were designed to provide a glimpse of the enormous range of nursing related questions that can be addressed when standardized terminologies are implemented widely in documentation and communication systems that are interoperable on three levels and acceptable to front line users.

FUTURE DIRECTIONS

In a recent IOM report on the *Future of Nursing: Leading the Change, Advancing Health* (IOM, 2010) the document stresses the important role nursing will play in leading the way to improved patient care. One of the four major goals in the report states "Effective workforce planning and policy making require better data collection and as an improved information infrastructure" (IOM, 2010 p. 3). The importance of SNLs within our current and future documentation will help address workforce demands, develop predictive models for high quality, safe, efficient and effective care, help cost out nursing services and document nursing's contribution to patient outcomes. For this to be realized, nursing must be visible within the EHR. This will require the use of standardized languages and educational preparation of nurses to document their Practice (Cronenwett et al., 2007; Cronenwett, Sherwood, & Gelman, 2009). While the use of nursing diagnosis, interventions and outcomes are predicated on good decision making and do not explain the full extent of nursing practice, they do offer some insight into the nature of patient care uniquely influenced by the nurse. The further development testing and refinement of nursing language and the advancement of disciplinary knowledge enhanced by research of the terms will expand our science and related knowledge base. The potential use of SNLs in randomized trials, population based studies and data mining with an established data base will extend nurses opportunities to contribute to deliver knowledge driven care. Qualitative studies that focus on understanding the meaning of a human experience self care (loss, resilience, etc.) can begin to isolate themes (concepts) and eventually lead to the naming of new phenomena of concern. Quantitative studies that focus on the study of phenomena can help validate phenomena, identify links and significant relationships between and among phenomena and generate care models with greater prediction, precision, control to improve care accuracy and comprehensiveness.

Use of a standardized and unified language internationally can increase cross culture/population studies of the phenomena, focus on instrument development to measure phenomena, generate intervention studies and lead to outcome/evidence-based studies (randomized clinical trial). With the consistent use of standardized language, administrative models can be developed to improve definitions and determinants of staffing ratios and patterns and integrate the level of provider with increase safe, efficient, cost-effective, and high-quality patient centric care.

REFERENCES

Abdellah, F. (1969). The nature of nursing service. *Nursing Research, 18,* 390–393.

Amundsen, H. (2010). *A computer-assisted method for developing nursing workload measurement terms.* Paper presented at the AENTDE/NANDA international Conference, Madrid, Spain.

Anderson, C., Keenan, G., & Jones, J. (2009). Using bibliometrics to support your selection of a nursing terminology set (CE Offering). *Computers, Informatics, Nursing (CIN), 27,* 82–92.

American Nurses Association. (2004). *A social policy statement.* Washington, DC: Author.

American Nurses Association. (2006). *ANA recognized terminologies and data element sets.* Retrieved from http://nursingworld.org/npii/terminologies.htm

American Pain Society. (2000). *Pain guidelines.* Retrieved from http://www.painbalance.org/guidelines-1003197398

Aspinall, M. (1979). Use of a decision tree to improve accuracy of diagnosis. *Nursing Research, 28,* 182–185.

Aspinall, M. J. (1976). Nursing diagnosis: The weak link. *Nursing Outlook, 24,* 433–437.

Avant, K. (1990). The art and science of nursing diagnosis development. *Nursing Diagnosis, 1*(2), 51–56.

Baernholdt, M., & Lang, N. M. (2003). Why an ICNP? Links among quality, information, and policy. *International Nursing Review, 50,* 73–78.

Baumberger, D., Buchmann, D., Gilles, A., Kuster, B., & Lehmann, T. (2010, May). *The linkage of NANDA-I and nursing workload measurement.* Paper presented at AENTDE/NANDA International Conference, Madrid, Spain.

Berger, S. (2008, November). *Validation studies on NANDA-I diagnoses: Methodological demands, overview of studies, and critical evaluation.* Paper presented at the NNN conference, Miami, Florida.

Brannon, L. A., & Carson, K. L. (2003). The representative heuristic: Influence on nurses' decision making. *Applied Nursing Research, 16,* 201–204.

Canham, D., Mao, C. L., Yoder, M., Connolly, P., & Dietz, E. (2008). The Omaha System and quality measurement in academic nurse-managed centers: Ten steps for implementation. *Journal of Nursing Education, 47,* 105–110.

Carlson, J. (2006). Abstract: Consensus validation process: A standardized research method to identify and link the relevant NANDA, NIC and NOC terms for local populations. *International Journal of Nursing Terminologies & Classification, 17,* 23–24.

Carlson, J. (2010, May). *Capturing professional nursing practice in an outpatient setting by using linked NANDA-I diagnoses, NIC interventions, and NOC outcomes in an electronic nursing documentation system (FNDS).* Paper presented at the AENTDE-NANDA International conference, Madrid, Spain.

Carlson-Catalano, J., & Lunney, M. (1995). Quantitative methods for clinical validation of nursing diagnoses. *Clinical Nurse Specialist: The Journal of Advanced Nursing Practice, 9,* 306–311.

Carlson-Catalano, J., Lunney, M., Paradiso, C., Bruno, J., Luise, B., Martin, T., . . . Pachter, S. (1998). Clinical validation of ineffective breathing pattern, ineffective airway clearance, and impaired gas exchange. *Image: Journal of Nursing Scholarship, 30,* 243–248.

Carnevali, D. L., & Thomas, M. J. (1993). *Diagnostic reasoning and treatment decision making.* Philadelphia: Lippincott.

Carroll-Johnson, R. M. (1990). *Classification of nursing diagnoses: Proceedings of the ninth conference.* Philadelphia, PA: Lippincott.

Center for Nursing Classification and Clinical Effectiveness. (n.d.). *Center for Nursing Classification and Clinical Effectiveness.* Retrieved from http://www.nursing.uiowa.edu/excellence/nursing_knowledge/clinical_effectiveness/index.htm

Cianfrani, K. L. (1984). The influence of amounts and relevance of data on identifying health problems. In M. J. Kim, G. K. McFarland, & A. M. McLane (Eds.), *Classification of nursing diagnosis: Proceedings of the fifth national conference* (pp. 150–161). St. Louis, MO: C.V. Mosby.

Clancy, T. R., Delaney, C. W., Morrison, B., & Gunn, J. K. (2006). The benefits of standardized nursing languages in complex adaptive systems such as hospitals. *Journal of Nursing Administration, 36,* 426–434.

Clark, J., & Lang, N. M. (1991). An international classification of nursing practice. *International Nursing Review, 39*(4), 1–4

Corcoran, S. A. (1986). Task complexity and nursing expertise as factors in decision making. *Nursing Research, 35*(2), 107–112.

Craig, J. L. (1986). Types of statements made by nurses as first impressions of patient problems. In M. E. Hurley (Ed.), *Classification of nursing diagnosis: Proceedings of the sixth conference* (pp. 245–255). St. Louis, MO: C.V. Mosby.

Cronenwett, L., Sherwood, G., Barnsteiner, J., Disch, J., Johnson, J., Mitchell, P., . . . Warren, J. (2007). Quality and safety education for nurses. *Nursing Outlook, 55*(3), 122–131.

Cronenwett, L., Sherwood, G., & Gelman, S. B. (2009). Improving quality and safety education: The QSEN learning collaborative. *Nursing Outlook, 57*(6), 304–312.

Cruz, D. M., Pimenta, C. M., & Lunney, M. (2009). Improving critical thinking and clinical reasoning with a continuing education course. *Journal of Continuing Education in Nursing, 40*(3), 121–127.

Delaney, C. (2006). Terminology minimum data set. Delaney@umn.edu

del Bueno, D. (2005). A crisis in critical thinking. *Nursing Education Perspectives, 26,* 278–282.

del Bueno, D. J. (2001). Buyer beware: The cost of competence. *Nursing Economics, 19*(6), 251–257.

Dochterman, J., & Jones, D. (2003). *Unifying nursing languages* (p. 59). Washington, DC: American Nurses Association.

Dochterman, J., & Jones, D. (2007). Unifying nursing language: Communicating nursing practice. In C. Alliata Roy & D. Jones (Eds.), *Nursing knowledge development and clinical practice* (pp. 215–232). New York, NY: Springer.

Dochterman, J., Titler, M., Wang, J., Reed, D., Pettit, D., Mathew-Wilson, M., . . . Kanak, M. (2005). Describing use of nursing interventions for three groups of patients. *Journal of Nursing Scholarship, 37,* 57–66.

Dunn-Lopez, K., & Keenan, G. (2010). Collaboration between nurses and physicians: Need for a broader view. In J. C. McCloskey & H. K. Grace (Eds.), *Current issues in nursing* (8th ed.). St. Louis, MO: Mosby.

Dykes, P., Kim, H. E., Goldsmith, D. M., Choi, J., Esumi, K., & Goldberg, H. S. (2009). The adequacy of ICNP version 1.0 as a representational model for electronic nursing assessment documentation. *Journal of American Medical Informatics Association, 16*(2), 238–246

Ebright, P., Patterson, E., Chalko, B., & Render, M. (2003). Understanding the complexity of registered nurse work in acute care settings. *Journal of Nursing Administration, 33,* 630–638.

Faster Cures. (2006). *Ensuring the inclusion of clinical research in the nationwide health information network.* Retrieved from http://www.fastercures.org/objects/pdfs/meetings/FC_AHRQ-NCRR_report.pdf

Feeg, V. D., Saba, V. K., & Feeg, A. N. (2008). Testing a bedside personal computer Clinical Care Classification System for nursing students using Microsoft Access. *Computers Informatics, Nursing, 26,* 339–349.

Ferhing, R. J. (1986). Validating diagnostic labels: Standardized methodology. In M. E. Hurley (Ed.), *Classification of nursing diagnosis: Proceedings of the sixth conference* (pp. 113–120). St. Louis, MO: Mosby.

Ferhing R. J. (1987). Methods to validate nursing diagnosis. *Heart and Lung, 16,* 625–629.

Ferrario, C. G. (2003). Experienced and less experienced nurses' diagnostic reasoning: Implications for fostering students' critical thinking. *International Journal of Nursing Terminologies & Classification, 14,* 41–52.

Flanagan, J., & Jones, D. (2009). High frequency nursing diagnosis following same-day knee arthroscopy. *International Journal of Nursing Terminologies and Classifications, 20*(2), 89–95.

Fredette, S. L., & O'Neill, E. S. (1987). Can theory improve diagnosis? An examination of the relationship between didactic content and the ability to diagnose in clinical practice. In A. M. McLane (Ed.), *Classification of nursing diagnosis: Proceedings of the seventh conference* (pp. 423–435). St. Louis, MO: C.V. Mosby.

Gebbie, K., & Lavin, M. A. (Eds.). (1975). *Classification of nursing diagnosis: Proceedings from the first national conference.* St. Louis, MO: Mosby.

Gordon, M. (1980). Predictive strategies in diagnostic tasks. *Nursing Research, 29,* 39–45.

Gordon, M., & Sweeney, M. A. (1979). Methodologic problems and issues in identifying and standardizing nursing diagnoses. *Advances in Nursing Science, 2,* 1–16.

Gordon, M. (1987). *Nursing diagnosis: Process and application.* New York, NY: McGraw Hill, Inc.

Gordon, M. (1989). Qualitative research in nursing diagnosis: A reaction paper, Nursing Education. *Nursing Diagnosis Research Methodologies,* NANDA (pub) St. Louis.

Gordon, M. (1994). *Nursing diagnosis: Process and application* (3rd ed.). St Louis: Mosby.

Gordon, M., & Sweeney, M. A. (1979). Methodologic problems and issues in identifying and standardizing nursing diagnosis. *Advances in Nursing Science, 2*(1) 1–15.

Hasegawa, T., Ogasawara, C., & Katz, E. C. (2007). Measuring diagnostic competency and the analysis of factors influencing competency using written case studies. *International Journal of Nursing Terminologies and Classifications, 18,* 93–102.

Hayakawa, S. I., & Hayakawa, A. R. (1990). *Language in thought and action.* New York, NY: Harcourt.

Hendrich, A., Chow, M., Skierczynski, B. A., & Lu, Z. (2008). A 36 hospital time and motion study: How do medical-surgical nurses spend their time? *The Permanente Journal, 12*(3), 25–34.

Hicks, F. D., Merritt, S. L., & Elstein, A. S. (2003). Critical thinking and clinical decision making in critical care nursing: A pilot study. *Heart & Lung, 32*(3), 169–180.

HIMSS. (2010). Electronic health record (EHR). Retrieved from http://www.himss.org/ASP/topics_ehr.asp

HL7 EHR Interoperability Work Group. (February 7, 2007). *Coming to terms: Scoping interoperability for health care.* HL3 Workgroup

Holden, G. W., & Klingner, A. M. (1988). Learning from experience: Differences in how novice vs. expert nurses diagnose why an infant is crying. *Journal of Nursing Education, 27,* 23–29.

Hoskins, L. (1989a).Clinical validation methodologies for nursing diagnosis research. In R. M. Carroll Johnson (Ed.), *Classification of nursing of nursing diagnosis: Proceedings of the eighth conference* (pp. 126–131). Philadelphia, PA: Lippincott.

Hoskins, L. (1989b). Tool development: reliability and related statistics. Response to Padilla. In *Monograph of the International Conference on Research Methods for Validating Nursing Diagnosis* (pp. 196–206). Philadelphia, PA: Lippincott

Hughes, K. K., & Young, W. B. (1990). The relationship between task complexity and decision-making consistency. *Research in Nursing & Health, 13,* 189–197.

Hyeoun-Ae, P., Hardiker, N., Bartz, C., Coenen, A. (2005). ICNP Tutorial Version—College of Nursing Seoul National University, Seoul Korea.

Institute for Healthcare Improvement. (nd). *Protecting 5 Million Lives from harm.* Retrieved from http://www.ihi.org/IHI/Programs/Campaign/Campaign.htm?TabId=1

Institute of Medicine. (2000). *To err is human: Building a safer health system.* Washington, DC: National Academy Press.

Institute of Medicine. (2003a). *Health professions education: A bridge to quality.* Washington, DC: National Academies Press.

Institute of Medicine. (2003b). *Key capabilities of an electronic health record.* Washington, DC: National Academies Press.

Institute of Medicine. (2004). *Keeping patients safe: Transforming the work environment of nurses.* Washington, DC: National Academies Press.

Institute of Medicine. (October, 2010). *The future of nursing: Leading change, advancing health.* Washington, DC: National Academies Press.

Jenkins, H. M. (1985). A research tool for measuring perceptions of clinical decision making. *Journal of Professional Nursing, 1*(4), 221–229.

Jenny, J. (1995). Advancing the science of nursing. In M. Ranz & P. M. Le Mone (Eds.), *Classification of nursing diagnosis: Proceedings of the eleventh conference* (pp. 126–131). Philadelphia, PA.

Joint Commission. (2008). *2009 national patient safety goals hospital program.* Retrieved from http://www.jointcommission.org/PatientSafety/NationalPatientSafetyGoals/09

Johnson, M., Bulechek, G. M., Butcher, H. K., Dochterman, J. M., Mass, M., Moorhead, S., & Swanson, E. (2006). *NANDA, NOC, and NIC Linkages.* St. Louis, MO: Mosby.

Johnson, M., Maas, M., & Moorhead, S. (1997–2002). *Evaluation of nursing-sensitive outcomes measures.* #1RO1NR03437-0, National Institute of Nursing Research, National Institutes of Health.

Jones, D. (2007). A synthesis of philosophical perspectives for knowledge development. In C. Roy & D. Jones (Eds.) *Nursing knowledge development and clinical practice* (pp. 163–176). New York: Springer.

Junnola, T., Eriksson, E., Salantera, S., & Lauri, S. (2002). Nurses' decision-making in collecting information for the assessment of patients' nursing problems. *Journal of Clinical Nursing, 11,* 186–196.

Kautz, D., Kulper, T. A. Pesut, D. J., & Williams, R. L. (2006). Using NANDA, NIC and NOC (NNN): Language for clinical reasoning with outcome-present-stare-test (OPT) model. *International Journal of Nursing Terminologies and Classifications, 17,* 129—138.

Kautz, D. D., & Horn, E. R. (2008). An exemplar of the use of NNN language in developing evidenced-based practice guidelines. *International Journal of Nursing Terminologies and Classifications, 19,* 14–19.

Keenan, G. (2004–2008). HIT (Health Information Technology) support for safe nursing 1 R01 HS015054-01-HHS PHS, Agency of Health Research and Quality (AHRQ).

Keenan, G. (2009). AHRQ Final Report, HIT Support for Safe Nursing Care. 1 R01 HS015054-01-HHS PHS.

Keenan, G., Barkauskas, V., Johnson, M., Maas, M., Moorhead, S., & Reed, D. (2003e). Establishing the validity, reliability, and sensitivity of NOC in adult care nurse practitioner clinics. *Outcomes Management, 7*(2), 74–83.

Keenan, G., Falan, S., Heath, C., & Treder, M. (2003a). Establishing competency in the use of NANDA, NOC, and NIC terminology. *Journal of Nursing Measurement, 11* (2), 183–196.

Keenan, G., Stocker, J., Geo-Thomas, A., Soporkar, N., Barkauskas, V., & Lee, J. (2002). The HANDS project: Studying and refining the automated collection of a cross-setting clinical data set. *Computers, Informatics, Nursing, 20*(3), 89–100.

Keenan, G., Stocker, J., Barakauskas, V., Johnson, M., Maas, M., Moorhead, S., & Reed, D. (2003b). Establishing the validity, reliability, and sensitivity of NOC in home care settings. *Journal of Nursing Measurement, 11*(2), 135–155.

Keenan, G., Stocker, J., Barkauskas, V., Treder, M., & Heath, C. (2003c). Toward integrating a common nursing data set in home care to facilitate monitoring outcomes across settings. *Journal of Nursing Measurement, 11*(2), 157–169.

Keenan, G., Stocker, J., Barkauskas, V., Treder, M., & Heath, C. (2003d). Toward collecting a standardized nursing data set across the continuum: Case of adult care nurse practitioner settings. *Outcomes Management, 7*(3), 113–120.

Keenan, G., Tschannen, D., & Wesley, M. (2008). Standardized nursing terminologies can transform practice. *Journal of Nursing Administration, 38*, 103–106.

Keenan, G., & Yakel, E. (2005). *Promoting safe nursing care by bringing visibility to the disciplinary aspects of interdisciplinary care.* Proceedings of American Medical Informatics Association Fall 2005 Conference, Washington DC. (Winner Harriet Werley Award for Top Nursing Informatics Paper.)

Keenan, G., Yakel, E., & Tschannen, D., Mandeville, M. (2008). Documentation and the nurse care planning process. In R. Hughes (Ed.), *Patient safety and quality: An evidence based handbook for nurses.* AHRQ Publication No. 08-0043), Agency for Healthcare Research and Quality, Rockville, MD., Chapter 49, http://www.ahrq.gov/qual/nurseshdbk/docs/KeenanG_DNCPP.pdf

Keenan, G., Yakel, E., & Tschannen, D. (2008). Documentation and the nurse care planning process. In Hughes, R. (Ed). *Patient safety and quality: An evidence-based handbook for nurses.* Washington, DC: Agency for Health Research and Quality.

Keenan, G., Yakel, E., Tschannen, D., Ford, Y., Wilkie, D., Sorokin, O., & Szalacha, L. The (Under Review, 2010). HANDS model: Maintaining a consistent big picture of the patient's situation. *Journal of the American Medical Informatics Association.*

Keenan, G. M., Tschannen, D., & Ford, Y. (2010, May). *The effective use of NANDA, NOC and NIC in the HANDS Sharer handoff.* Paper presented at the AENTDE/NANDA-International conference, Madrid, Spain.

Kim, M. J. (1990). In R. M. Carroll Johnson (Ed.), *Classification of nursing diagnoses: Proceedings of the ninth conference.* Philadelphia, PA: Lippincott.

Konno, R., Otake, Y., Suzuki, K., & Emoto, E. (2000). *A study on accuracy of nursing diagnoses (the second report): Comparison of pre-educational and post-educational groups.* Paper presented at the sixth conference of the Japan Society of Nursing Diagnosis.

Kritek, P. (1978). The generation and classification of nursing diagnosis: Toward a theory of nursing. *Image, 10*(2), 33–40.

Lasater, K., & Nielsen, A. (2009). The influence of concept-based learning activities on students' clinical judgment development. *Journal of Nursing Education, 48*, 441–446.

Lenz, E. R., Wolfe, M. L., Shelley, S. I., & Madison, A. S. (1986). Clinical specialty preparation and nurses' interpretation of client situations. *Western Journal of Nursing Research, 8,* 431–444.

Levin, R. F., Lunney, M., & Krainovich-Miller, B. (2004). Improving diagnostic accuracy using an evidenced-based nursing model. *International Journal of Nursing Terminologies & Classification, 15,* 114–122.

Leviss, J., Gugerty, B., Kaplan, B., Keenan, G., Ozeran, L., & Silverstein, S. (Eds.). (2010). *Hit or miss: Lessons learned from health information technology.* Bethesda, MD: AHIMA Press.

Lunney, M. (1992). Divergent productive thinking factors and accuracy of nursing diagnoses. *Research in Nursing & Health, 15,* 303–311.

Lunney, M. (2008). Critical need to address accuracy of nurses' diagnoses. *Online Journal of Issues in Nursing, 13*(1). Retrieved from www.nursingworld.org/MainMenuCategories/ANAMarketplace/ANAPeriodicals/OJINTableofContents/vol132008/No1Jan08/ArticlePreviousTopic/AccuracyofNursesDiagnoses.aspx

Lunney, M. (2009). *Critical thinking to achieve positive health outcomes: Nursing case studies and analyses* (2nd ed.). Ames, IA: Wiley-Blackwell.

Lunney, M., McCaffrey, P., & Umbro, S. (2010). *Action research to identify nursing diagnoses, patient outcomes, and nursing interventions for end of life care.* Paper presented at the AENTDE/NANDA International Conference, Madrid, Spain.

Lunney, M., Delaney, C., Duffy, M., Moorhead, S., & Welton, J. (2005). Advocating for standardized nursing languages in electronic health records. *Journal of Nursing Administration, 35,* 1–3.

Lunney, M., Karlik, B. A., Kiss, M., & Murphy, P. (1997). Accuracy of nurses' diagnoses of psychosocial responses. *Nursing Diagnoses, 8*(4), 157–166.

Lunney, M., McGuire, M., Endozo, N., & McIntosh-Waddy, D. (2010). Consensus validation identifies relevant nursing diagnoses, nursing interventions, and health outcomes for people with traumatic brain injuries. *Rehabilitation Nursing, 35,* 161–166.

Lunney, M., Parker, L., Fiore, L., Cavendish, R., & Pulcini, J. (2004). Feasibility of studying the effects of using NANDA, NIC and NOC on children's health outcomes. *CIN: Computers, Informatics, Nursing, 22,* 316–325.

Lyon, B. (1990). Getting back on track: Nursing's autonomous scope pf practice. *Clinical Nurse Specialist, 19*(1), 28–33.

Martin, K. S. (2005). *The Omaha System: A key to practice, documentation, and information management* (Reprinted 2nd ed.). Omaha, NE: Health Connections Press.

Martin, K. S., & Scheet N. (1992). *The Omaha System.* Philadelphia, PA: W.B. Saunders.

Matthews, C. A., & Gaul, A. L. (1979). Nursing diagnosis from the perspective of concept attainment and critical thinking. *Advances in Nursing Science, 2,* 17–26.

McCaffrey, M., & Ferrell, B. R. (1997). Nurses' knowledge of pain assessment and management: How much progress have we made? *Journal of Pain Symptom Management, 14,* 175–188.

Mc Farlane, A. (1990). In R. M. M. Carroll-Johnson (Ed.), *Classification of nursing diagnoses: Proceedings of the ninth conference.* Philadelphia: Lippincott.

Melnyk, B. M., & Fineout-Overholt, E. (2005). *Evidence-based practice in nursing & healthcare: A guide to best practice.* Philadelphia, PA: Lippincott Williams & Wilkins.

Moorhead, S., Johnson, M., Maas, M., & Swanson, E. (2008). *Nursing outcomes classification* (4th ed.). St. Louis, MO: Mosby Elsevier.

Minthorn, C., & Lunney, M. (in press). Participant action research with bedside nurses to identify NANDA International, NIC and NOC categories for hospitalized diabetics. *Applied Nursing Research.*

Mrayyan, M. T. (2005). The influence of standardized languages on nurses' autonomy. *Journal of Nursing Management, 13,* 238–241.

Muller-Staub, M., Lavin, M. A., Needham, I., & van Achterberg, T. (2006a). Nursing diagnoses, interventions and outcomes-application and impact on nursing practice: Systematic review. *Journal of Advanced Nursing, 56*(5), 514–531.

Muller-Staub, M., Lavin, M. A., Needham I., & van Achterberg, T. (2006b). Meeting the criteria of a nursing diagnosis classification: Evaluation of ICNP, ICF, NANDA and ZEFP. *International Journal of Nursing Studies, 44*, 702–713.

Müller-Staub, M., Lunney, M., Lavin, M. A., Needham, I., Odenbreit, M., & van Achterberg, T. (2010). Psychometric properties of Q-DIO, an instrument to measure the quality of documented nursing diagnoses, interventions and outcomes (German). *Pflege, 23*, 119–128.

Muller-Staub, M., Needham, I., Odenbreit, M., Lavin, M. A., & van Achterberg. (2007). Improved quality of nursing documentation: Results of a nursing diagnoses, interventions, and outcomes implementation study. *International Journal of Nursing Terminologies and Classifications, 18*, 5–17.

Muller-Staub, M., Needham, I., Odenbreit, M., Lavin, M. A., & van Achterberg. (2008). Implementing nursing diagnostics effectively: cluster randomized trial. *Journal of Advanced Nursing, 633*, 291–301.

NANDA International. (2009). *Nursing diagnoses: Definitions and classification, 2009–2011.* Philadelphia, PA: Wiley-Blackwell.

National Committee on Vital and Health Statistics. (2010). *Toward enhanced information capacities for health: An NCVHS concept paper.* Retrieved from http://www.ncvhs.hhs.gov/100526concept.pdf

Odenbreit, M. (2010, May). *An electronic nursing documentation expert system based on NNN.* Paper presented at AENTDE/NANDA-International conference, Madrid, Spain.

Olsson, S., Lymberts, A., & Whitehouse, D. (2004). European Commission activities in health. *International Journal of Circumpolar Health, 63*, 310–316.

O'Neill, E. S., Dluhy, N. M., & Chin, E. (2005). Modeling novice clinical reasoning for a computerized decision support system. *Journal of Advanced Nursing, 49*, 68–77.

O'Neill, E. S., Dluhy, N. M., Hansen, A. S., & Ryan, J. R. (2006). Coupling the N-CODES system with actual nurse decision-making. *CIN: Computers, Informatics, Nursing, 24*, 28–34.

Paans, W., Sermeus, W., Nieweg, R., van der Schans, C. P. (2009). Development of a measurement instrument for nursing documentation in the patient record. *Studies in Health Technology and Informatics, 146*, 297–300.

Paans, W., Sermeus, W., Nieweg, R. M., van der Schans, C. P. (2010, May). *Knowledge, knowledge sources, and reasoning skills as influencing factors on the accuracy of nursing diagnoses in hospital practice: A randomized study.* Paper presented at the AENTDE/NANDA-International Conference, Madrid, Spain.

Paans, W., Sermeus, W., Nieweg, R. M., van der Schans, C. P. (2010a). D-Catch instrument: development and psychometric testing of a measurement instrument for nursing documentation in hospitals. *Journal of Advanced Nursing, 66*, 1388–1400.

Paans, W., Sermeus, W., Nieweg, R. M., & van der Schans, C. P. (2010b). Prevalence of accurate nursing documentation in patient records. *Journal of Advanced Nursing,* Aug 23 [Epub ahead of print].

Palese, A., De Silvestre, D., Valoppi, G., & Tomietto, M. (2009). A 10-year retrospective study of teaching nursing diagnosis to baccalaureate students in Italy. *International Journal of Nursing Terminologies and Classifications, 20*(2), 64–74.

Pinnell, N. L., Spies, M. A., & Myers, J. L. (October, 1992). *Measurement of diagnostic ability of nurses using the Lunney Scoring Method for Rating Accuracy of Nursing Diagnosis.* Paper presented at the nineteenth Annual research Conference, St. Louis University, St. Louis, MO.

Pesut, D. J., & Herman, J. (1998). OPT: Transformation of nursing process for contemporary practice. *Nursing Outlook, 46*(1), 29–36.

Potter, P., Boxerman, S., Wolf, L., Marshall, J., Grayson, D., Sledge, J., & Evanoff, B. (2004). Mapping the nursing process: A new approach for understanding the work of nursing. *Journal of Nursing Administration, 34*, 101–109.

Potter, P., Wolf, L., Boxerman, S., Grayson, D., Sledge, J., Dunagan, C., & Evanoff, B. (2005). Understanding the cognitive work of nursing in the acute care environment. *Journal of Nursing Administration, 35*, 327–335.

Puntillo, K., Neighbor, M., O'Neil, N., & Nixon, R. (2003). Accuracy of emergency nurses in assessment of patients' pain. *Pain Management Nursing, 4*(4), 171–175.

Rotegaard, A. K., & Ruland, C. M.(2009). Representation of patients' health asset concepts in the International Classification of Nursing Practice (ICNP). *Study of Health Technology Information, 146*, 314–319.

Ruland, C. M., & Bakken, S. (2003). Developing, implementing, and evaluating decision support systems for shared decision making in patient care: A conceptual model and case illustration. *Journal of Biomedical Informatics, 35*, 313–321.

Rutherford, M. A. (2008). Standardized nursing language: What does it mean for nursing? practice? *The Online Journal of Issues in Nursing (OJIN)*. Retrieved from http://www.nursingworld.org/MainMenuCategories/ANAMarketplace/ANAPeriodicals/OJIN/TableofContents/vol132008/No1Jan08/ArticlePreviousTopic/StandardizedNursingLanguage.aspx

Saba, V. K. (1997). Why the home health care classification is a recognized nursing nomenclature. *Computers in Nursing, 15*(2 Suppl.), S69–S76.

Saba, V. K., & Taylor, S. L. (2007). Moving past theory: use of a standardized, coded nursing terminology to enhance nursing visibility. *Computers Informatics Nursing, 25*, 324–331.

Simpson, R. (2007). ICNP: The language of worldwide nursing. *Nursing Management,* February, 2007, 15–18.

Smith, M., & McCarthy, M. P. (2010). Disciplinary knowledge in nursing education: Going beyond the blueprints. *Nursing Outlook, 58*(1), 44–51.

Spies, M. A., Myers, J. L., & Pinnell, N. (1994). Measurement of diagnostic ability of nurses using the Lunney scoring method for rating accuracy of nursing diagnosis. In Carroll-Johnson RM (Ed.), *Classification of nursing diagnoses: Proceedings of the tenth conference held on April 25–29, 1992 in San Diego, CA* (pp. 352–353). Philadelphia, PA: Lippincott.

Swan, B. A., Lang, N. A., & McGinley, A. (2004). Access to quality health care: Links between evidence, nursing language, and informatics. *Nursing Economics, 22*(6), 325–332.

Instruction on the diagnostic process: An experimental study. In M. J. Kim & D. A. Moritz (Eds.), *Classification of nursing diagnoses: Proceedings of the third and fourth National Conferences* (pp. 145–152). New York, NY: McGraw Hill.

Tanner, C. A., Padrick, K. P., Westfall, U. E., & Putzier, D. J. (1987). Diagnostic reasoning strategies of nurses and nursing students. *Nursing Research, 36*, 258–263.

Thiele, J. E., Baldwin, J. H., Hyde, R. S., Sloan, B., & Strandquist, G. A. (1986). An investigation of decision theory: What are the effects of teaching cue recognition? *Journal of Nursing Education, 25*, 319–324.

Thiele, J. E., Holloway, J., Murphy, D., Pendarvis, J., & Stucky, M. (1991. Perceived and actual decision making by novice baccalaureate students. *Western Journal of Nursing Research, 13*, 616–626.

Thoroddsen, A., & Enfors, M. (2007). Putting policy into practice: Pre and posttests of implementing standardized languages for nursing documentation. *Journal of Clinical Nursing, 16*, 1826–1838.

Warren, J. J., & Coenen, A. (1998). International Classification for Nursing Practice (ICNP): Most-frequently asked questions. *JAMIA, 5*, 335–336.

Warren, J., Welton, J. M., & Halloran, E. J. (2005). Nursing diagnoses, diagnosis-related group, and hospital outcomes. *Journal of Nursing Administration, 35*(12), 541–549.

Westendorf, J. J. (2007). Utilizing the Perioperative Nursing Data Set in a surgical setting. *Plastic Surgery Nursing, 27*, 181–184.

Westfall, U. E., Tanner, C. A., Putzier, D., & Padrick, K. P. (1986). Activating clinical inferences: A component of diagnostic reasoning. *Research in Nursing & Health, 9*, 269–277.

Westra, B. L., Delaney, C. W., Konicek, D., & Keenan, G. (2008). Nursing standards to support the electronic health record. *Nursing Outlook, 56*, 258–266.

Whitley, G. (1996). Nursing diagnosis research: Forging ahead. *Nursing Diagnosis, 7*(1), 40–41.

CHAPTER 11

Results of an Integrative Review of Patient Classification Systems

DiJon R. Fasoli and Kathlyn Sue Haddock

ABSTRACT

This chapter presents the findings of an integrative review of the literature to identify current practices related to patient classification systems (PCSs). We sought to determine if there was a "gold standard" PCS that could be adopted or adapted for use by nurse leaders in practice. Sixty-three articles reporting studies related to PCS, Patient Acuity Systems or Workload Management Systems from 1983 to 2010 and applicable for inpatient medical/surgical settings were reviewed. Generally, we found that many of the criticisms of earlier PCSs are still evident: (1) difficulties with measuring workload remain an overarching theme throughout the literature; (2) definitions and descriptions of nursing work continue to be deemed inadequate; (3) there is insufficient evidence of reliability and validity testing of PCSs; and (4) there is still a need to identify nursing sensitive performance indicators and outcomes. We identified characteristics of promising PCSs, but concluded that no consensus exists about PCSs. We suggest that any approach to predicting staffing should seek to be parsimonious, minimize additional workload, be based on expert nurse judgment, be a true reflection of nursing work, and include indicators that measure patient complexity, required nursing care, available resources, and relevant organizational attributes.

The views expressed in this article are those of the authors and do not necessarily reflect the position or policy of the Department of Veterans Affairs or the United States government.

INTRODUCTION

Nurse staffing has become a critical element in the efforts to ensure patient safety and improve outcomes. In theory, the formula is "simple economics"—match patient demand to nurse supply. However, in practice, the solution is far from simple. Each side of the equation is multifaceted, with environmental or system factors adding an additional layer of complexity. Patient classification systems (PCSs) are tools designed to categorize patient needs to determine nursing resources required for care in a given setting. PCSs have been used for at least 50 years but were criticized early in their application for being narrowly focused on physiological dimensions of care and for lacking precision, reliability and validity (Aydelotte, 1973). Today, though the research on PCSs is still limited and there is little consensus on what constitutes a quality PCS (Harper & McCully, 2007), PCSs continue to be used in many hospitals and in states where minimum nurse staffing ratios have been mandated (Upenieks, Kotlerman, Akhavan, Esser, & Ngo, 2007).

It was in this context that nurse researchers recognized the need to conduct a systematic review of the literature to identify current practices related to PCSs. The purpose of the review was to determine if there was a "gold standard" PCS that could be adopted or adapted for use by nurse leaders in practice. Ultimately, we were limited to performing an integrative review due to the lack of randomized controlled studies available for analysis.

BACKGROUND OF PATIENT CLASSIFICATION SYSTEMS

The historical context influencing the need for and development of PCSs is important for understanding our review. We begin with a seminal report presented at a National Institutes of Health conference that convened 45 nurse staffing research experts, Aydelotte (1973) credited Connor and the Johns Hopkins Operation Group with the first major effort to group patients into categories. Connor's PCS used factors associated with nursing problems to create a PCS based on direct patient care elements (Connor, 1960). According to Aydelotte, subsequent studies built on this work and PCS variable choices were fairly consistent: patient self-care capability, patient characteristics related to sensory deprivation, illness acuity, specific nursing care requirements, skill level of personnel, and geographic location or status in hospital. In her extensive review of the literature, Aydelotte recovered 41 sources in the literature referring to classification schemes, and concluded the following about PCSs:

- Schemes were developed primarily along physiological dimensions of care
- Schemes lacked precision and reliability, in terms of categorization of patients

- There was little testing of validity
- Staffing methodologies frequently relied upon PCSs

In 1983, diagnosis-related groups (DRGs) were introduced by Medicare. DRGs had a major impact on how hospitals were reimbursed by Medicare for inpatient care, changing from a per-patient fee-based system to a prospective reimbursement system based on patient classification by medical diagnosis. DRGs classify patients into major diagnostic categories (by major body system), then by diagnostic group (based on patient diagnosis, surgical procedure and other clinical information). PCSs became relevant as a means to categorize patients and their resource use, especially important in times of cost-containment. Many PCSs were introduced at this time, with accrediting organizations mandating some form of classification. Advancements in biomedical informatics and computer technology resulted in the movement from manual PCS calculations to computer-generated PCS models (Malloch & Conovaloff, 1999).

Edwardson and Giovanetti (1994) provided another extensive review of the workload management system (WMS) literature, covering the period between 1977 and 1992. They referred to major reviews of the literature conducted prior to their contribution (i.e., Aydelotte, 1973; Giovanetti, 1978; Young, Giovannetti, Lewison, & Thoms, 1981). They concluded that three major approaches to WMS were identified in the literature: (1) the use of patient profile instruments (prototype evaluations based on patient groups (e.g., DRGs), (2) the use of critical indicators of care (i.e., factor evaluation systems with differences between systems based on selection and number of indicators), and (3) nursing task-time systems. It is outside the scope of this systematic review to provide a detailed description of specific PCSs. We refer readers to O'Brien-Pallas, Meyer, and Thomson (2005) for a comprehensive table of more commonly used WMSs.

With the availability of improved informatics, PCS approaches have moved towards statistical methods, for example, weighting variables using regression analysis (Hughes, 1999). The literature from Canada, U.S., and Australia display trends toward the measurement of nursing work and its impact on nursing-sensitive indicators, that is, structure, process and outcome indicators that reflect nursing care (e.g., nurse staffing, nursing interventions, and pressure ulcers [patient outcome]) and create optimum staffing models (in terms of mix and number of staff; Lang, Hodge, Olson, Romano, & Kravitz, 2004; McGillis Hall et al., 2003; Upenieks et al., 2007). Another trend in the literature is toward optimum staffing ratios based on a combination of patient classification, nurse resource assessment, and a professional assessment of optimal nursing care. These measures have been used in a system developed in Finland (Fagerstrom & Rainio, 1999; Rainio & Ohinmaa, 2005; Rauhala & Fagerstrom, 2004, 2007).

TABLE 11.1

Whittemore and Knafl (2005) Modified Strategies to Enhance Rigor

Review Stage	Adaptation
Problem identification	Identify conflicting evidence on PCSs
Focused literature search	Focused on PCSs and workload management systems related to hospital settings
Data evaluation	Incorporated quality ratings
Data analysis	Data abstraction, data comparison, and conclusion drawing

Whittemore and Knafl modified Cooper's (1998) research review stages for an integrative review.

METHODS

We began our review with a clarification of what a PCS is and what it measures. A PCS is used to match staffing resources with patient needs. PCSs are also referred to as patient acuity systems or WMSs. Unless specifically named, we simplified the terminology by referring to the majority of classification systems as PCSs. A PCS measures the severity of illness and the intensity of care required by the patient (Brennan & Daly, 2009). Brennan refers to acuity at four levels— non–patient related, client-related, provider-related, and system-related. In this framework, a PCS is a measure of system-related acuity and must account for patient, provider and system factors. We used this categorization in the data abstraction and analysis processes to classify PCS indicators reported in the literature.

In order to capture the breadth and scope of the use of PCSs, an integrative review was conducted. An integrative review is a broad research method used when a comprehensive understanding of both theoretical and empirical literature is needed (Whittemore & Knafl, 2005). We used strategies outlined by Cooper (1998) and modified and demonstrated by Whittemore and Knafl to enhance the rigor of the review, as shown in Table 11.1. The last stage in the integrative review is the reporting of results. We are making our findings accessible to nurses in multiple roles, which Kirkevold (1997) suggests is necessary to enhance both the science and practice of nursing.

We conducted a review of the literature focused on patient classification or acuity systems and workload measurement systems, concentrating on three goals:

- To identify systematic reviews of the literature on *patient classification/acuity systems*

- To identify validated *staffing models*
- To *identify classification variables* from the literature that should be considered in a staffing model

To capture these elements, we adapted a framework used to evaluate an Emergency Department PCS (Williams & Crouch, 2006). Though specific to the Emergency Department, Williams and Crouch's adaptation of a conceptual framework for *evaluation* of a PCS by De Groot (1989a) was pertinent. De Groot (1989b) identified six critical factors for selection of a PCS:

- Validity—the tool accurately and adequately predicts individual patient care requirements
- Reliability—the tool consistently predicts patient care requirements
- Simplicity/efficiency—the tool is clear, concise and efficient in terms of including the critical indicators of care
- Utility—the tool is simple, efficient, and able to be incorporated into the patient's medical record
- Objectivity—the acuity rating measure is clear and can be verified
- Acceptability (to nurses)—the tool should allow subjectivity based on clinical judgment

These factors were used as our review criteria. In addition, we incorporated two other factors suggested by De Groot to be critical elements for *both design and implementation* of PCS: involvement of nurse experts in the tool development and evidence that there is recognition that nursing work is more than a sum of tasks.

We searched a variety of electronic sources, including Medline, CINAHL, Social Sciences Citation Index, and Embase. Terms, and combinations of terms, included nurse(ing) workload or work load, nurse intensity or staff or skill mix, patient acuity or classification or identification system, staff or plan or team or teams or teamwork or ratio, and benchmark or best practice. Searches of the Cochrane Database of Systematic Reviews and Biosis (biological abstracts) databases yielded no matches for systematic reviews related to patient classification or patient acuity systems. The search included only English language articles published since 1983 that focused on the adult population and were applicable to general inpatient medical/surgical settings, primarily from the United States, Canada, Great Britain, and Australia. An exception was made for work from Finland because of the methodological rigor evidenced in the articles. Additional articles were retrieved from reference lists of articles meeting the inclusion criteria. See Figure 11.1 for an example of the search strategy used with Medline. The search was originally conducted in 2007 and updated for this review in July 2010, using the same criteria.

Set	Items	Description
S2	281	(NURS? (N2) (WORKLOAD? OR WORK()LOAD? OR INTENSITY) (N5) (MEASUR? OR METHOD? OR ANALY?))/TI,AB,DE,ID,GS
S3	9769	(PATIENT? (N2) ACUITY OR CLASSIF? OR INDENT?)(N2) (SYSTEM?)/ TI,AB,DE,ID
S4	890	(NURS? (N5) STAFF?) (N10) PLAN?/TI,AB,DE,ID,GS
S5	28	(S2 OR S4) AND S3
S6	27	S5/ENG
S7	141	NURS? (N5) SKILL? (N5) MIX/TI,AB,DE,ID,GS
S8	150520	PATIENT? (N3) (CARE OR CENTERED)/TI,AB,DE,ID,GS
S9	47124	S8 (N5) (STAFF? OR PLAN? OR TEAM OR TEAMS OR TEAMWORK OR RATIO?)/TI,AB,DE,ID,GS
S10	35	(S2 OR S7) AND S9
S11	6	(S2 OR S7) (N15) S9
S12	60	S6 OR S10
S13	60	RD (unique items)

FIGURE 11.1 Example of search strategy used for Medline.

EVIDENCE ABSTRACTION

The original literature search yielded 367 unduplicated titles. From this output, 168 abstracts of interest were reviewed and 99 articles were retrieved based on the inclusion criteria. Fifty-seven were selected for final review and data were entered into the evidence tables. The updated search resulted in an additional six articles, for a total of 63 articles (see Figure 11.2). We abstracted the following information from each publication, as applicable:

- Author/year/country (of study or first author)
- Number of studies reviewed (for systematic reviews)
- Clinical area (where PCS was utilized)
- For theoretical articles—purpose or study design, informational value
- For empirical articles—study design, sample, measure, factor type (i.e., client, nurse/provider, or system)

All publications were reviewed independently by two reviewers. Quality was evaluated using three methods. For comparative reviews of more than two systems, a quality rating methodology for systematic reviews (Oxman, 1994; Oxman & Guyatt, 1991) was employed, as adapted by both Furlan et al. (2001) and Schuldheis, Carney, Helfand, Olds, and Shekelle (2006). Second, all studies were reviewed using criteria suggested by Whittemore and Knafl (2005), assessing methodological quality, theoretical rigor, evidence of validity/reliability, representativeness, and informational value. Finally, all studies were rated using a

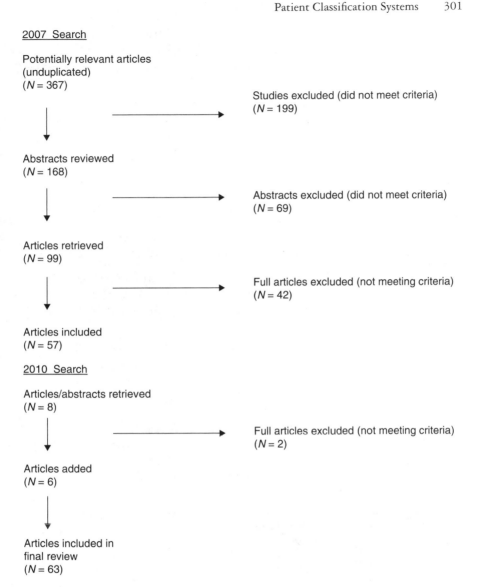

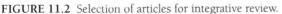

FIGURE 11.2 Selection of articles for integrative review.

simple assessment of rigor and relevance. We achieved inter-rater agreement of 80%, initially. Studies not achieving inter-rater agreement were reviewed by a third reviewer and the majority decision was used.

Our review resulted in 31 theoretical and 32 empirical studies with most (94%) rated as at least of medium quality. Information abstracted from these publications was entered into tables and categorized as empirical or theoretical.

The articles were further divided within the tables based on the three review goals and an added section for related background information. Eight articles were classified as reviews of multiple systems or offered comparative information between PCSs. Twenty-three articles focused on one or two specific PCSs. Eleven studies addressed specific variables relevant to workload measurement. The remaining 21 publications discussed relevant information, including outcomes and expert opinion that are important to the discussion of future WMSs (see Table 11.2).

TABLE 11.2
Articles Reviewed

	Empirical (First Author, Year, Country)	Theoretical (First Author, Year, Country)
Goal 1: Review of Multiple PCS	Phillips 1992 (US) O'Brien-Pallas1992 (CA) Carr-Hill 1995 (UK) Seago 2002 (US)	Arthur 1994 (UK) Edwardson 1994 (US) Hughes 1999 (UK) O'Brien-Pallas 2005 (CA)
Goal 2: Identify Validated Staffing Models	Sherrod 1984 (US) Prescott 1991 (US) Finnigan 1993 (US)* Campbell 1997 (UK)* Diers 1997 (US) O'Brien-Pallas 1997 (CA) Fagerstrom 1999 (FI) Botter 2000 (US)* Van Slyck 2001 (US)* Holcomb 2002 (US)* Rauhala 2004 (FI) Gran-Moravec 2005 (US)* Rainio 2005 (FI) Brewer 2006 (US)* Rauhala 2007 (FI)	Giovannetti 1990 (US)* Dunn 1995 (US) Malloch 1999 (US) Averill 2000 (US)* Walsh 2003 (US)* Curley 2004 (US)* Beglinger 2006 (US) Harper 2007 (US)
Goal 3: Identify Variables to Be Considered in a Staffing Model	Halloran 1985 (US) Mark 1992 (US) Mark 2000 (US) Doran 2002 (CA) Doran 2006 (CA) Berkow 2007 (US) Minnick 2009 (US) Beswick 2010 (US)	Kelleher 1992 (US) Brooten 2006 (US) Hyun 2008 (US)

TABLE 11.2

Articles Reviewed   (Continued)

	Empirical (First Author, Year, Country)	Theoretical (First Author, Year, Country)
Other Relevant Information and Evolving Concepts	Minnick 1998 (US) Bowles 2000 (US) McGillis Hall 2003 (CA) Rauhala 2007 (FI) Upenieks 2007 (US)	Alward 1983 (US) Halloran 1987 (US) Hernandez 1996 (CA) Needham 1997 (UK) Grobe 2001 (CA) Doran 2001 (CA)* McGillis Hall 2003 (CA) Currie 2004 (UK) Lang 2004 (US) Moody 2004 (US) Lankshear 2005 (UK) Tourangeau 2006 (CA) McGillis Hall 2006 (CA) Gerdtz 2007 (AUS)* Needleman 2007 (US)* Brennan 2009 (US)

Only first author's name is used; see complete citation in reference list. Asterisk indicates that reference is included only in the reference list, not in text.

Articles only loosely met criteria for applying to the various categories. There were no statistically quantified systematic reviews that met our criteria, and only four studies were both a comparison of more than one PCS and empirical (Carr-Hill & Jenkins-Clarke, 1995; O'Brien-Pallas, Cockerill, & Leatt, 1992; Phillips, Castorr, Prescott, & Soeken, 1992; Seago, 2002). A few empirical studies, addressing a specific PCS, met our criteria for validation and reliability (O'Brien-Pallas, Irvine, Peereboom, & Murray, 1997; Rauhala & Fagerstrom, 2004; Sherrod, 1984).

RESULTS

Goal 1: Identify Systematic Reviews of Patient Classification/ Acuity Systems

In the eight studies meeting the criteria of a review of more than one PCS, there were no empirically based systematic reviews evaluating multiple PCSs. However, as noted previously, the early work of Ayedolotte (1973), Giovannetti (1978), and Edwardson and Giovannetti (1994) did provide useful overviews of the state of the art in PCSs. Similarly, a more recent review (O'Brien-Pallas et al., 2005) examined the literature on nursing workload management methods and productivity. Though we attempted to do a rigorous systematic review of empirical studies, none of the studies provided sufficient data to be combined statistically.

We were particularly interested in studies providing evidence of validity and reliability. As discussed in the background section, Edwardson and Giovannetti (1994) conducted a systematic literature review of WMSs for the years between 1977 and 1992. They concluded that little objective and validated information was known about WMSs. They also showed that WMSs lacked validity and stability over time. In two studies of less theoretical and methodological rigor, authors came to similar conclusions about overall reliability and validity. Arthur and James (1994) created a classification of existing nurse demand measurement methods, consisting of consensus, top down management and bottom up management approaches. They regarded such systems as facilitators of staffing rather than prescriptions for staffing levels. In a review of commonly used methods of assessment, Hughes (1999) looked at nursing workload assessment methods in the United Kingdom, classifying them into three approaches based on (1) nursing activity, (2) patient dependency, or (3) the use of statistical methods to predict future staffing needs based on various clinical indicators. Hughes concluded that there were no theoretically rigorous and reliable measures of workload management in use. Several studies addressed comparability between systems. In empirical reviews of multiple models, three studies, published from 1992 to 1995, compared multiple PCSs or WMSs. Philips, Castorr, Prescott, and Soeken (1992) observed systems at four hospitals and found that three systems (Patient Intensity for Nursing Index [PINI], Medicus, and GRASP), varied in the way that nursing resource use was measured. For example, hours of care in Medicus and Grasp are derived from estimates of time and motion studies, whereas PINI uses a nurse's estimate of actual care delivered. Authors cited the need for standardization so that comparisons could be done for calculating nursing costs. Though a less rigorous study, Carr-Hill and Jenkins-Clarke (1995) achieved similar results when comparing three different types of WMS utilized in the United Kingdom (dependency type, task oriented, and a care planning approach). O'Brien-Pallas, Cockerill, and Leatt (1992) also found that systems were not comparable, but they concluded that with standardization of required hours of care estimated across systems, comparisons could be made between workload estimates of the GRASP, PRN, and Medicus systems. In a comparison of summative and critical incident PCSs, Seago (2002) found no difference in the predictive validity between the two types of PCS, each over-predicting and underpredicting staffing equally. Seago concluded that though

PCSs are likely necessary, they might not be sufficient in accurately measuring required resources.

O'Brien-Pallas, Meyer, and Thomson (2005) provided an excellent review of workload and productivity, in a manuscript examining the quality of work environments for nurses. Definitions and theory behind the study of nursing workload and productivity, as well as influencing factors (patient characteristics, care provider characteristics, staffing patterns, and organization of care) were discussed. They linked nursing workload and productivity to outcomes and covered related issues, that is, reliability and validity, measure equivalence, and productivity measures. They determined, as did we, that the literature on PCSs tends to be descriptive studies of single hospital WMSs, thereby significantly limiting the generalization of the findings. A major contribution of their review is a discussion and tabular presentation of five relatively common workload measurement systems that authors determined to have evidence of reliability and validity testing, that is, GRASP, PINI, Medicus, PRN, and the Environmental Complexity Scale. They also examined the use of Management Information System data, which is already a part of Canadian routine reporting. Similar to our findings, they concluded there is no existing gold standard of nursing workload measurement and cited the need for multiple measures capturing the complexity of factors.

Goal 2: Identify Validated Staffing Models

Of 15 *empirical* articles on specific PCSs retrieved, only seven studies were reviewed as having sufficient reliability and validity to be considered of high quality. These validated studies addressed five different PCSs: Army Classification Instrument (Sherrod, 1984), PINI (Prescott et al., 1991), Project Nursing in Research 80 (PRN 80; O'Brien-Pallas et al., 1997), RAFAELA/PAONCIL (Rainio & Ohinmaa, 2005; Rauhala & Fagerstrom, 2004, 2007) and Resource Information Management System (RIMS; Diers & Bozzo, 1997). Eight *theoretical* studies discussed specific PCS models used in a unique setting.

In a high quality study by Diers and Bozzo (1997), DRGs were weighted by nursing intensity, thus using existing management tools and integrating with the hospital information system without having to use a supplemental PCS. The resulting PCS, RIMS, was designed to develop a patient acuity system using existing data. The study used an expert panel to classify DRGs into six clusters or categories with similar nursing care requirements, establishing the amount of nursing time for an average day for an average patient within the cluster for a particular area of care (e.g., inpatient, ICU, pediatrics). The approach was validated against actual nursing care hours provided per patient. This method may be a relatively cost-effective, feasible approach to retrospective analysis of nursing requirements, though it requires further development of the categorical measures and then testing for reliability and validity.

O'Brien-Pallas, Irvine, Peereboom, and Murray (1997) recognized the variability and complexity of measuring nursing workload. They included four key variables in their model: patient-nursing condition (measured by nursing diagnosis), medical complexity (measured by the Canadian version of DRGs), medical severity (i.e., length of stay) and environmental complexity (i.e., unanticipated and delayed events, multiple and long procedures, and caregiving-team characteristics). A major contribution of this study is the Unit Factor scale, which incorporated both nurse characteristics and indirect care and the extra demands placed on nurses by the dynamic and unpredictable nature of caring for a *group* of patients.

A group of hospitals in Finland have implemented and validated an optimum staffing model, the RAFAELA PCS, which is based on initials of the research team who developed the system. The system consists of a combination of a PCS, a nurse resource assessment, and a professional assessment of optimal nursing care (Fagerstrom & Rainio, 1999; Rainio & Ohinmaa, 2005; Rauhala & Fagerstrom, 2004). In a study to examine the relative impact of their PCS and nonpatient factors on assessment of nursing workload, investigators found that the PCS explains about 45% of the variation in workload assessment compared to 11% of the perceived assessment of nursing workload by nonpatient factors (administration, staff resources, mental stress, and inter- and intra-unit cooperation; Rauhala & Fagerstrom, 2007).

In a particularly relevant, though less rigorous descriptive review, Dunn et al. (1995) described the Expert Panel Method for Nurse Staffing and Resource Management that was implemented in the U.S. Veterans Health Administration in the early 1990s. Expert panels were used to identify staffing requirements for direct and nondirect nursing care activities. Using a structure-process-outcome framework, experts assessed patient dependency on nursing care, nurse and patient demographics, and organizational factors such as affiliation and physical layout. The Expert Panel Method was cited as a critical tool to determine staffing needs in other studies as well (Beglinger, 2006; Diers & Bozzo, 1997; Malloch & Conovaloff, 1999).

Several articles provided useful guidance for the development and testing of future models. Alward (1983) outlined elements of an ideal PCS and compared it with real PCSs of her day, highlighting the need for ongoing review of validity and reliability. She proposed an alternative approach using a factor evaluation tool and assignment of nursing hours based on current nursing budget. In a review of the literature, Hernandez and O'Brien-Pallas (1996) provided an overview of the types of validity and factors that affect reliability, as they apply to

WMSs. Authors concluded that reliability and validity are more often addressed at implementation of a PCS, but are ignored as an ongoing requirement of PCS use. Minnick and Pabst (1998) further reported that in the presence of WMS, understaffing occurs due to failure to re-validate WMSs. In terms of validity, Halloran and Vermeersch (1987) concluded that there was much variability in nurse staffing research, especially in the areas of data collection and analysis, resulting in barriers to comparability between models and systems.

Issues with reliability and validity of specific PCSs abound in the literature. One study provides an informative overview of the intractability of problems associated with PCS (McGillis Hall et al., 2006). Investigators interviewed Canadian nurse decision-makers, users and stakeholders of WMS tools and processes to understand issues related to nurse staffing. They concluded PCSs are not used for staffing decisions because they are not responsive enough to changes in staffing needs, they lack validity and reliability, and they often call for greater staffing than what organizations can provide. Additionally, though PCSs may be valuable for other purposes, such as long-term staffing corrections and trend analysis, respondents reported that they are not reflective of real nursing work. Respondents reported nurse-staffing decisions are more realistically made intuitively, based on experience and professional judgment, or within financial constraints.

Goal 3: Identify Variables to Be Considered in a Staffing Model

Several general concepts to consider in developing a PCS model emerged from the literature:

- more variables are not necessarily better (Edwardson & Giovannetti, 1994);
- simplicity is desirable (Alward, 1983; Hughes, 1999);
- existing measures should be used where possible (Diers & Bozzo, 1997; Kelleher, 1992);
- specific variables to be considered should include indicators of patient-related, nurse-specific and organizational characteristics (Beswick, Hill, & Anderson, 2010; Minnick & Mion, 2009; O'Brien-Pallas et al., 2005).

This set of studies examined specific indicators of nursing workload. A variety of variables were identified in the literature. Consistent with our definition and operationalization of a PCS as a measure accounting for patient, provider and system level factors, we categorized the variables accordingly. Table 11.3 provides a representative sampling of specific indicators, classified as client, nurse/provider, or system-level (unit or hospital) variables, that were used in PCSs and reported in the literature.

TABLE 11.3

Variables from the Literature to Consider in a Staffing Model, Classified as Patient, Nurse, or Organizational Indicators

Patient	Nurse	Unit/Organization
Complexity (nursing diagnosis, DRGs)	Education	Stability/maturity
	Experience—total	Volume
Severity (length of stay)	Experience—unit	Patient turnover (admissions/
Dependency/functional status	Skill mix	discharges/transfers)
Activities of daily living/		Interdisciplinary relationships/
Transports		communication
Age		Support services
Patient care needs		Unit complexity/variation (in
• Observational needs		patient type and treatment)
• Obesity		Autonomy/work environment
• Postdischarge needs		Protocol-driven care
• Psychosocial needs		Multitasking (high frequency/low volume)

Noting that PCSs did not adequately reflect nursing work and the lack of comparability between systems, Kelleher (1992) advocated for standardizing PCSs and using validated measures as proxies for nursing acuity, including measures of functional status, severity of illness, and psychosocial health. Bowles (2000) suggested that a PCS could be designed using the following four patient-related domains: (1) environmental problems, (2) psychosocial problems, (3) physiological problems, and (4) health related behaviors. In an attempt to identify the indicators of nursing work, the Rush-Medicus PCS tool was used to estimate nursing time and explain nursing workload (Halloran, 1985). Halloran estimated the effect of patient nursing condition (based on nursing diagnosis), patient medical condition (based on DRGs), and patient demographics on nursing workload. Patient age, sex, and race explained 4.3% of the variation. Nursing diagnosis predicted twice as much variation in nursing care time as DRGs, suggesting that nursing care is better described by nursing diagnoses than by physician diagnoses.

Mark, Salyer, and Wan (2000) examined market, hospital and nursing unit characteristics as predictors of nursing unit skill mix in a multisite cross-sectional observational study of 67 hospitals participating in the ORNA (Outcomes Research in Nursing Administration) project. Higher skill mix (i.e., registered nurses [RNs] to total staff) was predicted by higher use of technology services, a higher percentage of managed care admissions, and lower hospital patient volume. The complexity of patient need and support service availability did not have an effect. Though results are subject to measurement limitations, findings from this study suggest that hospital characteristics (e.g., managed care admissions and high technology services) were more important predictors of nursing skill mix than either market or nursing unit characteristics.

Similarly, in an earlier study, Mark (1992) found no difference among team, primary, and case management care delivery models except in continuity of patient assignments. This suggests that continuity of patient assignment, rather than care delivery model, may be a better indicator of staffing need.

In a study examining the factors that affect nursing role performance, Doran, Sidani, Keatings, and Doidge (2002) tested the Nursing Role Effectiveness Model (NREM). The model examined patient, nurse, and unit structural variables and how they affect patients' perceptions of nursing effectiveness. Nursing role performance mediated the effect of structural variables on outcomes, indicating the need to consider processes of care. In a follow-up study, the nursing sensitive outcome measures and the instruments and methods used to measure outcomes in the NREM, were further tested and validated (Doran et al., 2006).

A number of unit attributes have been deemed relevant for staffing. Berkow, Jaggi, Fogelson, Katz, and Hirschoff (2007) conducted structured interviews with nurse executives to understand how workforce planning research is being incorporated into staffing decisions in practice. Fourteen unit attributes (e.g., variation in patients or treatment, high-risk patients, and technology) were identified. Nurse executives rated their importance in determining how staffing decisions are made relative to nurse-to-patient ratios, RN education, RN experience, and support staff level. Researchers found challenging situations and unit attributes were used to make decisions about staffing more than specific unit type (i.e., pediatrics, medical-surgical, intermediate care, and emergency department). Similarly, unit turbulence (admissions, discharges, and transfers) and acuity should be included when predicting staffing (Beswick et al., 2010; Minnick & Mion, 2009; Spetz & Phibbs, 2008; Unruh & Fottler, 2006). Indicators of indirect care, such as documentation, patient transport, and interdisciplinary communication, have also been cited as factors to be included in staffing models (Harper & McCully, 2007; Hyun, Gakken, Douglas, & Stone, 2008; Upenieks et al., 2007).

OTHER RELEVANT INFORMATION AND EVOLVING CONCEPTS

We identified emerging themes in our integrative review that relate to predicting nurse staffing. These concepts go beyond the scope of the current state of the science on PCSs, and accordingly, beyond the scope of this project. However, we mention them briefly in our discussion, as evolving concepts for further investigation and consideration, when implementing, designing or evaluating PCSs.

At the foundation of the problems with nursing workload measurement is the lack of a *standardized language* to describe and communicate what it is that nurses do. Needham (1997) described the use of instruments that assess patient dependency as a compromise solution, based on "soft data," for workload measurement. Kelleher (1992) suggested that many of the instruments used to measure nursing work in the past have not adequately described nursing work. Grobe (2001) described the problems with capturing nurses' work as evidence of a need for a nursing language and a need to capture reliable and valid data that both focuses on intensity and complexity of care.

Nurse dose is another concept being examined for its potential impact on the quality of health care delivery. Nurse dose refers to the amount of nursing care provided (Brooten & Youngblut, 2006). The three necessary components include dose (number or amount of nurses), nurse (education, expertise, and experience), and the host response of both patients and the organization. Nurse effectiveness at the patient level is determined by acceptability of the nurse to the patient's beliefs, values, and culture. At the organizational level, nurse effectiveness is influenced by the organization's culture and willingness to give the nurse autonomy and control of practice (Brooten & Youngblut, 2006).

As practice moves toward validating the effectiveness of PCSs to predict nurse-staffing needs, it will be ever more critical to examine *nursing-sensitive outcomes* in staffing models. Our search resulted in several studies addressing outcomes associated with nurse staffing. For example, in a systematic review of international literature related to nursing workforce and patient outcomes, resulting in 22 studies of variable quality, Lankshear, Sheldon, and Maynard (2005) concluded that higher nurse staffing and richer skill mix may be associated with improved patient outcomes. However, in a review of the literature examining the relationship between perceptions of quality of care and differences in nurse staffing, skill mix and autonomy, Currie and Kerrin (2004) argued that the research on patient satisfaction is presently insufficient for drawing conclusions. Nurse staffing characteristics were identified as one of the strongest predictors of mortality in a study synthesizing the published research exploring determinants of mortality for acute hospitalized patients, from 1986 to 2004 (Tourangeau, Cranley, & Jeffs, 2006). Finally, in a study examining work overload, an increased nursing workload was positively associated with increased absenteeism (Rauhala et al., 2007).

As noted in the introduction, mandated *minimum nurse–patient staffing ratios* are emerging as a driving force behind the need for PCSs (Upenieks et al., 2007) and, therefore, are mentioned here. Minimum nurse–patient staffing ratios refer to the minimum number of licensed nurses (including RNs and Licensed Practical Nurses or Licensed Vocational Nurses) required to care for a specific number of patients. At the state level, these ratios may be mandated through legislation or regulation, set by holding hospitals accountable for determining appropriate staffing ratios, or monitored by requiring hospitals to disclose staffing ratios. A systematic literature review on minimum nurse–patient staffing ratios (Lang et al., 2004) resulted in 43 studies on minimum nurse–patient ratios. The review reported little support for specific minimum nurse–patient ratios. The authors concluded that the following variables also needed to be considered for staffing requirements: patient acuity, skill mix, nurse competence, nursing process variables, technology sophistication, and institutional support of nursing. In a more recent study of nurse staff ratios in Australia (Gerdtz & Nelson, 2007), authors critiqued minimum nurse–patient ratios and compared them to the Patient Dependency System (a form of PCS). They concluded that minimums should be set for the number of nurses per ward, not per patient, allowing for manager discretion; they reported that there is little evidence to support minimum nurse–patient ratios and that neither ratios nor patient dependency systems account for skill mix. In a study of minimum unit-specific staffing ratios, Upenieks et al. (2007) concluded that minimum staffing ratios did not reflect variability in patient needs or nurse activities across similarly staffed units.

Finally, the work being done on *nursing productivity* adds to our understanding of relevant indicators to include in staffing models. In a nursing productivity framework proposed by McGillis Hall et al. (2003) authors recommended using nursing knowledge indicators (e.g., education, experience, career development, autonomy, organizational trust and commitment, and employee satisfaction) and organizational support to predict nursing productivity. Other variables related to nursing care that should be considered include system indicators (e.g., nursing costs, turnover, absenteeism, and nursing replacement, orientation and education costs) and patient indicators (e.g., patient safety and satisfaction). Moody (2004) described a fully integrated model of a nursing productivity index, including patient intensity, nurse staffing, dependability (error rates), institutional resources, negotiated patient outcomes, durability, and provider outcomes that gives an additional perspective for consideration.

CONCLUSION

The purpose of this paper was to present the methods and results of an integrative review related to PCSs because of the impact on staffing methodologies. Generally, we found that many of the criticisms of earlier PCSs are still evident. For example, (1) difficulties with measuring workload remain an overarching theme throughout the literature; (2) definitions and descriptions of nursing work continue to be deemed inadequate; (3) there is insufficient evidence of reliability and validity testing of PCSs, and (4) there is still a need to identify nursing-sensitive performance indicators and outcomes. More recent systems have expanded the dimensions included in classification schemes beyond primarily physiological patient characteristics to incorporate patient complexity and nursing and organizational attributes.

Staffing continues to be at the forefront of efforts to ensure patient safety and to provide quality care for hospitalized patients. We need valid and reliable tools to plan, implement, and evaluate staffing processes. In our integrative review, we have attempted to provide an update on the evidence related to PCSs. We identified characteristics of promising PCSs, and, in the end, our work supported AHRQ's conclusion that no consensus exists about PCSs (Agency for Healthcare Research and Quality, 2007).

In conclusion, perhaps there is no "one size fits all" patient classification scheme, and the best approach to predicting staffing is one based on sound design principles of

- parsimony
- minimal additional workload requirement
- a basis in expert nurse judgment
- true reflection of nursing work
- indicators that measure patient complexity, optimal required nursing care, available resources, and relevant organizational attributes.

This integrative review serves to reflect the significant work that has been done to develop a "gold standard" for patient classification. Although we have been unable to find such a system, much of the groundwork has been laid for future work. Given the knowledge gained from previous studies, future work should focus on evaluating staffing approaches and processes to identify the core variables that will assist in the development of result-oriented staffing models. Future work will be needed in partnership with nurse leaders in practice settings to test the predictability of linking the staffing models with outcomes.

ACKNOWLEDGMENT

The authors thank the efforts of their research team, Maureen Festa, MLS, and Barbara Weatherford, PhD, RN, for helping to conduct the literature search, retrieve papers, assess the quality of the evidence, and to abstract the data from the final set of papers. This material is based upon work supported by the Department of Veterans Affairs, Veterans Health Administration, Office of

Research and Development, Health Services Research and Development (RRP 07-336: Assessing Evidence for Nurse Staffing to Improve Patient/Organizational Outcomes, Haddock, 2007).

REFERENCES

Agency for Healthcare Research and Quality. (2007). *Nurse Staffing and Quality of Patient Care: Evidence Report/Technology Assessment Number 151.* Rockville, MD: AHRQ.

Alward, R. (1983). Patient classification systems: The ideal vs. reality. *Journal of Nursing Administration,* 14–19.

Arthur, T., & James, N. (1994). Determining nurse staffing levels: A critical review of the literature. *Journal of Advanced Nursing, 19*(3), 558–565.

Averill, C. B., & Fairbrother, M. B. (2000). Developing a statewide patient classification system. *Nursing Administration Quarterly, 24*(4), 29–35.

Aydelotte, M. (1973). *Nurse staffing methodology: A review and critique of selected literature* (No. NIH 73-433): Superintendent of Documents, U.S. Government Printing Office.

Beglinger, J. E. (2006). Quantifying patient care intensity: An evidence-based approach to determining staffing requirements. *Nursing Administration Quarterly 30*(3), 193–202.

Berkow, S., Jaggi, T., Fogelson, R., Katz, S., & Hirschoff, A. (2007). Fourteen unit attributes to guide staffing. *Journal of Nursing Administration, 37*(3), 150–155.

Beswick, S., Hill, P. D., & Anderson, M. A. (2010). Comparison of nurse workload approaches. *Journal of Nursing Management, 18*(5), 592–598.

Botter, M. L. (2000). The use of information generated by a patient classification system. *Journal of Nursing Administration, 30*(11), 544–551.

Bowles, K. H. (2000). Patient problems and nurse interventions during acute care and discharge planning. *Journal of Cardiovascular Nursing, 14*(3), 29–41.

Brennan, C. W., & Daly, B. J. (2009). Patient acuity: A concept analysis. *Journal of Advanced Nursing, 65*(5), 1114–1126.

Brewer, B. (2006). Is patient acuity a proxy for patient characteristics of the AACN synergy model for patient care? *Nursing Administration Quarterly, 30*(4), 351–357.

Brooten, D., & Youngblut, J. M. (2006). Nurse dose as concept. *Journal of Nursing Scholarship, 38*(1), 94–99.

Campbell, T., Taylor, S., Callaghan, S., & Shuldham, C. (1997). Case mix type as a predictor of nursing workload. *Journal of Nursing Management, 5*(4), 237–240.

Carr-Hill, R. A., & Jenkins-Clarke, S. (1995). Measurement systems in principle and in practice: The example of nursing workload. *Journal of Advanced Nursing, 22*(2), 221–225.

Connor, R. (1960). *A hospital inpatient classification system.* Unpublished doctoral dissertation, The Johns Hopkins University, Baltimore, MD.

Cooper, H. (1998). *Synthesizing research: A guide for literature reviews* (3rd ed.). Thousand Oaks, CA: Sage Publications.

Curley, M. A. Q. (2004, August/September). Origins of the synergy model. *Excellence in Nursing Knowledge.* Retrieved October 22, 2010, from Publisher URL.http://www.nursingknowledge.org/

Currie, G., & Kerrin, M. (2004). The limits of a technological fix to knowledge management: Epistemological, political and cultural issues in the case of intranet implementation. *Management Learning, 35,* 9–29.

De Groot, H. A. (1989a). Patient classification system evaluation: Essential system elements: part 1. *Journal of Nursing Administration, 19*(6), 30–35.

De Groot, H. A. (1989b). Patient classification system evaluation: System selection and implementation: part 2. *Journal of Nursing Administration, 19*(7), 24–30.

Diers, D., & Bozzo, J. (1997). Nursing resource definition in DRGs. RIMS/Nursing Acuity Project Group. *Nursing Economics, 15*(3), 124–130, 137.

Doran, D. I., Sidani, S., Keatings, M., & Doidge, D. (2002). An empirical test of the nursing role effectiveness model. *Journal of Advanced Nursing, 38*(1), 29–39.

Doran, D. I., Sidani, S., Watt-Watson, J., Laschinger, H., & Hall, L. M. (2001). *A methodological review of the literature of nursing-sensitive outcomes.* Paper presented at the Symposium: Nursing & Health Outcomes Project Toronto, Canada.

Doran, D. M., Harrison, M. B., Laschinger, H., Hirdes, J. P., Rukholm, E., Sidani, S.,... Tourangeau, A. E. (2006). Nurse sensitive outcomes data collection in acute care and long-term-care settings. *Nursing Research, 55*(2S), S75–S81.

Dunn, M. G., Norby, R., Cournoyer, P., Hudec, S., O'Donnell, J., & Snider, M. D. (1995). Expert panel method for nurse staffing and resource management. *Journal of Nursing Administration, 25*(10), 61–67.

Edwardson, S., & Giovannetti, P. (1994). Nursing workload measurement systems. *Annual Review of Nursing Research, 12*(1), 95–123.

Fagerstrom, L., & Rainio, A. K. (1999). Professional assessment of optimal nursing care intensity level: A new method of assessing personnel resources for nursing care. *Journal of Clinical Nursing, 8*(4), 369–379.

Finnigan, S., Abel, M., Dobler, T., Hudon, L., & Terry, B. (1993). Automated patient acuity. *Journal of Nursing Administration, 23*(5), 62–71.

Furlan, A., Clarke, J., Esmail, R., Sinclair, S., Irvin, E., & Bombardier, C. (2001). A critical review of reviews on the treatment of chronic low back pain. *Spine, 26*(7), E155–E162.

Giovannetti, P. (1978). *Patient classification systems in nursing: A description and analysis. Nurse Planning Information Series*: National Technical Information Service, 5285 Port Royal Road, Springfield, VA. 22161.

Giovannetti, P., & Johnson, J. M. (1990). A new generation patient classification system—ARIC (allocation, resource identification and costing). *Journal of Nursing Administration, 20*(5), 33–40.

Gran-Moravec, M. B., & Hughes, C. M. (2005). Nursing time allocation and other considerations for staffing. *Nursing and Health Sciences, 7*, 126–133.

Grobe, S. (2001, March 15–16). *Capturing nurses work.* Paper presented at the Symposium: Nursing and Health Outcomes Project, Toronto, Canada.

Halloran, E. J. (1985). Nursing workload, medical diagnosis related groups, and nursing diagnoses. *Research in Nursing & Health, 8*(4), 421–433.

Halloran, E. J., & Vermeersch, P. E. (1987). Variability in nurse staffing research. *The Journal of Nursing Administration, 17*(2), 26–34.

Harper, K., & McCully, C. (2007). Acuity systems dialogue and patient classification system essentials. *Nursing Administration Quarterly, 31*(4), 284–299.

Hernandez, C. A., & O'Brien-Pallas, L. L. (1996). Validity and reliability of nursing workload measurement systems: Review of validity and reliability theory. *Canadian Journal of Nursing Administration, 9*(3), 32–50.

Holcomb, B. R., Hoffart, N., & Fox, M. H. (2002). Defining and measuring nursing productivity: A concept analysis and pilot study. *Journal of Advanced Nursing, 38*(4), 378–386.

Hughes, M. (1999). Nursing workload: An unquantifiable entity. *Journal of Nursing Management, 7*, 317–322.

Hyun, S., Gakken, S., Douglas, K., & Stone, P. W. (2008). Evidence-based staffing: Potential roles for informatics. *Nursing Economics, 26*(3), 151.

Kelleher, C. (1992). Validated indexes: Key to nursing acuity standardization. *Nursing Economics,* 10(1), 31–37.

Kirkevold, M. (1997). Integrative nursing research—An important strategy to further the development of nursing science and nursing practice. *Journal of Advanced Nursing,* 25(5), 977–984.

Lang, T. A., Hodge, M., Olson, V., Romano, P. S., & Kravitz, R. L. (2004). Nurse-patient ratios—A systematic review on the effects of nurse staffing on patient, nurse employee, and hospital outcomes. *Journal of Nursing Administration,* 34(7–8), 326–337.

Lankshear, A. J., Sheldon, T. A., & Maynard, A. (2005). Nurse staffing and healthcare outcomes: A systematic review of the international research evidence. *Advances in Nursing Science,* 28(2), 163–174.

Malloch, K., & Conovaloff, A. (1999). Patient classification systems, Part 1: The third generation. *The Journal of Nursing Administration,* 29(7–8), 49–56.

Mark, B. (1992). Characteristics of nursing practice models. *Journal of Nursing Administration,* 22(11), 57–63.

Mark, B. A., Salyer, J., & Wan, T. T. (2000). Market, hospital, and nursing unit characteristics as predictors of nursing unit skill mix: A contextual analysis. *The Journal of Nursing Administration,* 30(11), 552–560.

McGillis Hall, L., Doran, D., Baker, G., Pink, G., Sidani, S., O'Brien-Pallas, L., & Donner GJ. (2003). Nurse staffing models as predictors of patient outcomes. *Medical Care,* 41(9), 1096–1108.

McGillis Hall, L., Pink, L., Lalonde, M., Murphy, G. T., O'Brien-Pallas, L., Laschinger, H.,... Akeroyd, J. (2006). Decision making for nurse staffing: Canadian perspectives. *Policy, Politics & Nursing Practice,* 7(4), 261–269.

Minnick, A. F., & Mion, L. C. (2009). Nurse labor data: The collection and interpretation of nurse-to-patient ratios. *Journal of Nursing Administration,* 39(9), 377–381.

Minnick, A. F., & Pabst, M. K. (1998). Improving the ability to detect the impact of labor on patient outcomes. *Journal of Nursing Administration,* 28(12), 17–21.

Moody, R. C. (2004). Nurse productivity measures for the 21st century. *Health Care Management Review,* 29(2), 98–106.

Needham, J. (1997). Accuracy in workload measurement: A fact or fallacy? *Journal of Nursing Management,* 5(2), 83–87.

Needleman, J., Kurtzman, E. T., & Kizer, K. W. (2007). Performance measurement of nursing care: State of the science and the current consensus. *Medical Care Research and Review,* 64 (2 Suppl.), 10S–43S.

O'Brien-Pallas, L., Cockerill, R., & Leatt, P. (1992). Different systems, different costs? An examination of the comparability of workload measurement systems. *Journal of Nursing Administration,* 22(12), 17–22.

O'Brien-Pallas, L., Irvine, D., Peereboom, E., & Murray, M. (1997). Measuring nursing workload: Understanding the variability. *Nursing Economics,* 15(4), 171–182.

O'Brien-Pallas, L., Meyer, R., & Thomson, D. (2005). Workload and productivity. In L. M. Hall (Ed.), *Quality work environments for nurse and patient safety.* New Sudbury, MA: Jones and Bartlett.

Oxman, A. D. (1994). Systematic reviews: Checklists for review articles. *BMJ,* 309(6955), 648–651.

Oxman, A. D., & Guyatt, G. H. (1991). Validation of an index of the quality of review articles. *Journal of Clinical Epidemiology,* 44(11), 1271–1278.

Phillips, C. Y., Castorr, A., Prescott, P. A., & Soeken, K. (1992). Nursing intensity: Going beyond patient classification. *Journal of Nursing Administration,* 22(4), 46–52.

Prescott, P. A., Ryan, J. W., Soeken, K. L., Castorr, A. H., Thompson, K. O., & Phillips, C. Y. (1991). The Patient Intensity for Nursing Index: A validity assessment. *Research in Nursing & Health,* 14(3), 213–221.

Rainio, A. K., & Ohinmaa, A. E. (2005). Assessment of nursing management and utilization of nursing resources with the RAFAELA patient classification system—Case study from the general wards of one central hospital. *Journal of Clinical Nursing, 14*(6), 674–684.

Rauhala, A., & Fagerstrom, L. (2004). Determining optimal nursing intensity: The RAFAELA method. *Journal of Advanced Nursing, 45*(4), 351–359.

Rauhala, A., & Fagerstrom, L. (2007). Are nurses' assessments of their workload affected by non-patient factors? An analysis of the RAFAELA system. *Journal of Nursing Management, 15*(5), 490–499.

Rauhala, A., Kivimaki, M., Fagerstrom, L., Elovainio, M., Virtanen, M., Vahtera, J.,...Kinnunen, J. (2007). What degree of work overload is likely to cause increased sickness absenteeism among nurses? Evidence from the RAFAELA patient classification system. *Journal of Advanced Nursing, 57*(3), 286–295.

Schuldheis, S., Carney, N., Helfand, M., Olds, J., & Shekelle, P. (2006). *Assessment of the Evidence base for information systems and technology related to nursing practices and patient outcomes—Technical Report.* Department of Veterans Affairs, Office of Nursing Services, Washington, DC.

Seago, J. (2002). A comparison of two patient classification instruments in an acute care hospital. *Journal of Nursing Administration, 32*(5), 243–249.

Sherrod, S. M. (1984). Patient classification system: A link between diagnosis-related groupings and acuity factors. *Military Medicine, 149*(9), 506–511.

Spetz, J., & Phibbs, C. (2008). CPRS and BCMA through the rearview mirror—Retrospectively evaluating health IT implementations. On *VIREC Clinical Informatics Seminar* [HERC Slide presentation]. Washington, DC: US Department of Veterans Affairs, Health Services Research & Development.

Tourangeau, A. E., Cranley, L. A., & Jeffs, L. (2006). Impact of nursing on hospital patient mortality: A focused review and related policy implications. *Quality & Safety in Health Care, 15*(1), 4–8.

Unruh, L. Y., & Fottler, M. D. (2006). Patient turnover and nursing staff adequacy. *Health Services Research, 41*(2), 599–612.

Upenieks, V., Kotlerman, J., Akhavan, J., Esser, J., & Ngo, M. (2007). Assessing nursing staff ratios: Variability in workload intensity. *Policy, Politics & Nursing Practice, 8*(1), 7–19.

Van Slyck, A., & Johnson, K. R. (2001). Using patient acuity data to manage patient care outcomes and patient care costs. *Outcomes Management for Nursing Practice, 5*(1), 36–40.

Walsh, E. (2003). Get real with workload measurement. *Nursing Management, 2*, 38–42.

Whittemore, R., & Knafl, K. (2005). The integrative review: Updated methodology. *Journal of Advanced Nursing, 52*(5), 546–553.

Williams, S., & Crouch, R. (2006). Emergency department patient classification systems: A systematic review. *Accident and Emergency Nursing, 14*(3), 160–170.

Young, J. P., Giovannetti, P., Lewison, D., & Thoms, M. L. (1981). *Factors affecting nurse staffing in acute care hospitals: A review and critique of the literature. Nurse Planning Information Series 17.* Rockville, MD: Public Health Service (DHHS).

CHAPTER 12

An Integrative Review of Nursing Workforce Studies

Annette Tyree Debisette, Irene Sandvold,
Barbara Easterling, and Angela Martinelli

ABSTRACT

The purpose of this chapter is to present an analysis of selected published nursing workforce studies published between the years of 2005 and 2010. Thirteen nursing workforce studies were reviewed and analyzed using a modification of the method suggested by Ganong (1987). Nursing workforce studies were selected based on the following criteria: (1) the date of publication was between the years of 2005 and 2010; (2) the primary focus was on nurses working in practice; or, as students or faculty in nursing educational programs. When reviewed, the 13 studies (1) lacked uniform measures among databases; (2) lacked longitudinal studies that followed the respondent over time from the beginning of their career to retirement; (3) had response rates that contributed to small sample sizes or sampling frame that did not take into consideration all characteristics of interest; (4) lacked attention to an interdisciplinary mix of providers; and (5) implied the need for future study on intergenerational characteristics due to shifting demographics in the profession and nursing workforce.

The views expressed in this manuscript do not necessarily represent the views of the U.S. Department of Health and Human Services, United States Public Health Service, Food and Drug Administration, Health Resources and Services Administration or the National Institutes of Health, or the United States Government.

INTRODUCTION

The United States is in the midst of major reform in health care and changes in Medicare reimbursement. To further complicate this issue, the shortage of registered nurses (RNs) is expected to grow as baby boomers age and health care needs change. Compounding the problem is the fact that U.S. nursing programs are struggling to expand enrollment to meet the rising demand for care. Studies indicate that nursing school enrollments fail to match the projected demand for RNs and the shortage of nursing school faculty are restricting nursing program enrollments (www.aacn.nche.edu/Media/shortageresource.html; http://www.nln. org/governmentaffairs/hcreform_shortage_info.htm).

The American Nurses Association first surveyed RNs in 1949 to develop an understanding of the nursing workforce in terms of composition and distribution (American Nurses Association, 1949). Fifty-one years later, as nursing became one of the largest health professions, researchers continued to strive to understand the ever-changing context of the nursing profession. As the profession continues to change and grow in numbers, so have the variety of nursing educational programs, levels of credentialing, and roles for nurses. Moreover, the health care industry, laws and regulations guiding health care and health care reform are in continual fluctuation as steps are taken to implement the Patient Protection and Affordable Care Act, Public Law 111-148 (2010). As the health care industry and the market for nurses change, there continues to be a need to perform studies on all aspects of the nursing workforce. Interestingly, quite a number of bodies have conducted studies of the nursing workforce in the United States and abroad. Although there are differences in purpose for conducting studies, most use similar methodologies in surveying their populations of interest.

As the aging trend of the RN population remains a concern, so does the age of the U.S. population. As the U.S. population ages it does so with a variety of chronic and complex needs. The complexity of illness and care, along with insufficient workplace staffing leading to decreased quality and unfavorable patient outcomes has raised the level of stress that nurses endure. This stress, in turn, contributed to decreased job satisfaction and is driving many nurses to leave the profession; in turn impacting turnover and vacancy rates that are affecting access to health care. Now more than ever, nurse and policy makers are in need of valid and reliable data on which to plan for the future health care needs of our nation.

THE 2010 AFFORDABLE CARE ACT

The Affordable Care Act (ACA) authorized mechanisms and directed resources to gain additional data on the health care workforce, including nursing, through several mechanisms: National Health Care Workforce Commission, National

Center for Health Care Workforce Analysis, and State Health Workforce Development Centers.

National Health Care Workforce Commission

The ACA, P.L. 111-148, Section 5101, authorized the establishment of a National Health Care Workforce Commission and delegated its administration to the Comptroller General in the Government Accountability Office (GAO). The purpose of the Commission is to serve as a national resource for Congress, the President, States, and localities; communicate and coordinate with the Departments of Health and Human Services, Labor, Veterans Affairs, Homeland Security, and Education on related activities; and develop and commission evaluations of education and training activities to determine whether or not the demand for health care workers is being met, to identify barriers to improved coordination at the Federal, State, and local levels and to recommend ways to address such barriers, and to encourage innovations to address population needs, constant changes in technology, and other environmental factors. The Department of Health and Human Services will have a consulting role.

The Commission's data-collection functions are specified so that it can carry out the functions. It will use existing information, engage in or award grants/contracts for engaging in original research and development to study areas where there is inadequate information to make policy recommendations, and design procedures that make it possible for people to submit information for the Commission's use in making reports and recommendations.

The ACA broadly defined health care workforce and health professionals. More information on the National Commission for Health Care Workforce and its current membership can be found at www.gao.gov and in the ACA (ACA, 2010).

National Center for Health Care Workforce Analysis

Significant resources were authorized through the Affordable Care Act (ACA) to support Health Care Workforce Assessment (P.L. 111-148, article Section 5103, Section 761 of the PHS Act). The National Center for Health Care Workforce Analysis was established to address the National Health Care Workforce Commission to address the development of information describing the health professions workforce, analyze workforce related issues, and provide information for decision-making regarding future directions in health professions and nursing programs in response to societal and professional needs in coordination with the National Health Workforce Commission.

The Center has been established to provide for the development of information on the health care workforce and workforce related issues, evaluation, develop and publish performance measures and benchmarks; and to establish, maintain, and publicize a national Internet registry of grants awarded and a database to collect data from longitudinal evaluations. The National Center will work in collaboration with Federal agencies and relevant professional and educational organizations or societies on linking data. This Center will support State and Regional Centers for Workforce Analysis to collect, analyze and report data on programs to the public, provide technical assistance, and support longitudinal evaluations on individuals who have received education, training or financial assistance from programs funded through Title VII of the PHS Act.

State Health Care Workforce Development Grants

A health care workforce development grant program has been established as authorized in ACA, Section 5102, to support State partnerships for comprehensive planning and to carry out activities leading to comprehensive workforce development strategies at the State and local levels. Twenty-five State Planning grants were funded by the end of FY 2010 and one implementation grant received funding. This program is carried out in consultation with the National Health Care Workforce Commission. One of the many activities involves the responsibility to collect, assess, and report on data on the performance benchmarks selected by the State partnership and Health Resources and Services Administration (HRSA) for implementation activities carried out by the partnership and to participate in HRSA's evaluation and reporting activities. More information can be obtained through www.bhpr@hrsa.gov.

SURVEY METHODS

McLaughlin and Marascuilo (1990) discussed the benefit of using surveys to describe the profession of nursing at different points and times. According to McLaughlin and Marascuilo, "major federal and state policies directly stem from survey data funded both by governmental and private sources. It should be apparent that crucial decisions that specifically affect nurses are made on the basis of information collected from surveys" (p. 88). Survey methods are modified depending upon the purpose of the study and variables of interest. Survey studies can provide critical data to the nursing profession about demographics such as residence, employment, age, and gender and can be used by governmental agencies toward policy decisions and development. These studies are useful in explaining a real-time view of the nursing workforce to legislators, policy makers, and state and local authorities. In addition, findings often provide scientific rationale for nurse researchers and faculty seeking funding for research or for professional training grants.

Burns and Grove (1993) define *survey* as "a method of data collection used to describe a phenomenon by collecting data using questions or personal interviews." Early survey methods used standardized approaches to collect data from individuals and groups by using paper-and-pencil questionnaires, in-person interview, or via postal mail or telephone. Within the last decade, a number of novel methods and technologies have been developed to speed and improve data collection. Such methods include, ecological momentary assessment (EMA; e.g., interactive voice response technology, cell phones, and text messaging) for capturing real-time data, electronic mailing, Internet-based surveys. In addition, methods such as Web-mining software of social networking sites can be used to capture social network information among nurses and other health care providers.

For the purpose of this integrative review, the authors operationally defined the term *studies* as a research survey that examined a phenomenon to advance knowledge of particular phenomenon or explained a particular phenomenon under study through the use of a survey research methodology. Whittemore and Knafl (2005) quoted Broome in their definition of integrative review as "a specific review method that summarizes past empirical or theoretical literature to provide a more comprehensive understanding of a particular phenomenon or healthcare problem." They further discussed the benefits of integrative reviews to advance nursing science in areas of research practice and policy. Table 12.1 lists a few examples of published nursing workforce studies supported by U.S. federal agencies.

TABLE 12.1

Examples of Published Nursing Workforce Data Sets Supported by Federal Agencies

Agency	Study Author and Year
Agency for Healthcare Research and Quality (ARHQ)	Stanton & Rutherford, 2004
Bureau of Labor Statistics (BLS)	Bureau of Labor Statistics, 2010
Centers for Disease Control (CDC) and National Center for Health Statistics (NCHS)	Squillace, Remsburg, Bercovitz, Rosenoff, & Branden, 2007
Health Resources Administration (HRSA)	HRSA, 1977–2010
Tri-Service Nursing Research Program (TSNRP) Department of Defense (DOD)	DeJong, Benner, Benner, Kenny, Kelley, Bingham, & Debisette, 2010

Professional nursing associations perform annual or periodic surveys on their active and inactive members and on nurses in specialty and/or advanced nursing practices and schools of nursing. Table 12.2 lists examples of published nursing workforce studies supported by professional nursing associations.

National and State regulatory bodies, such as the National Council of State Boards of Nursing (NCSBN), State Workforce Commissions, and the Commission on Graduates of Foreign Nursing Schools (CGFNS) have also performed studies. The National Council of State Boards of Nursing (NCSBN) is a not-for-profit organization whose function is to serve as an organization in which boards of nursing act and counsel together on common issues surrounding the public health, safety and welfare, including the development of licensing examinations in nursing.

The National Forum of State Nursing Workforce Centers is comprised of nurse workforce entities from various Sates. The forum strives to assure an adequate supply of qualified nurses to meet health care demands in the United States. The forum also supports the advancement of new, as well as existing nurse workforce initiatives, shares best practices in nursing workforce research, workforce planning, workforce development, and formulation of workforce policy (Cleary et al., 2010).

The Commission on Graduates of Foreign Nursing Schools (CGFNS) is a nonprofit organization whose purpose includes outreach to nurses and other

TABLE 12.2

Examples of Publications From Professional Associations That Perform Surveys on Their Respective Memberships and Specialty Practices

Professional Association	Study Author and Year
American Association of Colleges of Nursing (AACN)	Fang, Tracy, & Bednash, 2010
American Association of Nurse Anesthetists (AANA)	Merwin, Stern, Jordan, & Bucci, 2009
American Academy of Nurse Practitioners (AANP)	Goolsby, 2009
American College of Nurse-Midwives (ACNM)	Sipe, Fullerton, & Schuiling, 2009
National League for Nursing (NLN)	Kaufman, 2007
National Organization of Nurse Practitioner Faculties (NONPF)	Fang, Tracy, & Bednash, 2010
National Association of Clinical Nurse Specialists (NACNS)	Fang, Tracy, & Bednash, 2010

health care professionals worldwide. CGFNS is an international authority on education, registration and licensure for RNs and other health professionals.

Institute of Medicine (IOM)

As an independent, nonprofit organization with a mission to serve as an advisor to the nation to improve health, the Institute of Medicine (IOM) recently published a consensus report on *The Future of Nursing: Leading Change, Advancing Health* (Robert Wood Johnson Foundation [RWJF], 2011). This effort was collaboration between the IOM and the RWJF Initiative on the Future of Nursing. www.iom.edu.

Robert Wood Johnson Foundation

The RWJF works to improve the health of Americans through a goal of helping society to transform for the better. The organization is a major leader with the IOM in the Initiative on the Future of Nursing, an initiative to transform nursing for the future.

In 2008, the RWJF launched a two-year initiative to respond to the need to assess and transform the nursing profession. The IOM appointed the Committee on the RWJF Initiative on the Future of Nursing. Four key messages were developed by the Committee that structured the recommendations presented in the report. Of the four key messages developed by the Committee, one emphasizes that "effective workforce planning and policy making requires better data collection and information infrastructure." The other three key messages are as follows:

- Nurses should practice to the full extent of their education and training
- Nurses should achieve higher levels of education and training through an improved education system that promotes seamless academic progression and,
- Nurses should be full partners with physicians and other health care professionals, in redesigning health care in the United States. (RWJF, 2011)

The National Health Care Workforce Commission will help identify the demand for health care workers, and the National Center for Workforce Analysis will support workforce data collection and analysis. The IOM recommends that these programs place a priority on systematic monitoring of the supply of health care workers, review data and methods needed to make accurate predictions of workforce needs, and coordinate collection of data on the health care workforce at the State and regional levels. The report also emphasizes the need for timely data and that these data be publicly accessible. Work has begun, led by IOM, toward action steps to achieve these recommendations www.iom.edu/nursing.

INTERAGENCY COLLABORATIVE ON
NURSING STATISTICS

The Interagency Collaborative on Nursing Statistics (ICONS) is an alliance of organizations that promotes research efforts related to nurses, nursing education, and the nursing workforce www.iconsdata.org. The organization serves to support the generation of nursing workforce data, information, and research to drive evidence-based policy decision making about the nursing workforce and nursing education.

Theoretical Framework

The authors used a modification of the framework identified in the paper written by Lawrence H. Ganong's (1987) titled *Integrative Reviews of Nursing Research*. In the 1987 study, Ganong conducted an integrative review of 17 nursing research articles from four nursing research journals. Ganong identified 10 standard steps in the review process. The steps are listed below in the following order:

1. Formulate the purpose of the review and develop related questions to be answered by the review or hypotheses to be tested.
2. Establish tentative criteria for inclusion of studies in the review such that as data are gathered criteria may be changed on substantive or methodological grounds.
3. Conduct a literature search making sampling decisions if the number of studies located is large.
4. Develop a questionnaire with which to gather data from studies.
5. Identify rules of inference to be used in data analyses and interpretation.
6. Revise criteria for inclusion into the questionnaire as needed.
7. Read the studies used in the questionnaire to gather data.
8. Analyze data in a systematic fashion.
9. Discuss and interpret data.
10. Report the review as clearly and completely as possible.

The modification of Ganong's framework for purposes of this integrative review included the following seven steps:

1. Formulated the purpose.
2. Established criteria for inclusion of studies.
3. Conducted a literature search.
4. Developed questions to gather data.
5. Read the studies and reviewed the material according to the questions identified.
6. Analyzed the data in a systematic fashion.
7. Discussion and interpretation of data.

1. Purpose

The initial purpose of this literature review was to review all available nursing workforce studies that could be found in the literature. This review included data sets held by Federal, State, and local government agencies and data sets owned by professional nursing associations. All studies presented different information about nurses or nursing personnel germane to the population being studied. The initial review using specified search terms yielded 247,704 articles and data sets. After the initial search, the authors decided to include only studies that included primary source data, which resulted in 13 published databases.

2. Criteria for Inclusion

The criteria for review were as follow: data sets published in English, in the United States between the years of 2005 and 2010.

3. Literature Search

The authors conducted a literature search using a variety of digital archives of biomedical, psychological, nursing, allied health and life sciences journal literature (see Appendix). The database type ranged from general reference collections to specially designed, subject-specific databases for public, academic, medical, corporate and school libraries. Specifically, the archives used were PubMed, Ebscohost (Cumulative Index to Nursing and Allied Health Literature [CINAHL], Academic Search Complete, Business Source Complete and PsycINFO) and Google. PubMed Central (PMC) is the U.S. National Institutes of Health (NIH) free digital archive of that comprises more than 20 million citations for biomedical literature from MEDLINE, life science journals, and online books. CINAHL is the most comprehensive resource for nursing and allied health literature. While starting out as a single bibliographic database, CINAHL has expanded to offer four databases including two full-text versions. CINAHL is owned and operated by EBSCO Publishing. EBSCOhost is a company that offers a variety of proprietary full text databases and popular databases from leading information providers. PsycINFO provides systematic coverage of the psychological literature from the 1800s to the present. The database also includes records from the 1600s and 1700s. An essential tool for researchers, PsycINFO combines a wealth of content with precise indexing so you can get just what you need easily. PsycINFO contains bibliographic citations, abstracts, cited references, and descriptive information to help you find what you need across a wide variety of scholarly publications in the behavioral and social sciences.

Once we selected our archives, we limited our keyword search. The keywords listed below were used alone or in multiple combinations:

a. Nursing staff OR nurses
b. Workforce OR manpower OR staffing

   c. Development AND United States

   d. Data set OR survey

A search of public Internet sites from Federal agencies, State and local nursing groups, nursing workforce commissions, independent research groups, nongovernmental organizations, and professional nursing associations also produced links to research and data resources. Follow-up telephone calls were made to organizations that did not appear in results of the literature review of published databases from the years of 2005 to 2010.

4. Questions Used to Gather Data

   a. Source of data set.

   b. Title of data set.

   c. Population sampled and size.

   d. Discussion of primary data.

   e. Major findings.

   f. Limitations.

5. Studies Reviewed

   a. Thirteen published data sets between the years of 2005 and 2010 met the inclusion criteria for review. The authors used the framework to guide the examination of the publication for; source of data set, title of data set, population sampled and size, discussion of primary data, major findings, and limitations, if any.

6. Analyzed Data in a Systematic Fashion

Table 12.3 lists the 13 studies in this review according to four questions: source, title of data set, date(s), and population sampled.

7. Discussion and Interpretation of Data

This integrative review reported on published data sets from two federal sources and five professional nursing associations between the years of 2005 and 2010. The federal data sets published primary data to the Internet and all of the professional nursing associations published primary source data in a refereed journal article.

   The National Sample Survey of Registered Nurses (NSSRN, 2008; HRSA, 2010) and the Occupational Employment Statistics, Occupational Employment and Wages of Registered Nurses (OES, 2009; BLS, 2010) were the largest in terms of number of observations. The NSSRN examined the supply, composition, and distribution of RNs in national and State levels to describe the population of licenced RNs in the United States (HRSA, 2010).

TABLE 12.3

Table of Selected Nursing Workforce Datasets Published Between 2005 and 2010

Source (Dates)	Title of Data Set	Population Sampled
U.S. Department of Labor, Bureau of Labor Statistics. (2009). *Occupational Employment Statistics. Occupational Employment and Wages, May 2009. 29–1111 Registered Nurses.* Retrieved November 22, 2010, from http://www. bls.gov/oes/current/oes291111.htm	Occupational Employment Statistics	Employers of Registered Nurses
Health Resources and Services Administration (HRSA, 2010). *The Registered Nurse Population. Findings from the 2008 National Sample Survey of Registered Nurses.* Retrieved November 22, 2010, from http://bhpr.hrsa.gov/ healthworkforce/rnsurvey/2008/nssrn2008.pdf	The Registered Nurse Population: Findings from the 2008 National Sample Survey of Registered Nurses	Registered Nurses
American Association of Colleges of Nursing (AACN). Fang, D., Tracy, C., & Bednash, G.D. (2010). *2009–2010 Enrollment and graduations in baccalaureate and graduate programs in nursing.* Washington, DC: American Association of Colleges of Nursing.	2009–2010 Enrollment and Graduations in Baccalaureate and Graduate Programs in Nursing (in joint effort with National Organization of Nurse Practitioner Faculties and the National Association of Clinical Nurse Specialists).	Baccalaureate and Higher Degree Programs/Institutions; AACN Member Schools
American Association of Colleges of Nursing (AACN). Fang, D., Tracy, C., & Bednash, G.D. (2009). *2008–2009 Salaries of Instruction and Administrative Nursing Faculty in Baccalaureate and Graduate Programs in Nursing.* Washington, DC: American Association of Colleges of Nursing.	2008–2009 Salaries of Instructional and Administrative Nursing Faculty	Baccalaureate and Higher Degree Programs/ Institutions; Member Schools and Non-Member Schools

(Continued)

TABLE 12.3

Table of Selected Nursing Workforce Datasets Published Between 2005 and 2010   (Continued)

Source (Dates)	Title of Data Set	Population Sampled
American Association of Nurse Anesthetists (AANA). Merwin, E., Stern, S., & Jordan, L. (2006). Supply, demand and equilibrium in the market for CRNAs. AANA Journal, 74(4), 287–293.	Supply and Demand Models AANA Membership, Certification, Student Enrollment, and Longitudinal Annual Survey Data Demand for surgeries estimated from the Area Resources File (Health Resources and Services Administration)	Certified Nurse Anesthetists (CRNA)
American Association of Nurse Anesthetists (AANA). Survey of program directors and faculty (First Survey) (2006, 2007). Merwin, E., Stern, S., & Jordan, L. (2008). Salaries, recruitment, and retention for CRNA faculty—Part 1. AANA Journal, 76(2), 89–93.	Survey of Program Directors and Faculty (First Survey) (2006, 2007)	CRNAs that were associated with teaching programs.
American Association of Nurse Anesthetists (AANA). Merwin, E., Stern, S., & Jordan, L. (2008). Clinical faculty: major contributions to the education of new CRNAs–Part 2. AANA Journal 76(3), 167–171.	American Association of Nurse Anesthetists 2004 Practice Profile Database	Clinical Faculty; All Non-Faculty CRNAs; Academic Faculty
American Association of Nurse Anesthetists (AANA). Merwin, E., Stern, S., Jordan, L., & Bucci, M. (2009). New estimates for CRNA vacancies. AANA Journal 77(2), 121–129.	2007 Survey of hospitals and ambulatory surgical centers, and the American Hospital Association 2006 Annual Survey	Administrators of Hospitals and Ambulatory Surgical Centers

Reference	Data Source	Population
American Academy of Nurse Practitioners (AANP). Goolsby, M. J. (2009b). 2009 AANP membership survey. *Journal of the American Academy of Nurse Practitioners, 21*, 618–622.	2009 AANP Membership Survey	AANP Full Members
American Academy of Nurse Practitioners (AANP). Goolsby, M. J. (2009a). 2008 AANP National NP Compensation Survey. *Journal of the American Academy of Nurse Practitioners, 21*, 186–188.	2008 AANP National NP Compensation Survey	AANP Full Members and Non-Members
American College of Nurse-Midwives (ACNM). Schuiling, K. D., Sipe, T.A., & Fullerton, J. (2010). Findings from the analysis of the American College of Nurse-Midwives' Membership Surveys: 2006–2008. *Journal of Midwifery & Women's Health, 55*(4), 299–307.	American College of Nurse-Midwives' Membership Surveys: 2006–2008 / American College of Nurse-Midwives Annual Core Data Survey	ACNM Members
Sipe, T. A., Fullerton, J. T., Schuiling, K. D. (2009). Demographic profiles of Certified Nurse-Midwives, Certified Registered Nurse Anesthetists, and Nurse Practitioners: Reflections on implications for uniform education and regulation. *Journal of Professional Nursing, 25*(3), 178–185.	Membership Databases from American College of Nurse-Midwives, American Association of Nurse Anesthetists and the American Academy of Nurse Practitioners	Certified Nurse Midwives, Nurse Midwives, Nurse Midwives, Nurse Practitioners, Certified Registered Nurse Anesthetists.
National League for Nursing (NLN). Kaufman, K. (2007). Nurse Educators: Findings from the NLN/Carnegie national survey with implications for recruitment and retention. *Nursing Educator Perspectives, 28*(3), 164–167. Kaufman, K. (2007). Compensation for Nurse Educators: Findings from the NLN/Carnegie National Survey with Implications for Recruitment and Retention. *Nursing Education Perspectives, 28*(4), 223–225.	NLN: Carnegie National Survey of Nurse Educators Carnegie National Survey of Nurse Educators: Compensation, Workload, and Teaching Practice (2006)	Nurse Educators/Faculty in Schools of Nursing; NLN Members and Non-Members

The BLS OES (2010) published employment and wage statistics of RNs in national and state profiles.

Of the 13 databases with published findings between the years of 2005 and 2010, each had a unique purpose and was unrelated to the other in terms of design and methodology. Overall, studies were designed to answer specific questions most often related to the needs of the professional organization. In other words, studies were designed to better understand the membership through data. In this review, the unit of measurement ranged from the individual RN or advanced practice nurse (HRSA, 2010) to baccalaureate and higher degree nursing programs (Fang, Tracy, & Bednash, 2010). All 13 studies were descriptive in research design and described characteristics for the population under study. Associations conducted surveys in scheduled frequencies; some yearly, others did not mention how often. In two instances, there was collaboration among professional associations with data sharing or use of membership data. The American Association of Colleges of Nursing collected data in joint effort with the National Organization of Nurse Practitioner Faculties and the National Association of Clinical Nurse Specialists (Fang et al., 2010). Sipe et al. (2009) used secondary data sets to compare membership survey results from three groups of advanced practice nurses (American College of Nurse-Midwives; American Association of Nurse Anesthetists; and American Academy of Nurse Practitioners) to survey results from the NSSRN (2004). Merwin et al. (2006) used data from existing models to determine current trends in supply, demand, and equilibrium in the employment market for Certified Registered Nurse Anesthetists (CRNA).

The sample size of databases ranged from 55,171 to 72 observations. The 55,171 observations were from RNs (HRSA, 2010) while the lowest of 72 observations was from anesthesia programs (Merwin, Stern, & Jordan, 2008).

Response rates were variable and impacted the sample size of each database. AACN reported an 87.7% response rate to the enrollment and graduation survey (Fang et al., 2010) while the NSSRN reported 62.4 % response rate (HRSA, 2010). High levels of satisfaction were also noted among NPs responding to the AANP member survey (Goolsby, 2009b). This study reported that the NPs viewed their professional organization as satisfying which says that the services provided by AANP are viewed positively.

Four studies addressed issues of relevance to nurse faculty such salary, recruitment and retention, role of clinical faculty, and salaries of administrative nursing faculty (Fang et al., 2009; Merwin et al., 2008; Kaufman, 2007). Two surveys collected solely demographic information from its members (Goolsby, 2009; Schuiling, Sipe, & Fullerton, 2010). Two focused on supply and demand issues and vacancies in the CRNA workforce (Merwin et al., 2006; Merwin, Stern, Jordan, & Bucci, 2009). Goolsby (2009a) discussed findings from the American Academy of Nurse Practitioners Annual Compensation Survey.

Only one survey, the ACNM membership survey, included nonnurse members in their database. The ACNM membership survey included members of the professional association that were nonnurses certified midwives (CMs) which were small in the number of survey respondents (Schuiling, Sipe, & Fullerton, 2010). This was also corroborated with limitations identified by (Sipe, Fullerton, & Schuiling, 2009). Two surveys included nonmembers in data collection.

The length of time that lapsed from the beginning of data collection to the end of data collection was a factor for some studies. The data-collection time frame varied from a 2-week period to 1 calendar year (Goolsby, 2009b; Schuiling, 2010). All of the studies were time limited and did not follow the respondent over an extended period of years possibly attributed to the costs entailed in longitudinal studies.

The age of the nurse was a demographic in many studies (add in). For CRNA, retirements rates and age at retirement were a concern for supply predictions and an additional concern was the high exit rate from workforce when nurses were in their late 20s and early 30s (Merwin, Stern, & Jordan, 2006). HRSA (2010) found the older age groups of nurses (50–54 years old) representing 16.2% of RNs in the nursing workforce (HRSA, 2010). The average age of nursing faculty continues be in the 50s (Fang, Tracy, & Bednash, 2009; Kaufman, 2007) suggesting that both clinically based nurses and nursing faculty will face retirements in the very near future. A concern is the intergenerational divide between older nurses and younger nurses and bridging this gap for the transfer of knowledge and skills in academic and practice environments. Impending retirements and the younger age of the nursing profession (HRSA, 2010) implies an important need to plan for intergenerational transition programs to bridge the age divide between retiring nurses and new entrants. Socialization among generational nurse groups can be built into curricula.

Geographic location was found to be important in the CRNA Vacancy survey to project demand in rural and metropolitan areas (Merwin, Stern, Jordan, & Bucci, 2009). They found a higher need for hospital CRNAs; however, the increase in need reported may in part be related to changes in survey methodology. Other databases included geographic locations of where RNs and advanced practice nurses practiced (Goolsby, 2009b; HRSA, 2010; Schuiling, Sipe, & Fullerton, 2010).

CONCLUSION

The purpose of this chapter was to present an analysis of selected published nursing workforce studies published between the years of 2005 and 2010. Thirteen nursing workforce studies were reviewed and analyzed using a modification of the method suggested by Ganong (1987). Overall the studies lacked uniform observations among data sets; lacked longitudinal studies that followed the nurses from the beginning of their career to retirement; had response rates that contributed to small sample sizes; lacked attention to an interdisciplinary mix of providers; and implied the need for future study on intergenerational characteristics due to shifting demographics in age. Sample sizes on advanced practice nurses for each specialty were not large enough to enable data that could inform workforce planning and policy development at the county and local level. Many professional association surveys used their membership list as the sampling list instead of using the universe of individuals credentialed for the full scope of practice in that specialty.

The majority of data sets contained only descriptive data with no qualitative observations. Descriptive exploratory research provides insights for refining research questions. Qualitative and qualitative research with triangulation allows for validation while deepening and widening the ability to understand the phenomenon in question. Such work can be useful in depicting a more realistic picture and a more compelling story when trying to predict future workforce needs and communicate with policy makers and educational and funding institutions. In the future, multidisciplinary, interdisciplinary, and interprofessional approaches to research are needed to better execute meaningful research designs, address measurement issues, develop new data-collection techniques, and analyze data. How the research is designed depends on the central research questions. For workforce studies, future designs might focus on methods for archiving and disseminating complex data sets, especially longitudinal data sets, data sets including social network data, and data sets including geographic identifiers. Geographic identifiers not only protect the identities of study participants but also allow others, who were not part of the original research team, to use the data sets.

In reviewing several sources from the National Institutes of Health, the authors identified a variety of new methods that would be appropriate for the workforce studies. Developing and validating research instruments and questions are vitally important for collecting reliable information and have obvious impact on data validity and reliability. For example, data-collection instruments and questions developed for a particular age, gender, or group of nurses may not be valid for other groups. Specific consideration of the processes underlying potential bias in self-report data collection remains a measurement issue. Such processes include perceptual, cognitive, cultural, demographic, motivational, and affective influences on self-report data. Measurement issues that may impact workforce studies might include the development of instruments or technologies that measure behavior objectively or reduce self-report burden. Measurement issues in using technology such as computer-assisted data collection, web-based technology, and personal digital assistants (PDAs) are also relevant. Other issues for consideration include the following:

- Methodology for validating Geographic Information System (GIS) data obtained from different sources.
- Methodology to capture the behaviors of nurses in clinical settings.
- Development of measures for evaluating quality of work life and refinement of existing measures through longitudinal studies and across various disease states.

Data-collection techniques are the tools and procedures scientists use for implementing research designs and obtaining measurements. Methods for collecting research data have an important impact on data validity and reliability. For example, studies have suggested that use of self-administered instruments can facilitate the reporting of sensitive or illegal behaviors. Innovative methodologies can also open the door to the collection of new or more complex types of data. Recent developments in computer-assisted interviewing have permitted more complex question sequences in survey research and the development of hand-held "beepers" programmed for data entry have permitted the collection of time-specific data on activities. In addition, implicit measures have allowed researchers to examine processes of which people themselves have been unaware. In addition, more research is needed to understand how various methods work in diverse populations of nurses and how they can be modified to address the specific needs of populations. Potential innovations for data-collection techniques include, but are not limited to, the following:

- Data-collection techniques featuring unobtrusive, user-friendly, wearable devices and those utilizing WiFi technology that improve measurement of behavioral phenomena in the real-world setting in which they typically occur and at the moment when the phenomena of interest actually occurs (i.e., ecological momentary assessment).
- New methods for qualitative research; methods for validating narrative or text-based analyses; techniques for validating and replicating findings from qualitative research, including, collection strategies, development of coding protocols, and techniques that facilitate the integration and validation of qualitative and quantitative measurement.

- Methods to reduce sampling, survey, and item nonresponse bias in research studies, including techniques to reduce attrition in longitudinal studies and to improve response rates on sensitive items.
- Techniques for collecting contextual data (e.g., workforce composition, peer-group characteristics, geographic and environmental information) and for operationalizing the boundaries and/or reach of particular social, economic, physical, and cultural contexts.

Analytic methods encompass the concepts and techniques used in analyzing data and interpreting and reporting results. The goal of new and improved analytic methods is to improve estimation, hypothesis testing, and causal modeling based on scientific data. Challenges include developing techniques that distinguish underlying regularities from the noise created by variability and imprecise measurement; developing causal inferences from nonexperimental data; improving both the internal validity and external validity (generalizability) of measures and studies; and developing appropriate analytic techniques for use with new kinds of data and new approaches to research. Examples of topics within analytic methods include, but are not limited to, the following:

- Research to improve the analysis of longitudinal data, in particular, the analysis of correlated data, the modeling of different sources of error, and techniques for dealing with missing data at various levels of aggregation.
- Methodological research to improve the analysis of complex survey data, including the statistical modeling of nonresponse and other survey errors.
- Analytic methods for integrating evidence from qualitative and quantitative research, such as research examining the complex relationships among multiple sources of information on a single construct.
- Expanding current psychometric methodologies to handle the types of data collected in workforce studies, for example, multidimensional data, shorter scales, non–normal score distributions, mixed-response format, and complex survey structure.
- Improvements or new approaches to nonlinear analysis, for example, systems dynamic modeling, agent-based modeling, network analysis, and other simulation techniques.

REFERENCES

American Association of Colleges of Nursing, Nursing Faculty Shortage Fact Sheet. Accessed March 24, 2011, from http://www.aacn.nche.edu/media/FactSheets/FacultyShortage.htm
American Nurses Association. (1949). *Inventory of Professional Registered Nurses*. New York, NY: Author.

Bureau of Labor Statistics, Occupational Employment Statistics. (2009, May). *Occupational employment and wages 29–1111 registered nurses.* Retrieved from http://www.bls.gov/oes/current/oes291111.htm#nat

Burns, N., & Grove, S. K. (1993). *The practice of nursing research, conduct, critique & utilization* (2nd ed.). Philadelphia, PA: W. B. Saunders.

Cleary, B. L., Hassmiller, S. B., Reinhard, S. C., Richardson, E. M., Veenema, T. G., & Werner, S. (2010). Uniting states, sharing strategies: Forging partnerships to expand nursing education capacity. *American Journal of Nursing, 110*(1), 43–50.

DeJong, M., Benner, R., Benner, P., Richard, M., Kenny, D., Kelley, P.,...Debisette, A. T. (2010). Mass casualty and care in an expeditionary environment. *Journal of Trauma Nursing, 17*(1), 45–58.

Fang, D., Tracy, C., & Bednash, G. D. (2009). *2008–2009 Salaries of instruction and administrative nursing faculty in baccalaureate and graduate programs in nursing.* Washington, DC: American Association of Colleges of Nursing.

Fang, D., Tracy, C., & Bednash, G. D. (2010). *2009–2010 Enrollment and graduations in baccalaureate and graduate programs in nursing.* Washington, DC: American Association of Colleges of Nursing.

Ganong, L. H. (1987). *Integrative reviews of nursing research: Research in nursing and health.* New York, NY: Wiley Periodicals.

Goolsby, M. J. (2009a). 2008 AANP National NP Compensation Survey. *Journal of the American Academy of Nurse Practitioners, 21*, 186–188.

Goolsby, M. J. (2009b). 2009 AANP Membership Survey. *Journal of the American Academy of Nurse Practitioners, 21*, 618–622.

Goolsby, M. J. (2010). AANP research and education. *Journal of the American Academy of Nurse Practitioners, 22*, 279.

Institute of Medicine. (2011). *The future of nursing: Leading change, advancing health.* Washington, DC: The National Academies Press. Retrieved from http://www.rwjf.org/files/research/Future%20of%20Nursing_Leading%20Change%20Advancing%20Health.pdf

Interagency Collaborative on Nursing Statistics. (2008). *Nursing workforce data sources: Icons resource list.* Retrieved from http://www.iconsdata.org/research.htm

Kaufman, K. (2007). Introducing the NLN/Carnegie national survey of nurse educators: Compensation, workload, and teaching practice. *Nursing Education Perspectives, 28*(3), 164–167.

Kaufman, K. (2007). Compensation for nurse educators: Findings from the NLN/Carnegie national survey with implications for recruitment and retention. *Nursing Education Perspectives, 28*(4), 223–225.

McLaughlin, F., & Marascuilo, L. (1990). *Advanced nursing and health care research: Quantification approaches.* Philadelphia, PA: W. B. Saunders.

Merwin, E., Stern, S., & Jordan, L. (2006). Supply, demand, and equilibrium in the market for CRNAs. *AANA Journal, 74*(4), 287–293.

Merwin, E., Stern, S., & Jordan, L. (2008). Salaries, recruitment, and retention for CRNA faculty—Part 1. *AANA Journal, 76*(2), 89–93.

Merwin, E., Stern, S., & Jordan, L. (2008). Clinical faculty: major contributions to the education of new CRNAs—Part 2. *AANA Journal, 76*(3), 167–171.

Merwin, E., Stern, S., Jordan, L., & Bucci, M. (2009). New estimates for CRNA vacancies. *AANA Journal, 77*(2), 121–129.

National League for Nursing. (2010). *NLN Nurse Educator Shortage Fact Sheet.* Retrieved March 24, 2011, from http://www.nln.org/governmentaffairs/pdf/NurseFacultyShortage.pdf

Patient Protection and Affordable Care Act, Public Law 111–148. (2010). Retrieved from http://frwebgate.access.gpo.gov/cgi-bin/getdoc.cgi?dbname=111_cong_public_laws&docid=f:publ148.111.pdf

Squillace, M. R., Remsburg, R. E., Bercovitz, A., Rosenoff, E., & Branden, L. (2007, March). *An introduction to the National Nursing Assistant Survey* (Vital and Health Statistics, Series 1, No. 44). Washington, DC: National Center for Health Statistics. Retrieved from http://www.cdc.gov/nchs/data/series/sr_01/sr01_044.pdf

Schuiling, K. D., Sipe, T. A., & Fullerton, J. (2010). Findings from the Analysis of the American College of Nurse-Midwives' Membership Surveys: 2006–2008. *Journal of Midwifery & Women's Health, 55*(4), 299–307.

Sipe, T. A., Fullerton, J. T., & Schuiling, K. D. (2009). Demographic profiles of certified nurse-midwives certified registered nurse anesthetists, and nurse practitioners: Reflections on implications for uniform education and regulation. *Journal of Professional Nursing, 25*(3), 178–185.

Stanton, M. W., & Rutherford, M. K. (2004). *Hospital nurse staffing and quality of care.* Rockville, MD: Agency for Healthcare Research and Quality.

U.S. Department of Health and Human Services, Health Resources and Services Administration. (2010). *The registered nurse population: Findings from the 2008 National Sample Survey of Registered Nurses.* Retrieved from http://www.bhpr.hrsa.gov/healthworkforce/rnsurvey/2008/

Whittemore, R., & Knafl, K. (2005). The integrative review: Updated methodology. *Journal of Advanced Nursing, 52*(5), 546–553.

APPENDIX
Nursing Workforce Searches

PubMed
Search strategy:
(nursing staff OR nurses) AND (workforce OR manpower OR staffing) AND
development AND "United States" Limits: English, published in the last 5 years
115 results

Search strategy:
(nursing staff OR nursing) AND (workforce OR manpower OR staffing) AND
(**dataset OR survey**) AND "United States" Limits: English, published in the last
5 years
386 results

Ebscohost databases searched: CINAHL, Academic Search Complete, Business
Source Complete and PsycINFO

Search strategy:
(nursing staff OR nurses) AND (workforce OR manpower OR staffing) AND
development) and "United states"
Limiters – Scholarly (Peer Reviewed) Journals, Publication years 2005–2010
139 results

Search strategy:
(nursing staff OR nursing) AND (workforce OR manpower OR staffing) AND
(**dataset OR survey**) and "United states"
Limiters – Scholarly (Peer Reviewed) Journals, Publication years 2005–2010
164 results

Google
Search strategy:
nursing AND (dataset OR survey) AND (workforce OR manpower OR staffing)
site:.edu
Limits: Nov 2008–Nov 2010, English pages
79,900 results

Search strategy:
nursing AND (dataset OR survey) AND (workforce OR manpower OR staffing)
site:.org
Limits: Nov 2008–Nov 2010, English pages
167,000 results

Index

Note: Page references followed by "*f*" and "*t*" denote figures and tables, respectively.